Body Composition and Physical Health in Sports Practice

Body Composition and Physical Health in Sports Practice

Editor

Stefania Toselli

MDPI • Basel • Beijing • Wuhan • Barcelona • Belgrade • Manchester • Tokyo • Cluj • Tianjin

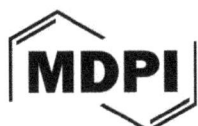

Editor
Stefania Toselli
Department of Biomedical and
Neuromotor Sciences
University of Bologna
Bologna
Italy

Editorial Office
MDPI
St. Alban-Anlage 66
4052 Basel, Switzerland

This is a reprint of articles from the Special Issue published online in the open access journal *International Journal of Environmental Research and Public Health* (ISSN 1660-4601) (available at: www. mdpi.com/journal/ijerph/special_issues/Body_Sports).

For citation purposes, cite each article independently as indicated on the article page online and as indicated below:

LastName, A.A.; LastName, B.B.; LastName, C.C. Article Title. *Journal Name* **Year**, *Volume Number*, Page Range.

ISBN 978-3-0365-1201-3 (Hbk)
ISBN 978-3-0365-1200-6 (PDF)

© 2021 by the authors. Articles in this book are Open Access and distributed under the Creative Commons Attribution (CC BY) license, which allows users to download, copy and build upon published articles, as long as the author and publisher are properly credited, which ensures maximum dissemination and a wider impact of our publications.

The book as a whole is distributed by MDPI under the terms and conditions of the Creative Commons license CC BY-NC-ND.

Contents

Stefania Toselli
Body Composition and Physical Health in Sports Practice: An Editorial
Reprinted from: *International Journal of Environmental Research and Public Health* 2021, 18, 4534,
doi:10.3390/ijerph18094534 1

José M. Sarabia, Carmen Doménech, Enrique Roche, Néstor Vicente-Salar and Raul Reina
Anthropometrical Features of Para-Footballers According to Their Cerebral Palsy Profiles and Compared to Controls
Reprinted from: *International Journal of Environmental Research and Public Health* 2020, 17, 9071,
doi:10.3390/ijerph17239071 5

Andrea Di Credico, Giulia Gaggi, Barbara Ghinassi, Gabriele Mascherini, Cristian Petri, Riccardo Di Giminiani, Angela Di Baldassarre and Pascal Izzicupo
The Influence of Maturity Status on Anthropometric Profile and Body Composition of Youth Goalkeepers
Reprinted from: *International Journal of Environmental Research and Public Health* 2020, 17, 8247,
doi:10.3390/ijerph17218247 19

Raquel Vaquero-Cristóbal, Mario Albaladejo-Saura, Ana E. Luna-Badachi and Francisco Esparza-Ros
Differences in Fat Mass Estimation Formulas in Physically Active Adult Population and Relationship with Sums of Skinfolds
Reprinted from: *International Journal of Environmental Research and Public Health* 2020, 17, 7777,
doi:10.3390/ijerph17217777 33

Jacek Trinschek, Jacek Zieliński and Krzysztof Kusy
Maximal Oxygen Uptake Adjusted for Skeletal Muscle Mass in Competitive Speed-Power and Endurance Male Athletes: Changes in a One-Year Training Cycle
Reprinted from: *International Journal of Environmental Research and Public Health* 2020, 17, 6226,
doi:10.3390/ijerph17176226 45

Marius Baranauskas, Valerija Jablonskienė, Jonas Algis Abaravičius, Laimutė Samsonienė and Rimantas Stukas
Dietary Acid-Base Balance in High-Performance Athletes
Reprinted from: *International Journal of Environmental Research and Public Health* 2020, 17, 5332,
doi:10.3390/ijerph17155332 59

Irina Kalabiska, Annamária Zsakai, Robert M. Malina and Tamas Szabo
Bone Mineral Reference Values for Athletes 11 to 20 Years of Age
Reprinted from: *International Journal of Environmental Research and Public Health* 2020, 17, 4930,
doi:10.3390/ijerph17144930 79

Ireneusz Cichy, Andrzej Dudkowski, Marek Kociuba, Zofia Ignasiak, Anna Sebastjan, Katarzyna Kochan, Slawomir Koziel, Andrzej Rokita and Robert M. Malina
Sex Differences in Body Composition Changes after Preseason Training in Elite Handball Players
Reprinted from: *International Journal of Environmental Research and Public Health* 2020, 17, 3880,
doi:10.3390/ijerph17113880 91

Silvia Stagi, Azzurra Doneddu, Gabriele Mulliri, Giovanna Ghiani, Valeria Succa, Antonio Crisafulli and Elisabetta Marini
Lower Percentage of Fat Mass among Tai Chi Chuan Practitioners
Reprinted from: *International Journal of Environmental Research and Public Health* **2020**, *17*, 1232, doi:10.3390/ijerph17041232 . . . . **99**

Stefania Toselli, Georgian Badicu, Laura Bragonzoni, Federico Spiga, Paolo Mazzuca and Francesco Campa
Comparison of the Effect of Different Resistance Training Frequencies on Phase Angle and Handgrip Strength in Obese Women: A Randomized Controlled Trial
Reprinted from: *International Journal of Environmental Research and Public Health* **2020**, *17*, 1163, doi:10.3390/ijerph17041163 . . . . **113**

Francesco Campa, Alessandro Piras, Milena Raffi, Aurelio Trofè, Monica Perazzolo, Gabriele Mascherini and Stefania Toselli
The Effects of Dehydration on Metabolic and Neuromuscular Functionality during Cycling
Reprinted from: *International Journal of Environmental Research and Public Health* **2020**, *17*, 1161, doi:10.3390/ijerph17041161 . . . . **123**

Marinella Coco, Andrea Buscemi, Claudia Savia Guerrera, Donatella Di Corrado, Paolo Cavallari, Agata Zappalà, Santo Di Nuovo, Rosalba Parenti, Tiziana Maci, Grazia Razza, Maria Cristina Petralia, Vincenzo Perciavalle and Valentina Perciavalle
Effects of a Bout of Intense Exercise on Some Executive Functions
Reprinted from: *International Journal of Environmental Research and Public Health* **2020**, *17*, 898, doi:10.3390/ijerph17030898 . . . . **133**

Ruben Francisco, Catarina N. Matias, Diana A. Santos, Francesco Campa, Claudia S. Minderico, Paulo Rocha, Steven B. Heymsfield, Henry Lukaski, Luís B. Sardinha and Analiza M. Silva
The Predictive Role of Raw Bioelectrical Impedance Parameters in Water Compartments and Fluid Distribution Assessed by Dilution Techniques in Athletes
Reprinted from: *International Journal of Environmental Research and Public Health* **2020**, *17*, 759, doi:10.3390/ijerph17030759 . . . . **145**

Gabriele Mascherini, Cristian Petri, Elena Ermini, Vittorio Bini, Piergiuseppe Calà, Giorgio Galanti and Pietro Amedeo Modesti
Overweight in Young Athletes: New Predictive Model of Overfat Condition
Reprinted from: *International Journal of Environmental Research and Public Health* **2019**, *16*, 5128, doi:10.3390/ijerph16245128 . . . . **159**

Francesco Campa, Catarina Matias, Hannes Gatterer, Stefania Toselli, Josely C. Koury, Angela Andreoli, Giovanni Melchiorri, Luis B. Sardinha and Analiza M. Silva
Classic Bioelectrical Impedance Vector Reference Values for Assessing Body Composition in Male and Female Athletes
Reprinted from: *International Journal of Environmental Research and Public Health* **2019**, *16*, 5066, doi:10.3390/ijerph16245066 . . . . **169**

Editorial

Body Composition and Physical Health in Sports Practice: An Editorial

Stefania Toselli

Department of Biomedical and Neuromotor Sciences, University of Bologna, 40126 Bologna, Italy; stefania.toselli@unibo.it

The assessment of the health status of athletes, at all ages, is an aspect of fundamental importance, and, in recent years, the analysis of body composition has become a fundamental and essential part in its evaluation, such as in the optimization of sports performance.

There are a number of techniques available for estimating body composition, all of which have advantages and disadvantages/limitations [1]. Factors such as the feasibility, cost, technical skill needed, level of accuracy, participant burden, radiation exposure, time taken, validation in an appropriate population, and availability of reference data have to be considered while choosing a suitable method [2].

Body composition can change according to sports practice and more generally by physical activity. It is to be considered that each particular sports discipline requires a specific type of training and activity, and this clearly affects athletes' body composition; therefore, it is not possible to apply a rigid notion of optimal body composition to every sport [3]. Strategies to achieve the best possible physique for each individual athlete and sports discipline form part of a comprehensive approach to maximize the performance of the athlete. For this purpose, recent studies conducted on athletes have highlighted the need of reference data for assessing the body composition of athletes of different sports, and with or without physical impairments [4,5]. In the absence of appropriate references for each sport category, researchers continue to use reference values from the general healthy population [6].

Monitoring and assessing body composition are important, since an adequate physique is a determinant of the athletic performance, success and health of athletes [7]. Attention should be given to preserving the long-term performance and health of the athlete, since physical stress during training and competitions may lead to body composition alterations, which can be detrimental to athletes. This can be achieved by carefully monitoring body composition parameters (fat mass, fat-free mass, hydration status and bone health), understanding the optimal physique for a given athlete, and avoiding potentially harmful practices that may lead to excessively rapid and/or extensive changes in body composition [3].

Finally, particular attention should be paid to young athletes and to their growth and development. Differences in body composition and performance occur in young athletes because of somatic maturation. Individual differences in biological maturity status and timing affect body size, physical fitness, and athletic aptitude in youths and are central to talent identification and development programs in many sports [8,9]. Fat-free mass (FFM) and total body water (TBW) are higher in early maturing athletes, and as a consequence, they present a lower fat percentage (%FM) and a better performance than late mature athletes [10]. This influences the selection—a particularly common scenario in elite teams is the selection of athletes with greater body dimensions and better physical performance, typical in more mature athletes [11,12].

In this Special Issue, titled "Body Composition and Physical Health in Sports Practice" in *IJERPH* [13], 14 papers were recently published on different topics related to body composition. Four papers are on methodological aspects, three papers provide specific reference values, one paper investigates the influence of maturity status on the anthropometric profile and body composition, and six are on the influence of physical exercise and sport practice on body composition and performances.

Concerning methodological aspects, one paper analyzes the usefulness of raw bioelectrical impedance (BI) parameters in assessing the water compartments and fluid distribution of athletes [14]. Assessing fluid balance to monitor the hydration status in athletes has received substantial interest for maximizing performance, and simple methods are required to assess water compartments and fluid distribution in athletes. The paper showed that raw BI parameters are useful predictors of total and extracellular pools, cellular hydration and fluid distribution in athletes. Another paper considered the specific bioimpedance vector analysis (specific BIVA) to screen and monitor the total body and regional body composition of middle-aged and elderly subjects and affirmed that it appears to be a suitable technique to evaluate the nutritional status and risk of morbidity in these subjects [15]. Body composition changes in different body districts and regional body composition provide relevant information for this purpose, since they allow a better understanding of the role of physical activity in different conditions, such as sarcopenia and obesity. One paper [16] focuses on the analysis of the differences between the formulas used to estimate fat mass and to establish the existing relationship with the body mass index and sums of skinfolds in kinanthropometry. Finally, one paper provides a new predictive model to determine when excess weight is due to excess fat mass [17]. This method could be useful for sports medicine physicians or athletic trainers as an additional assessment of young athletes during physical examinations.

Of the three papers regarding reference values for athletes, one was focused on the development reference values for male and female athletes using classic bioimpedance vector analysis (BIVA) [18]. The paper shows that vector distributions of endurance, velocity/power, and team-sport athletes differ from the general healthy population, and among themselves, due to their different body composition, and thus proposes different reference values. Another paper underlines the importance of bone health valuation of children and youth, given changes in bone mineral density (BMD) and content (BMC) during the course of growth and maturation [19]. In this paper, a reference for bone mineral density (BMD) and content (BMC) specific to young athletes of both sexes participating in several sports was proposed. This could be useful to understand bone development in young athletes and may inform training practices, leading to success in sport, facilitating the diagnosis of structural abnormalities in bone, and contributing to the prevention of skeletal injuries. The third paper provides reference scores on the anthropometric measures and body composition of international-level cerebral palsy (CP) para-footballers that can help sports coaches and physical trainers in the selection process, or to monitor the evolution of players' body composition [20]. Using these reference scores, coaches could monitor and guide their athletes' training to achieve the reference values of elite para-footballers.

A single paper investigates the influence of maturity status on anthropometric profile and body composition and confirms that the majority of the examined variables follow the physiological trend occurring during puberty [21]. The paper underlines the importance of monitoring the anthropometric profile and body composition of children and adolescents participating in sport, as an essential aspect to consider evaluating possible risk conditions and adopting effective countermeasures.

Six papers analyze the influence of physical exercise and sport practice on body composition and performance [22]. One paper focuses on the determination of the effects of dehydration on metabolic and neuromuscular functionality performance during a cycling exercise, pointing out that athletes exercising in a dehydrated state significantly decreased physical performances. This paper underlines the importance of following strategies to maintain a good hydration status during exercise and confirms the ability of BIVA to assess body fluid changes even in sports practice. Another paper details the effectiveness of physical activity interventions in obese subjects, comparing the effects of different weekly resistance training frequencies performed over a 24-week exercise program on phase angle (PA) and handgrip strength (HS) [23]. The paper pointed out that physical exercise performed three times a week promotes better adaptations in PA and HS when compared with the same program performed once a week in obese women. One paper demonstrates that the maximum oxygen uptake (VO2max) calculated per skeletal muscle mass (SMM) is not more useful than conventional VO2max measures to track longitudinal changes in competitive athletes, but it allows one to better distinguish between groups or individuals differing in training status [24]. The focus of another paper was on the examination of the effects of an exhaustive exercise on executive functions, since the effects of acute physical exercise on the cognitive performances of an adult individual are still under discussion [25]. The paper underlines the possibility that high levels of blood lactate induced by exhaustive exercise could adversely affect the executive functions, and stressed that, even with a reduction in quantity, the influences remain present even in older people. One paper refers to changes in estimated body composition prior to a season in elite female and male Polish handball players during a five-week preseason training camp and to sexual dimorphism in response to intensive preseason training [26]. Finally, one paper regards the determination of the dietary acid-base balance in competitive Lithuanian high-performance athletes, and the evaluation of the effect of the diets of athletes on NEAP (net endogenous acid production), muscle mass and body mineral content during a four-year Olympic cycle [27]. The paper showed that, regardless of the type of sport, the diets of Lithuanian high-performance athletes do not meet their requirements, underlying that the training of athletes in different sports needs to be very individualized in terms of the mesocycling of sports goals, including changes in the body composition, giving priority to the formation of eating habits.

In conclusion, the co-editor was satisfied with gathering 14 papers by leading international experts in nutritional status, body composition and exercise. This Special Issue demonstrates the importance of monitoring the health status of the athlete and how body composition assessment represents a fundamental and effective tool to meet this goal.

Conflicts of Interest: The author declares no conflict of interest.

References

1. Duren, D.L.; Sherwood, R.J.; Czerwinski, S.A.; Lee, M.; Choh, A.C.; Siervogel, R.M.; Chumlea, W.C. Body composition methods: Comparisons and interpretation. *J. Diabetes Sci. Technol.* **2008**, *2*, 1139–1146. [CrossRef]
2. Gatterer, H.; Schenk, K.; Burtscher, M. Assessment of human body composition: Methods and limitations. In *Body Composition: Health and Performance in Exercise and Sport*; Lukaski, H.C., Ed.; CRC Press-Taylor & Francis Group: Boca Raton, FL, USA, 2017; pp. 13–26.
3. Thomas, D.T.; Erdman, K.A.; Burke, L.M. American College of Sports Medicine joint position statement. Nutrition and Athletic Performance. *Med. Sci. Sports Exerc.* **2016**, *48*, 543–568. [CrossRef] [PubMed]
4. Micheli, M.L.; Pagani, L.; Marella, M.; Gulisano, M.; Piccoli, A.; Angelini, F.; Burtscher, M.; Gatterer, H. Bioimpedance and impedance vector patterns as predictors of league level in male soccer players. *Int. J. Sports Physiol. Perform.* **2014**, *9*, 532–539. [CrossRef]
5. Campa, F.; Toselli, S. Bioimpedance vector analysis of elite, subelite, and low-level male volleyball players. *Int. J. Sports Physiol. Perform.* **2018**, *13*, 1250–1253. [CrossRef] [PubMed]
6. Pollastri, L.; Lanfranconi, F.; Tredici, G.; Schenk, K.; Burtscher, M.; Gatterer, H. Body fluid status and physical demand during the Giro d'Italia. *Res. Sports Med.* **2016**, *24*, 30–38. [CrossRef]
7. Malina, R.M. Body composition in athletes: Assessment and estimated fatness. *Clin. Sports Med.* **2007**, *26*, 37–68. [CrossRef] [PubMed]
8. Burgess, D.J.; Naughton, G.A. Talent development in adolescent team sports: A review. *Int. J. Sports Physiol. Perform.* **2010**, *5*, 103–116. [CrossRef]
9. Malina, R.M.; Rogol, A.D.; Cumming, S.P.; Coelho-e-Silva, M.J.; Figueiredo, A.J. Biological maturation of youth athletes: Assessment and implications. *Br. J. Sports Med.* **2015**, *49*, 852–859. [CrossRef]
10. Toselli, S.; Marini, E.; Maietta Latessa, P.; Benedetti, L.; Campa, F. Maturity Related Differences in Body Composition Assessed by Classic and Specific Bioimpedance Vector Analysis among Male Elite Youth Soccer Players. *Int. J. Environ. Res. Public Health.* **2020**, *17*, 729. [CrossRef]
11. Malina, R.M. Children and adolescents in the sport culture: The overwhelming majority to the select few. *J. Exerc. Sci. Fit.* **2009**, *7* (Suppl. 2), S1–S10. [CrossRef]
12. Malina, R.M. Early sport specialization: Roots, effectiveness, risks. *Curr. Sports Med. Rep.* **2010**, *9*, 364–371. [CrossRef] [PubMed]

13. IJERPH | Special Issue: Body Composition and Physical Health in Sports Practice. Available online: https://www.mdpi.com/journal/ijerph/special_issues (accessed on 11 January 2021).
14. Francisco, R.; Matias, C.; Santos, D.; Campa, F.; Minderico, C.; Rocha, P.; Heymsfield, S.; Lukaski, H.; Sardinha, L.; Silva, A. The Predictive Role of Raw Bioelectrical Impedance Parameters in Water Compartments and Fluid Distribution Assessed by Dilution Techniques in Athletes. *Int. J. Environ. Res. Public Health* **2020**, *17*, 759. [CrossRef]
15. Stagi, S.; Doneddu, A.; Mulliri, G.; Ghiani, G.; Succa, V.; Crisafulli, A.; Marini, E. Lower Percentage of Fat Mass among Tai Chi Chuan Practitioners. *Int. J. Environ. Res. Public Health* **2020**, *17*, 1232. [CrossRef]
16. Vaquero-Cristóbal, R.; Albaladejo-Saura, M.; Luna-Badachi, A.; Esparza-Ros, F. Differences in Fat Mass Estimation Formulas in Physically Active Adult Population and Relationship with Sums of Skinfolds. *Int. J. Environ. Res. Public Health* **2020**, *17*, 7777. [CrossRef]
17. Mascherini, G.; Petri, C.; Ermini, E.; Bini, V.; Calà, P.; Galanti, G.; Modesti, P. Overweight in Young Athletes: New Predictive Model of Overfat Condition. *Int. J. Environ. Res. Public Health* **2019**, *16*, 5128. [CrossRef] [PubMed]
18. Campa, F.; Matias, C.; Gatterer, H.; Toselli, S.; Koury, J.; Andreoli, A.; Melchiorri, G.; Sardinha, L.; Silva, A. Classic Bioelectrical Impedance Vector Reference Values for Assessing Body Composition in Male and Female Athletes. *Int. J. Environ. Res. Public Health* **2019**, *16*, 5066. [CrossRef]
19. Kalabiska, I.; Zsakai, A.; Malina, R.; Szabo, T. Bone Mineral Reference Values for Athletes 11 to 20 Years of Age. *Int. J. Environ. Res. Public Health* **2020**, *17*, 4930. [CrossRef] [PubMed]
20. Sarabia, J.; Doménech, C.; Roche, E.; Vicente-Salar, N.; Reina, R. Anthropometrical Features of Para-Footballers According to Their Cerebral Palsy Profiles and Compared to Controls. *Int. J. Environ. Res. Public Health* **2020**, *17*, 9071. [CrossRef]
21. Di Credico, A.; Gaggi, G.; Ghinassi, B.; Mascherini, G.; Petri, C.; Di Giminiani, R.; Di Baldassarre, A.; Izzicupo, P. The Influence of Maturity Status on Anthropometric Profile and Body Composition of Youth Goalkeepers. *Int. J. Environ. Res. Public Health* **2020**, *17*, 8247. [CrossRef]
22. Campa, F.; Piras, A.; Raffi, M.; Trofè, A.; Perazzolo, M.; Mascherini, G.; Toselli, S. The Effects of Dehydration on Metabolic and Neuromuscular Functionality during Cycling. *Int. J. Environ. Res. Public Health* **2020**, *17*, 1161. [CrossRef]
23. Toselli, S.; Badicu, G.; Bragonzoni, L.; Spiga, F.; Mazzuca, P.; Campa, F. Comparison of the Effect of Different Resistance Training Frequencies on Phase Angle and Handgrip Strength in Obese Women: A Randomized Controlled Trial. *Int. J. Environ. Res. Public Health* **2020**, *17*, 1163. [CrossRef] [PubMed]
24. Trinschek, J.; Zieliński, J.; Kusy, K. Maximal Oxygen Uptake Adjusted for Skeletal Muscle Mass in Competitive Speed-Power and Endurance Male Athletes: Changes in a One-Year Training Cycle. *Int. J. Environ. Res. Public Health* **2020**, *17*, 6226. [CrossRef] [PubMed]
25. Coco, M.; Buscemi, A.; Guerrera, C.; Di Corrado, D.; Cavallari, P.; Zappalà, A.; Di Nuovo, S.; Parenti, R.; Maci, T.; Razza, G.; et al. Effects of a Bout of Intense Exercise on Some Executive Functions. *Int. J. Environ. Res. Public Health* **2020**, *17*, 898. [CrossRef] [PubMed]
26. Cichy, I.; Dudkowski, A.; Kociuba, M.; Ignasiak, Z.; Sebastjan, A.; Kochan, K.; Koziel, S.; Rokita, A.; Malina, R. Sex Differences in Body Composition Changes after Preseason Training in Elite Handball Players. *Int. J. Environ. Res. Public Health* **2020**, *17*, 3880. [CrossRef] [PubMed]
27. Baranauskas, M.; Jablonskienė, V.; Abaravičius, J.; Samsonienė, L.; Stukas, R. Dietary Acid-Base Balance in High-Performance Athletes. *Int. J. Environ. Res. Public Health* **2020**, *17*, 5332. [CrossRef] [PubMed]

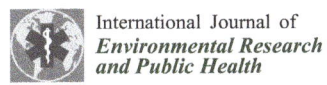

Article

Anthropometrical Features of Para-Footballers According to Their Cerebral Palsy Profiles and Compared to Controls

José M. Sarabia [1,2], Carmen Doménech [1], Enrique Roche [2,3,4], Néstor Vicente-Salar [2,3] and Raul Reina [1,*]

1. Sports Research Centre, Department of Sport Sciences, Miguel Hernández University, 03202 Elche, Spain; jsarabia@umh.es (J.M.S.); carmendomenechribes@live.com.mx (C.D.)
2. Alicante Institute for Health and Biomedical Research (ISABIAL Foundation), 03010 Alicante, Spain; eroche@umh.es (E.R.); nvicente@umh.es (N.V.-S.)
3. Department of Applied Biology-Nutrition, Institute of Bioengineering, Miguel Hernandez University, 03202 Elche, Spain
4. CIBER Fisiopatología de la Obesidad y Nutrición (CIBEROBN), Instituto de Salud Carlos III (ISCIII), 28029 Madrid, Spain
* Correspondence: rreina@umh.es; Tel.: +34-96-522-2443

Received: 25 September 2020; Accepted: 1 December 2020; Published: 4 December 2020

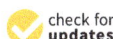

Abstract: Cerebral palsy (CP) football is a team para-sport practiced by para-athletes with eligible impairments of hypertonia, athetosis, and ataxia. This study aimed: (1) to describe the anthropometrical and body composition profiles of international CP para-footballers with different CP profiles (i.e., spastic diplegia, athetosis/ataxia, spastic hemiplegia, and minimum impairment); (2) to analyze the differences between both affected/nondominant and nonaffected/dominant sides; and (3) to compare the sample of international-level CP para-footballers ($n = 141$) with a sample of highly trained able-bodied footballers ($n = 39$). Anthropometric measures included four breadths, nine girths, and six skinfolds, while body composition was measured through fat mass (including Carter's, Faulkner's, and Withers' equations), muscle mass (Lee's equation), and bone mass (Rocha's and Martin's equations). This study found differences between the able-bodied footballers and the following impairment profiles: spastic diplegia (skinfolds); ataxia/athetosis (corrected calf of the nondominant side, and calf skinfolds for both sides); and spastic hemiplegia (all measurements excepting femur breadth, and thigh and ankle girths). No differences were found between para-athletes with minimum impairment and the able-bodied footballers. This study demonstrates that football players with or without physical impairments of hypertonia athetosis or ataxia may be considered homogeneous in shape when dominant size is compared. Besides, the study provides reference scores on anthropometric measures and body composition of international-level CP para-footballers that can help sports coaches and physical trainers to monitor physical fitness of their para-athletes.

Keywords: body composition; paralympics; para-sport; brain impairment; soccer; football

1. Introduction

In the field of sports, the assessment of body composition is an essential factor because it has been related to performance and even to success in a specific sport, in combination with other factors such as technical, tactical, physical, and psychological skills [1,2]. In the case of football, body composition is among the key fitness elements to football players' performance not only in adults but also in young football players [3]. While fat-free mass has been strongly correlated to strength and power performance [4], body fat might increase the injury risk [5] and negatively influence players' performance [6]. Hence, for football staff and researchers, a better understanding of the determinants of success—such as the specific anthropometric characteristics of the players—may be crucial for training and talent identification. Previous studies on able-bodied football players have disclosed significant differences in anthropometric and fitness measures between playing levels [7], across playing positions, and between age categories [8].

The body composition and anthropometrical characteristics of the para-athletes have also been previously described and in some cases related to performance in swimming [9–11], blind sports [11,12], track and field [11,13,14], wheelchair sports [15–17], or rowing [18]. However, most of these previous studies included a mixed pool of para-athletes with different types of impairment and from different para-sports. In addition, to the best of the authors' knowledge, the previous studies with cerebral palsy (CP) athletes only described the basic anthropometry measures (i.e., height, weight, and body mass index) [19,20] or somatotype [21]. Only the study by Yanci et al. [22] compared anthropometry measures with the physical performance (i.e., jump capacity), but body composition and anthropometrical characteristics of CP football players have not been previously described and compared to able-bodied football players.

CP football is a seven-a-side modality of football, played by ambulant athletes with CP or acquired brain injury. Para-footballers are classified into sport classes giving a special relevance to their CP profile and impairment severity. Over the last decades, CP football has used a functional classification system for their para-athletes developed by the Cerebral Palsy International Sports and Recreation Association (CPISRA) [23]. Specifically, those with moderate spastic diplegia, moderate athetoid or ataxic profile, and moderate spastic hemiplegia are grouped in FT5, FT6, or FT7, respectively. In addition, the mild forms of these impairments—also called "minimum impairment criteria" to be eligible for competing in this team para-sport—are classified together in the FT8 sport class [24].

The literature shows that both children and adults with CP tend to have below-average weight, linear growth, muscle mass, and fat mass compared with their peers [25–27]. Indeed, people with hemiplegia might show an increased bone loss and muscle atrophy, especially on the hemiplegic side [28] and more common in the upper body [29]. It has also been suggested that exercise may modify or reverse skeletal muscle abnormalities [30].

Knowing the anthropometric attributes of highly trained CP football players in relation to impairment/sport classes would provide the basis upon which practitioners could provide individualized practice, in an attempt to evaluate and develop the specific attributes and optimize players' performance. Thus, the aims of this study were (1) to describe the anthropometrical and body composition profiles of international CP football players for each CP profile; (2) to analyze the differences between both affected/nondominant and nonaffected/dominant sides; and (3) to compare them with a sample of highly trained able-bodied football players.

2. Materials and Methods

2.1. Participants

One hundred and forty-one footballers (age = 24.8 ± 6.3 years) with more than seven years of experience in football participated in the study (Table 1). Of those, 102 were international para-footballers from different countries who participated at the 2013 CPISRA Intercontinental Cup (Barcelona, Spain), a qualifying tournament for the 2015 CP-Football World Championships. These players were classified as spastic diplegia ($n = 8$), athetosis/ataxia ($n = 14$), spastic hemiplegia ($n = 64$), or minimum impairment ($n = 16$). The rest of the players were the control group (CG), that is, a group of 39 able-bodied footballers who were playing in the third Spanish football division. Prior to involvement in the investigation, all participants gave written informed consent after a detailed written and oral explanation of the potential risks and benefits resulting from participation in this study, as outlined in the Declaration of Helsinki (2013). Approval by the institutional review board (Office for Projects Evaluation, OEP) was obtained before the study began (Ref. DPS.RRV0.01.14).

Table 1. Characteristics of the sample and general body measurements.

Variable	Total Sample	Spastic Diplegia	Athetosis/ Ataxia	Spastic Hemiplegia	Minimum Impairment	Control Group
n	141	8	14	64	16	39
Laterality (R/L)	77/64	3/5	8/6	24/40	9/7	33/6
Ethnicity (CA/AF)	135/6	8/0	13/1	62/2	16/0	36/3
Training experience (year)	11 (6, 16)	12 (5, 15)	10 (10, 12)	10 (5, 14)	17 (5, 22)	15 (15, 16)
Age (year)	23 (20, 29)	23.5 (18, 33.3)	24.5 (19.8, 34)	23 (21, 30)	26.5 (21.3, 38.3)	22 (20, 23)
Weight (kg)	70.9 (64, 76.7)	63.4 (60.1, 73.3) [†]	68.1 (62.2, 73)	67.3 (62.4, 75) [††]	73.6 (69.4, 78.7) [†]	74.5 (69.3, 80)
Height (cm)	176 (172, 181)	171.5 (168.3, 178.8)	173 (170.8, 179.3) [†]	174 (172, 178.9) [††]	179 (170.4, 183.8)	181 (176, 184)
BMI (kg·m^{-2})	22.6 (21.5, 23.9)	21.9 (19.7, 24.4)	22.5 (20.4, 23.9)	22.1 (21, 23.7)	23.4 (21.6, 25.6)	23.2 (22.1, 24)

R = the right leg is dominant; L = the left leg is dominant; CA = Caucasian; AF = Afro-American. Data are delivered as median (25th and 75th percentiles). [†] significant difference with the control group $p < 0.05$; [††] significant difference with the control group $p < 0.01$.

2.2. Anthropometric Determinations

All variables were measured by a Level 2 anthropometrist certified by the International Society for the Advancement of Kinanthropometry (ISAK) with an individual technical error of measurement (TEM) of 0.76–0.39% for skinfolds and 0.12% for the remaining parameters. The errors were considered acceptable for ISAK standards (<7.5% for skinfolds and <1.5% for the remaining measurements). All measurements were made following the guidelines stated by ISAK [31] except for chest skinfold, which was according to Heyward and Stollarczyk [32]. The limb measurements were obtained for both body sides (except for neck girth and abdominal skinfold) in all the participants and taken in duplicate. An average of the two measurements was recorded.

The total body mass of each participant was measured in kilograms using a Tanita digital scale (model BC-601), breadths with a Holtain bicondylar caliper (Holtain, Crosswell, UK), girths with a metallic nonextensible tape (Lufkin, Sparks, NV, USA), and skinfolds with a Holtain Tanner/Whitehouse skinfold caliper (Holtain, Crosswell, UK). The following four breadths were measured: humerus, wrist, femur, and ankle. Regarding girths, six were measured: relaxed arm; flexed and tensed arm; neck; thigh; medial calf; and ankle. Finally, seven skinfolds were also measured: triceps (Tr); chest (Ch); subscapular (Sb); supraspinale (Sp); abdominal (A); thigh (Th); and medial calf (Ca). In addition, the corrected arm, thigh, and calf were calculated using the formula:

$$\text{Corrected Girth} = \text{Girth} - (\pi \text{ Skinfold}) \tag{1}$$

2.3. Body Composition

Three-component models of body composition were used, dividing fat-free mass into lean tissue mass and bone mineral content. Due to specific equations to calculate the different body mass types not having been developed for para-athletes with CP or other related neurological conditions, the equations recommended for athletes to calculate the components of body mass have been used [33]. Percentage of body fat mass was calculated using three different methods: Yuhasz's equation modified by Faulkner [34], Carter's equation [35], and calculating the body density with Withers' equations [36] and converting to body fat percentage using Siri's equation [37]. Percentage of bone mass was calculated according to two different equations: Rocha's [31] and Martin's [38] equations. Percentage of muscle mass was calculated from Lee's equation [39]. In addition, the following sums were considered for fat content calculations [40]:

- Three skinfolds

$$\sum 3Sk = Ch + A + Th \quad (2)$$

- Six skinfolds

$$\sum 6Sk = Tr + Sb + Sp + A + Th + Ca \quad (3)$$

- Upper body skinfolds

$$\sum UpSk = Tr + Sb \quad (4)$$

- Lower body skinfolds

$$\sum LowSk = Th + Ca \quad (5)$$

2.4. Body Proportionality

Body proportionality analyses were conducted using the Phantom stratagem proposed by Ross and Wilson [41], which has been previously applied in other sports with able-bodied athletes [42,43]. The Phantom is a unisex, bilaterally symmetrical conceptual model that was derived from reference data of men and women [44]. The Phantom-Z scores (Z-Scores) for each anthropometric variable were used to demonstrate the number and direction of standard deviations that each of the groups varied against the Phantom. Each variable was transformed in a Z-Score adjusting it to the Phantom size using the following equation:

$$Z\text{-Score} = (1/s) \, v \, [(170.18/h)^d - P] \quad (6)$$

where v is the size of any variable, 170.18 is the Phantom height constant, h is the subject's height, d is a dimensional exponent, P is the Phantom value for variable v, and s is the Phantom standard deviation value. These Z-Scores have a 0 mean, so a Z-Score higher than 0 means that the subject is proportionally greater than the Phantom, and Z-score lower than 0 means the opposite. This allows data standardization, providing a reference profile for each type of impairment and allowing future comparisons of individual scores with the results of this study.

2.5. Statistical Analyses

Statistical analysis was performed using the Statistical Package for Social Sciences (SPSS Inc., version 240.0 for Windows, Chicago, IL, USA). Statistical significance was set at the α-level of 0.05 for two-tailed tests. Distribution of the data was tested by using the Kolmogorov–Smirnov and the Shapiro–Wilk tests, and the Q–Q plot.

The results indicated that data were not normally distributed for the whole group or for the CP profiles (i.e., sport classes). For this reason, the median as central tendency measure and the interquartile range (25th and 75th percentiles) as a measure of the spread of the data have been considered in this study. Therefore, the nonparametric Wilcoxon test was used to detect significant differences between dominant and nondominant sides.

In addition, differences among the CP profiles were identified using the Kruskal–Wallis test and the Bonferroni correction in case of significant findings between groups. Finally, Friedman's comparisons were used to compare body fat mass equations and body bone mass equation between them inside each CP profile. When we found differences in Friedman's comparisons, we performed the Wilcoxon matched-pairs test for multiple analysis with Bonferroni's correction. Practical significance was assessed by calculating effect size (d) [45], according to the values suggested by Cohen [46]: above 0.8, between 0.8 and 0.50, between 0.50 and 0.2, and lower than 0.2 were considered as large, moderate, small, and trivial, respectively.

3. Results

3.1. Dominant vs. Nondominant Sides

Comparisons between the dominant and nondominant sides are shown in Tables 2 and 3. While spastic diplegia, minimum impairment, and control groups showed trivial differences in some anthropometrical data, the athetosis/ataxia group showed differences in girths, and the spastic hemiplegia group showed marked differences in all measures except for the trunk skinfolds.

3.2. Comparison with the Control Group

The comparisons between each CP group and the control group were made comparing Z-Scores. The Z-Scores are shown in Figure 1 and fully detailed in Table S1. All CP groups show differences in skinfolds of both sides of the body with the CG. In addition, the spastic hemiplegia group showed differences with the CG on many of the breadths and girths for the nondominant side.

3.3. Equation Comparison

Regarding body fat mass equations, Faulkner's equation was significantly different from Withers' and Carter's equations for spastic diplegia ($Z = 2.52$, $p = 0.012$, $d = 0.89$, for both comparisons), minimum impairment ($Z = 2.95$ and 3.52, $p < 0.001$, $d = 0.74$ and 0.88, respectively) and control group ($Z = 5.43$ and 5.44, $p < 0.001$, $d = 0.87$), while in the athetosis/ataxia group, it was significantly different only from Carter ($Z = 3.11$, $p = 0.002$, $d = 0.83$), and in the spastic hemiplegia group, all equations were significantly different from the others ($Z = 5.74$–6.94, $p < 0.0001$, $d = 0.72$–0.87).

Regarding body bone mass equations, both Rocha's and Martin's equations were significantly different for each group (spastic diplegia, $Z = 2.52$, $p = 0.012$, $d = 0.89$; athetosis/ataxia, $Z = 3.30$, $p = 0.001$, $d = 0.88$; spastic hemiplegia, $Z = 6.96$, $p < 0.001$, $d = 0.87$; minimum impairment, $Z = 3.52$, $p < 0.001$, $d = 0.88$; CG, $Z = 5.44$, $p < 0.001$, $d = 0.87$).

Table 2. Anthropometric measures and body composition of the four CP profiles and the able-bodied football players (control group).

	Spastic Diplegia (n = 8)		Athetosis/Ataxia (n = 14)		Spastic Hemiplegia (n = 64)		Minimum Impairment (n = 16)		Control Group (n = 39)	
	Dom	Non-Dom	Dom	Non-Dom	Dom	Non-Dom	Dom	Non-Dom	Dom	Non-Dom
Breadths (cm)										
Humerus	7.2 (6.8, 7.4) *	7 (6.4, 7.3)	7 (6.8, 7.5)	7.1 (6.8, 7.3)	7 (6.6, 7.3) **	6.6 (6.4, 6.9)	7 (6.6, 7.5)	6.9 (6.4, 7.2)	7.2 (7, 7.5) *	7.2 (6.9, 7.4)
Wrist	5.9 (5.6, 6.1)	5.9 (5.7, 6)	5.7 (5.5, 6.1) **	5.5 (5.2, 5.7)	5.6 (5.4, 5.9) **	5.4 (5.1, 5.6)	5.9 (5.5, 6)	5.6 (5.4, 5.8)	6 (5.8, 6.2)	5.9 (5.5, 6.1)
Femur	9.5 (9.3, 10)	9.7 (9.6, 10)	9.7 (9.4, 10)	9.7 (9.2, 9.8)	9.8 (9.5, 10.1) **	9.5 (9.3, 9.8)	10 (9.7, 10.3) **	9.9 (9.5, 10.1)	10.2 (10, 10.5) **	10.1 (9.7, 10.4)
Ankle	7.5 (7.3, 7.8)	7.4 (7.1, 7.5)	7.5 (7.3, 7.7)	7.5 (7.2, 7.8)	7.4 (7.2, 7.8) **	7.2 (7, 7.5)	7.4 (7.2, 7.8)	7.4 (7.1, 7.7)	7.6 (7.2, 8)	7.6 (7.2, 8)
Girths (cm)										
Relaxed arm	29.2 (26.3, 33.3)	27.8 (26.1, 32)	29.3 (27.6, 30.9) **	27.7 (26.3, 29.1)	29.6 (27.3, 30.6) **	26.9 (25.3, 28.6)	30 (28.1, 32.6)	29 (25.7, 32.9)	30.2 (29.3, 31.7)	30.2 (28.9, 32.1)
Flexed arm	32.4 (28.7, 33.8)	30.7 (28.7, 33.8)	30.6 (30.3, 33.7) *	29.5 (28.8, 31.7)	31.2 (29.8, 32.6) **	28.7 (27.4, 30.1)	33.3 (30.7, 34.7)	31.8 (27.8, 35)	33.3 (32.3, 34.8)	33.2 (31.3, 34.6)
Neck	370.0 (360.0, 37.9)		36.8 (35.4, 37.8)		36.5 (35.2, 37.7)		36.4 (35.9, 38.4)		37.2 (35.6, 38.3)	
Thigh	49.9 (49.6, 53.9)	50.2 (45.4, 52.6)	51.7 (49.8, 54.1) *	50.7 (48.3, 53.5)	53.7 (51.3, 56.3) **	50.6 (47.9, 53.7)	54.9 (52.7, 55.8)	54.2 (52.7, 55.2)	54.4 (53.3, 55.7)	54.2 (51.6, 56.2)
Calf	34.5 (31.5, 37.3)	32.5 (31.3, 35.7)	35.6 (35, 36.9) *	35.1 (34.2, 36)	36.8 (35, 38.2) **	34.2 (32.1, 35.7)	37.1 (36.1, 37.9)	37 (35.7, 38.6)	37.3 (35.9, 38.7)	37.3 (35.7, 38.8)
Ankle	21.4 (20.3, 22.7)	21 (20.6, 22.4)	22.7 (21.8, 23.2) *	22.2 (21.4, 22.6)	22.3 (21.4, 23.4) **	21.5 (20.7, 22.3)	22.3 (21.6, 23.2)	22.6 (21.3, 23)	22.7 (21.9, 23.1)	22.5 (21.9, 23.4)
Corrected arm	26.1 (23.5, 29.4)	25.1 (22.6, 27.2)	26.3 (24.9, 28) *	24.5 (23.9, 25.5)	26 (24.8, 27.7) **	23.5 (21.9, 24.9)	26.7 (25.5, 29.9)	26.2 (22.6, 29.8)	28 (26.5, 29.1)	28.2 (26.5, 29.9)
Corrected thigh	45.9 (42.6, 48.7)	44.3 (41, 47.3)	48 (46.4, 50)	47.2 (44.5, 48.9)	49.1 (47.1, 51.4) **	44.8 (43.1, 47.7)	50.2 (47.2, 51.1)	49.7 (47.6, 52.1)	51.5 (49.3, 52.4)	50.8 (49, 52.9)
Corrected calf	31.1 (28.2, 34.2)	28.7 (27.2, 31.9)	32.7 (31.7, 33.9)	31.9 (31.5, 33.4)	34 (32.6, 35.5) **	30.6 (28.1, 33.2)	34.8 (32.3, 35.4)	34.2 (33.1, 36.7)	35.8 (34.4, 36.9) *	35.3 (33.7, 37.1)
Skinfolds (mm)										
Triceps	8.8 (8.3, 10.8)	9.4 (8.1, 11.9)	8.5 (6.5, 10.1)	9.4 (7.1, 12.1)	9.3 (6.7, 11.9) **	10.4 (7.6, 13.6)	8.9 (7.2, 11.1)	9.9 (8.1, 12)	6.9 (6.3, 8.7)	7 (5.3, 8.4)
Subscapular	9.6 (8.9, 11.5)	9.9 (8.3, 11.1)	8.9 (7.8, 10.6)	9.2 (7.6, 11.3)	10 (8.2, 12.8)	10.2 (8.2, 12.5)	9.8 (8.7, 12.5)	10.2 (8.9, 13.3)	8.5 (7.1, 9.2)	7.6 (6.9, 8.6)
Chest	6.5 (5.6, 9.2)	7 (6.5, 7.5)	6.7 (5.8, 11.2)	7.2 (4.5, 10.9)	7.9 (5.7, 11.7)	8.1 (5.1, 11.8)	8.3 (6, 12)	8.4 (5.6, 11.3)	4.2 (2.9, 4.9)	4.1 (3.1, 4.6)
Supraspinale	7.7 (6.1, 120.0)	8.1 (7.6, 9.8)	7.7 (6.1, 11.3)	7.9 (5, 10.4)	8.6 (6.6, 11.7)	8.6 (6.7, 13.2)	9.9 (7.2, 12.4)	9.7 (6.5, 11.8)	6.3 (5.1, 7.4) *	5.6 (4.8, 7.1)
Abdominal	17.8 (11.5, 20.8)		15.4 (9, 25.2)		18 (10.2, 26.2)		19.3 (12.6, 29.7)		9.2 (7.4, 10.3)	
Thigh	13.4 (11.4, 200.0)	13.1 (11, 18.9)	11.9 (7.6, 17.3)	13.9 (8.1, 16.1)	13.7 (8.5, 17.7) **	15.8 (11.1, 22.4)	15 (10.5, 19.8)	14.7 (11.1, 16.6)	9.3 (7.6, 12)	9 (7.6, 11.1)
Calf	11.2 (8.5, 12.6)	10.5 (7.5, 15.5)	7.9 (6.6, 12.6)	9.2 (6.2, 11.4)	7.7 (5.9, 12) **	10.1 (7.1, 14.2)	7.7 (6.1, 12)	7.7 (6, 9.5)	4.9 (4.2, 5.9)	5.3 (4.3, 6.4)

Data are delivered as median (25th and 75th percentiles); Dom = dominant side of the body; Non-Dom = nondominant side of the body. * significant difference with the nondominant side $p < 0.05$, ** significant difference with the nondominant side $p < 0.01$.

Table 3. Body composition of the four CP profiles and the able-bodied football players (control group).

	Spastic Diplegia (n = 8)		Athetosis/Ataxia (n = 14)		Spastic Hemiplegia (n = 64)		Minimum Impairment (n = 16)		Control Group (n = 39)	
	Dom	Non-Dom	Dom	Non-Dom	Dom	Non-Dom	Dom	Non-Dom	Dom	Non-Dom
Fat mass (%)										
Carter's equation	9.6 (9, 11.6)	9.6 (9.3, 10.1)	9 (7.7, 11.3)	9.2 (7.6, 12.5)	9.7 (7.7, 120.0) **	10.5 (8.2, 13.1)	10.8 (8.9, 12.2)	10.4 (8.6, 11.9)	7.5 (6.6, 8.2)	7.1 (6.6, 8.1)
Faulkner's equation	12.7 (11.1, 13.8)	12.4 (11.7, 13.2)	12.1 (10.7, 14.5)	12.5 (10.2, 14.7)	13.1 (10.9, 15.2) **	13.4 (10.9, 15.5)	13.6 (11.7, 15.2)	13.3 (11.8, 15.8)	10.6 (9.9, 11.2) *	10.3 (9.6, 11.2)
Withers' equation	10 (9, 14)	10.2 (9.6, 12.2)	10 (8.1, 12.5)	9.8 (7.9, 13.8)	10.8 (8.3, 140.0) **	11.7 (8.7, 15.1)	11.9 (9.2, 16.1)	10.7 (9.2, 14.6)	6.7 (6.1, 7.6)	6.7 (6.1, 7.5)
∑3 Sk	36.1 (32.1, 51.2)	37.6 (34.6, 38.5)	37.4 (27.4, 50.2)	36.4 (23.1, 52.2)	38.9 (27.5, 54.4) **	41.1 (28.2, 57.9)	43.7 (33.8, 61.3)	41.1 (32.7, 56.5)	23 (18.9, 26.7)	22 (18.7, 26.1)
∑6 Sk	67.1 (60.7, 85.6)	66.4 (63.9, 71.4)	61.2 (49.1, 82.6)	63.3 (47.6, 94)	67.7 (48.8, 89.3) **	75.3 (53.6, 100.2)	78.4 (60.3, 91.6)	74.2 (57.6, 88.3)	46.5 (38.2, 53.1)	42.8 (38.5, 52.9)
∑Upper body Sk	18.7 (16.9, 20.9)	19 (18.2, 19.8)	17.4 (14, 19.9)	18.8 (14.8, 22.6)	19.6 (15.3, 25.7) **	21 (17.1, 25.8)	18.7 (17.6, 22.6)	21 (18.3, 24.1)	15.2 (13.9, 17.5) *	14.9 (12.6, 16.6)
∑Lower body Sk	24.1 (19.6, 33.8)	24.7 (19.9, 30)	19.8 (14.8, 32.7)	23.7 (15.7, 28.2)	22.1 (14.5, 31.2) **	25.7 (18.2, 36.3)	25.5 (16.5, 32)	23 (16.8, 25.1)	14.2 (12.2, 18.4)	14 (12.4, 16.2)
Muscle mass (%)										
Lee's equation	43.7 (42.2, 45.4)	41.3 (39.5, 43.6)	43.8 (41.9, 46.8) *	41.5 (38.9, 45.8)	44.8 (42.8, 47.9) **	39 (36, 42.3)	42.9 (41, 43.9)	41.8 (40.1, 43.3)	45.8 (44.4, 47.2)	45.5 (44.1, 47.2)
Bone mass (%)										
Rocha's equation	17.3 (16.7, 19.8)	17.6 (16.5, 19.7)	17.6 (16, 18.2) *	16.5 (15.3, 17.8)	17.5 (16, 18.6) **	16.3 (15.4, 17.4)	17.1 (16.1, 18.1) *	16.5 (15.2, 17.4)	17.6 (16.9, 18.4) *	17.1 (16.3, 17.9)
Martin's equation	14.4 (13.6, 15.4)	13.7 (12.8, 14.7)	13.6 (13.3, 14.6) **	13.5 (13.1, 14.1)	13.9 (12.6, 15) **	12.7 (12, 13.5)	13.7 (12.4, 14.3) **	12.3 (11.8, 13.5)	13.8 (13.3, 14.4) *	13.6 (12.8, 14)

Data are delivered as median (25th and 75th percentiles); Dom = dominant side of the body; Non-Dom = nondominant side of the body; ∑3 Sk = the sum of chest, abdominal, and thigh skinfolds; ∑6 Sk = the sum of triceps, subscapular, supraspinale, abdominal, thigh, and calf skinfolds; ∑Upper body Sk = the sum of triceps and subscapular skinfolds; ∑Lower body Sk = the sum of thigh and calf skinfolds. * significant difference with the nondominant side $p < 0.05$, ** significant difference with the nondominant side $p < 0.01$.

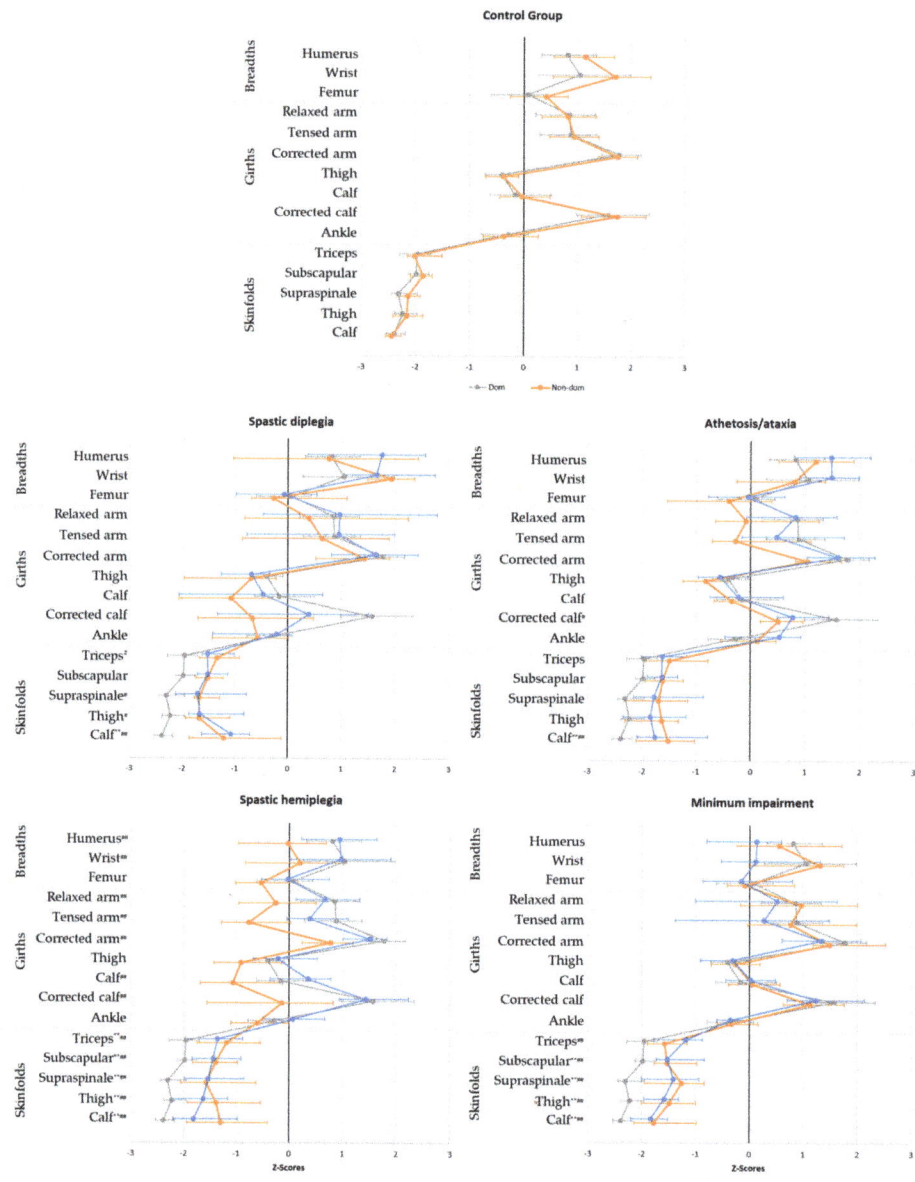

Figure 1. Z-Scores for dominant (dom) and nondominant (non-dom) sides of the body for each group and their comparison from the control group. ** significant difference between the control group and the dominant side $p < 0.01$, # significant difference between the control group and the nondominant side $p < 0.05$, ## significant difference between the control group and the nondominant side $p < 0.01$.

4. Discussion

Anthropometric and body composition parameters are of top importance in determining energy requirements [47] and are related with performance in sports [4]. However, there are still few studies describing body composition characteristics of athletes with a varied impairment and from different para-sports. The difficulty in collecting data is due to the different classes and degrees of impairment, which makes it challenging to establish a representative sample. Therefore, the main contributions of the current study are the descriptive anthropometrical data and proportionality characteristics for each impairment profile for elite CP footballers.

Previous studies have reported a broad range of fatness and leanness in adults with CP [26,48]. However, these studies have used a small and heterogeneous (i.e., different motor impairments and ambulation status) sample of sedentary people with CP, and in most cases with children. Only a few studies have studied the body composition of athletes with CP, but in most cases they mixed athletes with other different eligible impairments (e.g., vision impairment, limb deficiency), and they did not compare the results of para-athletes with an able-bodied group [10,11,14]. To the best of the authors' knowledge, only two previous studies have included only elite athletes with CP [13,21] but only Runciman [13] compared the six para-athletes included with a control group. Like this study, our results suggest that the anthropometrical measures and body composition of players with CP were closely matched to the able-bodied players in anthropometrical measures and body composition estimations. Although some differences in the affected/nondominant side appeared, these results are close to the average population (i.e., Z-Scores between −2 and 2).

In contrast with the fatness found in previous studies [26,48], all CP subgroups in the current study showed higher skinfolds than the CG. The authors hypothesize that this could be due to different nutritional habits and grades of training between groups [49]. While all players in the CG group were professional or semi-professional football players and included a considerable amount of off-field training (e.g., strength and aerobic training at the gym) and in some cases a nutritional controlled planning, the CP footballers were from different countries and, in some of them, this para-sport is not yet professionalized. In addition, the amount of the off-field training was in some cases reduced, mainly due to the impairment. Overall, able-bodied players were 6 kg heavier and 9 cm taller on average than the CP footballers, but with similar BMI for all groups (from 21.9 to 23.4 kg·m^2) and in the ranges showed by other studies [21]. In addition, the profiles for both types of footballers were similar in appearance when the dominant sizes were matched proportionally (Figure 1). This indicates that, whether through training or self-selection, specific proportionality characteristics dominate the preferred morphology for elite football players. The main difference (i.e., the body fat mass measure trough skinfolds) could be justified by the professionalism in physical preparation as shown by Ackland et al. [50] in canoe and kayak paddlers.

Moving to comparison for dominant and nondominant sides, any asymmetry was found in able-bodied footballers as supporting previous studies [51]. In addition, only one anthropometric measure was different between sides for the spastic diplegia subgroup (i.e., humerus breadth). This reveals the homogeneity of the impairment for both sides in these para-athletes. Even though this group showed a similar profile in proportionality to the CG, showing differences only in skinfolds, it is possible to see a high dispersion of calf data on both sides. While the median (25th and 75th percentiles) of the CG for the corrected calf was 1.74 (10.08, 2.27), dominant and nondominant sides of the spastic diplegia group were 0.4 (−1.34, 1.51) and −0.68 (−1.7, 0.49), respectively. This reflects the atrophy of the calf muscles [52]. However, the proportionality profile of girths in the lower limbs were like the CG despite the impairment, showing a similar effect of training in lower body. Still, the low number of players in this group and the high heterogeneity of the impairment prevent these data from showing a clear difference with the able-bodied players. However, the rest of the measures showed a very similar profile to the CG.

The athetosis/ataxia group showed higher anthropometric measures in the upper body (i.e., wrist breadth and relaxed, tensed, and corrected arm girth) and lower body (i.e., thigh, calf, and ankle girths) for the dominant side than for the nondominant side. Consequently, body muscle and bone mass percentages were higher when they were calculated with the dominant-side measures. However, no differences between sides were found for skinfolds and body fat mass percentage. The difficulty of the players with athetosis or ataxia to control their muscle tone and to reduce involuntary muscle activity [53] could be a consequence of this difference. Thus, we can see that the differences between tensed and relaxed arm for the dominant and nondominant sides were 1.3 cm and 1.8 cm, respectively, while it was higher and more homogeneous for both sides in the other groups. These increased girths result in a higher percentage of muscle mass when it is calculated for the dominant side of the body. When this group is compared with the CG, only corrected calf (for nondominant side) and calf skinfolds for both sides showed significant differences, suggesting that they may be due to the different training regimen between groups.

The spastic hemiplegia group showed the highest differences between sides of all groups. As expected, all anthropometrical measures were different between dominant and nondominant sides except the trunk skinfolds (i.e., subscapular, chest, and supraspinale skinfolds). Hence, estimations of body fat, muscle, and bone percentages were higher for the dominant side than for the nondominant side. By contrast, Runciman et al. [13] found symmetry in fat and bone mass in elite paralympic track sprinters with hemiplegia. However, they included only five athletes with hemiplegia and the tendency raises the suspicion of a trend to be different when the data are normalized by age (e.g., femoral neck Z-score was 0.40 ± 0.63 and 00.05 ± 0.91 for nonaffected and affected, respectively) [13]. In addition, the literature had shown a lower total bone and fat-free mass and a similar fat mass—measured with dual-energy X-ray absorptiometry—in people with CP compared with controls [54], reducing these differences when athletes with hemiplegia were compared with a control group [13]. In our results, the nondominant side of those with unilateral spasticity showed smaller breadths, girths, and muscle mass, and higher skinfolds and fat mass than the CG, but the dominant side was higher only in fat mass (i.e., skinfolds). Like previous studies [13], even though some measures were different from the CG, the Z-Scores of the current study were near to 0, showing a similar profile of average population. It was proposed that the differences reported in these individuals with CP were the result of low volumes of ambulation, and subsequent lower bone and muscle loading [55]. Hence, participation in sport activity could reduce these differences with able-bodied people.

Only one anthropometric measure was different between sides for the minimum impairment group (i.e., femur breadth). Even though this group was composed of players with different CP profiles, they showed no differences with the CG either for the dominant or the nondominant side. This reflects the low impact of impairment on these players, showing similar anthropometrical profiles to those of able-bodied football players. These results are in line with previous studies which compared the performance of this group of players with minimum impairment with a control group, showing similar sports performance [56], but also when comparing para-footballers with the different CP profiles included in this study [21].

The combination of these findings has an important implication for the necessity for people with CP to perform exercise [55]. It seems that elite athletes with CP who have undertaken physical exercise over many years may achieve similar adaptations to able-bodied athletes from the same sport. However, the finding that the anthropometrical measures were lower on the affected areas in these groups of athletes indicate that there may be an upper limit for the adaptations that occur and, as the differences showed by the minimum impairment and the other groups, this limit seems dependent on the grade of impairment.

Some limitations should be mentioned. Although the number of players with cerebral palsy included in the study is a good representation of elite CP footballers even for each impairment, the sample size of some groups is too small to achieve high statistical power. In addition, the equations used to estimate the body composition have not been previously validated in people with CP. For those reasons, results should be interpreted with caution.

5. Conclusions

This study was conducted with para-athletes from 12 different national teams that took part in a world-level competition. It has been demonstrated that there are no major differences between a group of able-bodied football players and the moderately impaired CP football sport profiles when the dominant size is measured and the data are relativized to the player's height beyond the fat mass. No differences were found between those para-athletes belonging to the sport class categorized as minimum (i.e., mild) impairment and the able-bodied football players. When comparing body sides, the most common profile in this para-sport (i.e., spastic hemiplegia) [57] was the group with more significant differences between dominant (i.e., nonaffected) and nondominant (i.e., affected) body sides, that is, all the variables measured excepting trunk skinfolds (i.e., subscapular, chest, and supraspinale skinfolds). Besides, this study demonstrates that football players with or without a physical impairment (i.e., hypertonia, athetosis, or ataxia) may be considered homogeneous in shape when dominant size is compared. This reflects the importance of measuring both or dominant side in people with CP and not only the right side as the recommendations for general populations say [31]. In addition, we provide reference scores of anthropometric measures and body composition scores of international-level CP footballers that can help sports coaches and physical trainers to monitor the physical fitness of their para-athletes. This study provides a proportionality profile to compare para-athletes' anthropometry which could help, for example, in the selection process—choosing players with the best match with the elite profile—or monitoring the evolution of players' body composition. Coaches would also monitor and guide their athletes' training to achieve the reference values of elite para-footballers.

Supplementary Materials: The following are available online at http://www.mdpi.com/1660-4601/17/23/9071/s1, Table S1: Z-Scores for dominant (dom) and nondominant (non-dom) sides of the body for each group and their comparison from the control group.

Author Contributions: Conceptualization, J.M.S. and R.R.; methodology, J.M.S. and C.D.; software, J.M.S.; validation, J.M.S., E.R., and N.V.-S.; formal analysis, J.M.S.; investigation, J.M.S., N.V.-S., and R.R.; resources, R.R.; data curation, C.D. and J.M.S.; writing—Original draft preparation, J.M.S. and C.D.; writing—Review and editing, J.M.S. and R.R.; visualization, R.R.; supervision, J.M.S.; project administration, R.R.; funding acquisition, R.R. All authors have read and agreed to the published version of the manuscript.

Funding: Data collection at the 2013 CPISRA Intercontinental Cup was supported by CPISRA. Transport was provided by the Spanish Paralympic Committee. This study was supported by the official funding agency for biomedical research of the Spanish government, Institute of Health Carlos III (ISCIII) through CIBEROBN CB12/03/30038), which is co-funded by the European Regional Development Fund. This study was supported by ISABIAL (grant number 190290).

Acknowledgments: The authors thank the Cerebral Palsy International Sports and Recreation Association (CPISRA) board members and their Football Committee for their support in the data collection during the 2013 CPISRA Intercontinental Cup. We also acknowledge players, coaches, and team managers who cooperated and participated in the data collection. We also thank Carmen Carpena for her support during data collection. CIBEROBN is an initiative of Instituto de Salud Carlos III, Spain.

Conflicts of Interest: The authors declare no conflict of interest.

References

1. Gil, S.M.; Gil, J.; Ruiz, F.; Irazusta, A.; Irazusta, J. Physiological and anthropometric characteristics of young soccer players according to their playing position: Relevance for the selection process. *J. Strength Cond. Res.* **2007**, *21*, 438–445. [CrossRef]
2. Rodríguez, F.J.R.; Flores, A.A.A.; Farias, T.Y.; Gutierrez, O.B.; Arce, P.L. Body composition and referential somatotype of physically active subjects. *Int. J. Morphol.* **2010**, *28*, 1159–1165. [CrossRef]
3. Munguía-Izquierdo, D.; Suárez-Arrones, L.; Di Salvo, V.; Paredes-Hernández, V.; Ara, I.; Mendez-Villanueva, A. Estimating fat-free mass in elite youth male soccer players: Cross-validation of different field methods and development of prediction equation. *J. Sports Sci.* **2019**, *37*, 1197–1204. [CrossRef]
4. Deprez, D.; Valente-Dos-Santos, J.; Coelho-E-Silva, M.J.; Lenoir, M.; Philippaerts, R.; Vaeyens, R. Longitudinal development of explosive leg power from childhood to adulthood in soccer players. *Int. J. Sports Med.* **2015**, *36*, 672–679. [CrossRef]
5. Kemper, G.L.J.; Van Der Sluis, A.; Brink, M.S.; Visscher, C.; Frencken, W.G.P.; Elferink-Gemser, M.T. Anthropometric injury risk factors in elite-standard youth soccer. *Int. J. Sports Med.* **2015**, *36*, 1112–1117. [CrossRef]
6. Nikolaidis, P.T. Association between body mass index, body fat per cent and muscle power output in soccer players. *Cent. Eur. J. Med.* **2012**, *7*, 783–789. [CrossRef]

7. Slimani, M.; Nikolaidis, P.T. Anthropometric and physiological characteristics of male soccer players according to their competitive level, playing position and age group: A systematic review. *J. Sports Med. Phys. Fit.* **2019**, *59*, 141–163. [CrossRef]
8. Torres-Luque, G.; Calahorro-Cañada, F.; Lara-Sánchez, A.J.; Garatachea, N.; Nikolaidis, P.T. Body composition using bioelectrical impedance analysis in elite young soccer players: The effects of age and playing position. *Sport Sci. Health* **2015**, *11*, 203–210. [CrossRef]
9. Dingley, A.A.; Pyne, D.B.; Burkett, B. Relationships between propulsion and anthropometry in paralympic swimmers. *Int. J. Sports Physiol. Perform.* **2015**, *10*, 978–985. [CrossRef]
10. Medeiros, R.M.V.; Alves, E.S.; Lemos, V.A.; Schwingel, P.A.; da Silva, A.; Vital, R.; Vieira, A.S.; Barreto, M.M.; Rocha, E.A.; Tufik, S.; et al. Assessment of body composition and sport performance of brazilian paralympic swim team athletes. *J. Sport Rehabil.* **2016**, *25*, 364–370. [CrossRef]
11. Lemos, V.D.A.; Alves, E.D.S.; Schwingel, P.A.; Rosa, J.P.P.; Da Silva, A.; Winckler, C.; Vital, R.; De Almeida, A.A.; Tufik, S.; De Mello, M.T. Analysis of the body composition of Paralympic athletes: Comparison of two methods. *Eur. J. Sport Sci.* **2016**, *16*, 955–964. [CrossRef] [PubMed]
12. Oliveira, G.L.; Oliveira, T.A.P.; Penello, F.M.; Fernandes Filho, J. Anthropometric characteristics and aerobic fitness of blind athletes of 5-a-side football. *Rev. Peru. Cienc. Act. Física Deporte* **2020**, *7*, 10.
13. Runciman, P.; Tucker, R.; Ferreira, S.; Albertus-Kajee, Y.; Micklesfield, L.; Derman, W. Site-specific bone mineral density is unaltered despite differences in fat-free soft tissue mass between affected and nonaffected sides in hemiplegic paralympic athletes with cerebral palsy: Preliminary findings. *Am. J. Phys. Med. Rehabil.* **2016**, *95*, 771–778. [CrossRef] [PubMed]
14. Juzwiak, C.R.; Winckler, C.; Joaquim, D.P.; Silva, A.; De Mello, M.T. Comparison of measured and predictive values of basal metabolic rate in brazilian paralympic track and field athletes. *Int. J. Sport Nutr. Exerc. Metab.* **2016**, *26*, 330–337. [CrossRef] [PubMed]
15. Flueck, J.L. Body composition in Swiss elite wheelchair athletes. *Front. Nutr.* **2020**, *7*. [CrossRef]
16. Keil, M.; Totosy de Zepetnek, J.O.; Brooke-Wavell, K.; Goosey-Tolfrey, V.L. Measurement precision of body composition variables in elite wheelchair athletes, using dual-energy X-ray absorptiometry. *Eur. J. Sport Sci.* **2016**, *16*, 65–71. [CrossRef]
17. Willems, A.; Thomas, T.A.; Keil, M.; Brooke-Wavell, K.; Goosey-Tolfrey, V.L. Dual-energy X-ray absorptiometry, skinfold thickness, and waist circumference for assessing body composition in ambulant and non-ambulant wheelchair games players. *Front. Physiol.* **2015**, *6*. [CrossRef]
18. Porto, Y.C.; Almeida, M.; De Sá, C.C.; Schwingel, P.A.; Zoppi, C.C. Anthropometric and physical characteristics of motor disabilited paralympic rowers. *Res. Sports Med.* **2008**, *16*, 203–212. [CrossRef]
19. Reina, R.; Sarabia, J.M.; Caballero, C.; Yanci, J. How does the ball influence the performance of change of direction and sprint tests in para-footballers with brain impairments? Implications for evidence-based classification in CP-Football. *PLoS ONE* **2017**, *12*, 1–16. [CrossRef]
20. Reina, R.; Iturricastillo, A.; Sabido, R.; Campayo-Piernas, M.; Yanci, J. Vertical and horizontal jump capacity in international cerebral palsy football players. *Int. J. Sports Physiol. Perform.* **2018**, *13*, 597–603. [CrossRef]
21. Gorla, J.; Nogueira, C.D.; Gonçalves, H.R.; De Faria, F.R.; Buratti, J.R.; Nunes, N.; do Rêgo, J.T.P.; Borges, M.; Vieira, I.B.; Roca, V.L. Composición corporal y perfil somatotípico de jugadores brasileños de fútbol siete con Parálisis Cerebral de acuerdo con la clasificación funcional. Contribución al deporte paralímpico. *Retos Nuevas Tendencias en Educación física Deporte y Recreación* **2019**, *35*, 326–328.
22. Yanci, J.; Los Arcos, A.; Grande, I.; Santalla, A.; Figueroa, J.; Gil, E.; Cámara, J. Jump capacity in cerebral palsy soccer players. *Int. J. Med. Sci. Phys. Act. Sport* **2014**, *14*, 199–211.
23. Durstine, J.L.; Moore, G.E.; Painter, P.L.; Roberts, S.O. *ACSM's Exercise Management for Persons with Chronic Diseases and Disabilities*, 3rd ed.; ACSM: Champaign, IL, USA, 2009.
24. Reina, R.; Elvira, J.; Valverde, M.; Roldán, A.; Yanci, J. Kinematic and kinetic analyses of the vertical jump with and without header as performed by para-footballers with cerebral palsy. *Sports* **2019**, *7*, 209. [CrossRef] [PubMed]
25. Oftedal, S.; Davies, P.S.W.; Boyd, R.N.; Stevenson, R.D.; Ware, R.S.; Keawutan, P.; Benfer, K.A.; Bell, K.L. Body composition, diet, and physical activity: A longitudinal cohort study in preschoolers with cerebral palsy. *Am. J. Clin. Nutr.* **2017**, *105*, 369–378. [CrossRef] [PubMed]

26. Hildreth, H.G.; Johnson, R.K.; Goran, M.I.; Contompasis, S.H. Body composition in adults with cerebral palsy by dual-energy X-ray absorptiometry, bioelectrical impedance analysis, and skinfold anthropometry compared with the 18O isotope-dilution technique. *Am. J. Clin. Nutr.* **1997**, *66*, 1436–1442. [CrossRef] [PubMed]
27. Snik, D.A.C.; de Roos, N.M. Criterion validity of assessment methods to estimate body composition in children with cerebral palsy: A systematic review. *Ann. Phys. Rehabil. Med.* **2020**. [CrossRef]
28. Iversen, E.; Hassager, C.; Christiansen, C. The effect of hemiplegia on bone mass and soft tissue body composition. *Acta Neurol. Scand.* **1989**, *79*, 155–159. [CrossRef]
29. De Brito, C.M.M.; Garcia, A.C.F.; Takayama, L.; Fregni, F.; Battistella, L.R.; Pereira, R.M.R. Bone loss in chronic hemiplegia: A longitudinal cohort study. *J. Clin. Densitom.* **2013**, *16*, 160–167. [CrossRef]
30. Hafer-Macko, C.E.; Ryan, A.S.; Ivey, F.M.; Macko, R.F. Skeletal muscle changes after hemiparetic stroke and potential beneficial effects of exercise intervention strategies. *J. Rehabil. Res. Dev.* **2008**, *45*, 261–272. [CrossRef]
31. Marfell-Jones, M.J.; Stewart, A.; De Ridder, J. *International Standards for Anthropometric Assessment*; International Society for the Advancement of Kinanthropometry: Potchefstroom, South Africa, 2012.
32. Heyward, V.H.; Wagner, D.R. *Applied Body Composition Assessment*; Human Kinetics: Champaign, IL, USA, 2004; ISBN 0736046305.
33. Alvero Cruz, J.R.; Cabañas Armesilla, M.D.; Herrero de Lucas, A.; Martinez Riaza, L.; Moreno Pascual, C.; Porta Manzañino, J.; Sillero Quintana, M.; Sirvent Belando, J.E. Protocolo de valoración de la composición corporal para el reconocimiento médico-deportivo. Documento de consenso del grupo español de cineantropometría de la federación española de medicina del deporte. *Rev. Arch. Med. Deporte* **2009**, *16*, 166–179.
34. Faulkner, J.A. Physiology of swimming. *Res. Q. Am. Assoc. Heal. Phys. Educ. Recreat.* **1966**, *37*, 41–54. [CrossRef]
35. Carter, J.L. Body composition of Montreal olympic athletes. In *Physical Structure of Olympic Athletes*; Carter, J.E.L., Ed.; Basel Karger Publishers: Basel, Switzerland, 1982; pp. 107–116.
36. Withers, R.T.; Craig, N.P.; Bourdon, P.C.; Norton, K.I. Relative body fat and anthropometric prediction of body density of male athletes. *Eur. J. Appl. Physiol. Occup. Physiol.* **1987**, *56*, 191–200. [CrossRef] [PubMed]
37. Siri, W.E. Body composition from fluid spaces and density: Analysis of methods. *Tech. Meas. Body Compos.* **1961**, *61*, 223–244.
38. Martin, A. Anthropometric assessment of bone mineral. In *Anthropometric Assessment of Nutritional Status*; Himes, J., Ed.; Wiley-Liss: New York, NY, USA, 1991; pp. 185–196.
39. Valensise, H.; Andreoli, A.; Lello, S.; Magnani, F.; Romanini, C.; De Lorenzo, A. Total-body skeletal muscle mass: Development and cross-validation of anthropometric prediction models. *Am. J. Clin. Nutr.* **2000**, *72*, 796–803. [CrossRef]
40. Garrido-Chamorro, R.; Sirvent-Belando, J.E.; González-Lorenzo, M.; Blasco-Lafarga, C.; Roche, E. Sumatorio de Pliegues Subcutáneos: Valores de Referencia para Atletas de Élite. *Int. J. Morphol.* **2012**, *30*, 803–809. [CrossRef]
41. Ross, W.D.; Wilson, N.C. A stratagem for proportional growth assessment. *Acta Paediatr. Belg.* **1974**, *28*, 169–182.
42. Bacciotti, S.; Baxter-Jones, A.; Gaya, A.; Maia, J. Body physique and proportionality of Brazilian female artistic gymnasts. *J. Sports Sci.* **2018**. [CrossRef]
43. Alacid, F.; Marfell-Jones, M.; Muyor, J.M.; López-Miñarro, P.A.; Martínez, I. Kinanthropometric comparison between young elite kayakers and canoeists. *Coll. Antropol.* **2015**, *39*, 119–124.
44. Ross, W.D. Kinanthropometry. In *Physiological Testing of the High-Performance Athlete*; Human Kinetics: Champaign, IL, USA, 1991.
45. Tomczak, M.; Tomczak, E. The need to report effect size estimates revisited. An overview of some recommended measures of effect size. *Trends Sport Sci.* **2014**, *1*, 19–25.
46. Cohen, J. *Statistical Power Analysis for the Behavioral Sciences*; Routledge: Abingdon, UK, 2013.
47. Portal, S.; Rabinowitz, J.; Adler-Portal, D.; Burstein, R.P.; Lahav, Y.; Meckel, Y.; Nemet, D.; Eliakim, A. Body fat measurements in elite adolescent volleyball players: Correlation between skinfold thickness, bioelectrical impedance analysis, air-displacement plethysmography, and body mass index percentiles. *J. Pediatr. Endocrinol. Metab.* **2010**, *23*, 395–400. [CrossRef]
48. Ferrang, T.M.; Johnson, R.K.; Ferrara, M.S. Dietary and anthropometric assessment of adults with cerebral palsy. *J. Am. Diet. Assoc.* **1992**, *92*, 1083–1086. [PubMed]
49. Oliveira, C.; Ferreira, D.; Caetano, C.; Granja, D.; Pinto, R.; Mendes, B.; Sousa, M. Nutrition and supplementation in soccer. *Sports* **2017**, *5*, 28. [CrossRef] [PubMed]

50. Ackland, T.R.; Ong, K.B.; Kerr, D.A.; Ridge, B. Morphological characteristics of Olympic sprint canoe and kayak paddlers. *J. Sci. Med. Sport* **2003**. [CrossRef]
51. Sanchis-Moysi, J.; Calbet, J.A.L. Ghost or real musculoskeletal asymmetries in football players? *Med. Sci. Sports Exerc.* **2016**, *48*. [CrossRef] [PubMed]
52. Oberhofer, K.; Stott, N.S.; Mithraratne, K.; Anderson, I.A. Subject-specific modelling of lower limb muscles in children with cerebral palsy. *Clin. Biomech.* **2010**, *25*, 88–94. [CrossRef]
53. Monbaliu, E.; De Cock, P.; Mailleux, L.; Dan, B.; Feys, H. The relationship of dystonia and choreoathetosis with activity, participation and quality of life in children and youth with dyskinetic cerebral palsy. *Eur. J. Paediatr. Neurol.* **2017**, *21*, 327–335. [CrossRef]
54. Chad, K.E.; McKay, H.A.; Zello, G.A.; Bailey, D.A.; Faulkner, R.A.; Snyder, R.E. Body composition in nutritionally adequate ambulatory and non-ambulatory children with cerebral palsy and a healthy reference group. *Dev. Med. Child Neurol.* **2000**. [CrossRef]
55. Verschuren, O.; Peterson, M.D.; Balemans, A.C.J.; Hurvitz, E.A. Exercise and physical activity recommendations for people with cerebral palsy. *Dev. Med. Child Neurol.* **2016**, *58*, 798–808. [CrossRef]
56. Reina, R.; Sarabia, J.M.; Yanci, J.; García-Vaquero, M.P.; Campayo-Piernas, M. Change of direction ability performance in cerebral palsy football players according to functional profiles. *Front. Physiol.* **2016**, *6*, 409. [CrossRef]
57. Cans, C. Surveillance of cerebral palsy in Europe: A collaboration of cerebral palsy surveys and registers. *Dev. Med. Child Neurol.* **2000**, *42*, 816–824. [CrossRef]

Publisher's Note: MDPI stays neutral with regard to jurisdictional claims in published maps and institutional affiliations.

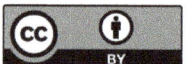

© 2020 by the authors. Licensee MDPI, Basel, Switzerland. This article is an open access article distributed under the terms and conditions of the Creative Commons Attribution (CC BY) license (http://creativecommons.org/licenses/by/4.0/).

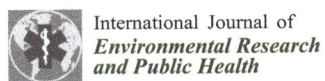
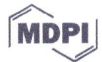

Article

The Influence of Maturity Status on Anthropometric Profile and Body Composition of Youth Goalkeepers

Andrea Di Credico [1], Giulia Gaggi [1], Barbara Ghinassi [1], Gabriele Mascherini [2], Cristian Petri [2], Riccardo Di Giminiani [3], Angela Di Baldassarre [1,*] and Pascal Izzicupo [1]

[1] Department of Medicine and Aging Sciences, University "G. D'Annunzio" of Chieti-Pescara, 66100 Chieti, Italy; andrea.dicredico@unich.it (A.D.C.); giulia.gaggi@unich.it (G.G.); b.ghinassi@unich.it (B.G.); izzicupo@unich.it (P.I.)
[2] Department of Experimental and Clinical Medicine, University of Florence, 50121 Firenze, Italy; gabriele.mascherini@unifi.it (G.M.); cristian.petri@unifi.it (C.P.)
[3] Department of Biotechnological and Applied Clinical Sciences, University of L'Aquila, 67100 L'Aquila, Italy; riccardo.digiminiani@univaq.it
* Correspondence: angela.dibaldassarre@unich.it

Received: 30 September 2020; Accepted: 6 November 2020; Published: 8 November 2020

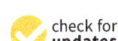

Abstract: The anthropometric profile assessment is an important aspect to consider during the growth stages of youth sport practitioners due to its usefulness in controlling maturity status and overall health. We performed an anthropometric profile evaluation in a sample of youth goalkeepers ($n = 42$) during a training camp, dividing them into three categories based on their years from peak height velocity (YPHV). We also checked if the selection of goalkeepers was associated with the birth quartile. The results showed that most of the participants' anthropometric parameters followed the normal trend according to the maturation stages. However, several subjects showed an overweight/obese condition and/or high waist circumference. Non-optimal values were found, mostly in the group of goalkeepers around the PHV. In addition, no selection based on birth quartile was seen. Therefore, the anthropometric profile and body composition of youth goalkeepers are physiologically affected by maturity status. However, several subjects were found to be overweight/obese and at cardiometabolic risk, suggesting that children and adolescents, although practicing sport, should pay attention to potentially contributing factors such as the attainment of the recommended levels of physical activity, lowering sedentary time, and adopt a healthy lifestyle.

Keywords: anthropometry; somatic maturation; body composition; cardiometabolic risk; youth athletes; soccer; obesity; physical health

1. Introduction

Anthropometry is a valuable technique for assessing the size, proportions, and composition of the human body [1]. Common anthropometric measurements include height, weight, skinfolds, and circumferences, frequently used as nutritional status indexes, health, and growth [2]. In particular, anthropometry and the derived body composition parameters are useful tools to evaluate both the children and adolescents at the different stages of growth [3]. In this regard, Mirwald et al. developed a formula to obtain the peak height velocity (PHV) [4]. PHV is defined as the maximum velocity of growth in stature or the growth spurt in height, and it represents a valid indicator of somatic maturity status [3]. Moreover, years from PHV (YPHV) are obtained subtracting the age of PHV from chronological age, and characterize a non-invasive method to assess the trend of maturity in children [4].

The anthropometric profile, body composition, and maturity status are parameters of great importance in sports [5–7]. For example, improved body composition in athletes is associated with greater strength [8] and cardiorespiratory fitness [9]. Furthermore, anthropometric variables and maturity are associated with team sports success, such as soccer [10]. For instance, in different soccer categories based on age groups, players in advanced maturation tend to be taller and heavier than others [11,12]. Furthermore, specific anthropometric characteristics represent a prerequisite to playing in different positions considering the different roles (e.g., defenders, forwards, and goalkeepers) [13].

Specifically, goalkeepers tend to be taller and heavier due to the specific requirements of their role. Thus soccer teams are inclined to select them, taking into account such anthropometric characteristics [14]. Accordingly, it seems that coaches and athletic trainers select youth athletes based on their date of birth, preferring those who are more advanced in growth, especially in high-level teams [15]. This phenomenon is known as the relative age effect (RAE), a condition in which the relative birth quarter distribution in a sample of athletes is not evenly distributed [16]. Indeed, in such a situation, the older athletes, born close to the beginning of the year, represent the majority of the team [17]. In contrast, these preferential choices are not evident within soccer teams of lower levels [18].

However, with the increasing adoption of unhealthy lifestyles (including the massive usage of electronic devices and social media), children and adolescents can spend a large amount of time in sedentary behaviors and fail to reach the recommended physical activity levels [19,20], despite sports participation [21]. Sedentary behaviors, physical inactivity, and incorrect nutritional habits are detrimental factors for overall health [22] and are responsible for increasing all-cause mortality [23] at all population levels [24]. Thus, examinations indicating pathological states such as obesity or cardiometabolic risk in children and adolescents participating in sport are valuable procedures [25]. In this regard, different parameters can be assessed. For example, body mass index (BMI) is extensively used to recognize subjects having excessive adiposity [4,26–28]. However, BMI usage has significant limitations, as it does not allow discrimination between fat mass (FM) and free fat mass (FFM) [27]. Thus, body FM and the percentage of fat mass (%FM) are usually assessed to overcome BMI limits. However, even the %FM alone does consider factors such as height and FFM [29]. In this regard, the fat mass index (FMI) and fat-free mass index (FFMI) are two useful estimates to use along with BMI, absolute FM, and %FM for assessing body composition using anthropometry [30].

Other valuable methods are skinfold and circumference measurements and the ratios between various anthropometric parameters [28,31,32]. Notably, the skinfold thickness is a valid anthropometric indicator of fatness because it is widely representative of adipose tissue [33]. Moreover, higher waist circumferences are associated with an increased health risk, and measures such as waist/height ratio represent a useful means to stratify cardiometabolic risk in the youth population, taking into account sex and age [34,35]. Given the importance of such measures, various references for children and adolescents exist [31,36]. Hence, performing periodic anthropometric assessments is of utmost importance in children and adolescents, particularly in a team sport context, where such analysis provides insight about the ideal predisposition for a specific role/position, performance, and health as well [37]. In particular, the assessment of maturity status allows considerations beyond the simple chronological age, body size, proportion, and composition.

Therefore, this observational study aimed to investigate how maturity status, based on YPHV, can influence the anthropometric profile and body composition of youth goalkeepers from different soccer teams, indicating the differences in the different stages of maturation. We also analyzed how the different anthropometric variables correlated with YPHV. Finally, we checked if maturity status could lead to the presence of RAE in the different groups.

2. Materials and Methods

2.1. Participants

Forty-two young male goalkeepers were recruited from different soccer teams during a training camp dedicated to youth goalkeepers. Participants were classified into three groups: pre-PHV ($n = 12$, age = 11.98 ± 0.93), circa-PHV ($n = 14$, age = 13.74 ± 0.74) and post-PHV ($n = 16$, age = 15.99 ± 0.72).

All participants were involved in soccer as goalkeepers from at least one year and performed 3 to 5 training sessions per week. The study was conducted in accordance with the Declaration of Helsinki. This study is part of a project of the Tuscany Region called "Sports Medicine to support regional surveillance systems"; it was approved by the Regional Prevention Plan 2014–2018 with the code O-Range18. Informed consent was obtained from all the participants before inclusion in the study.

2.2. Anthropometry and Body Composition

All the anthropometric measurements were performed by a certified specialist (i.e., a level 1 certification of the International Society for the Advancement of Kinanthropometry (ISAK)). Subjects wore light clothing and had fasted for at least 12 h before the assessments. Height was measured to the nearest 0.1 cm, and body weight was measured to the nearest 0.1 kg using a stadiometer with a balance-beam scale (Seca 200, Seca, Hamburg, Germany). Triceps and subscapular skinfolds were measured using a Cescorf skinfold caliper (Cescorf, Porto Alegre, Brazil). Arm span, waist circumferences (WC), and mid-arm circumference (MAC) were measured using a Cescorf anthropometric tape (Cescorf, Porto Alegre, Brazil). The percentage of fat-mass was calculated according to Slaughter [38] as follows:

$$Prepubescent\ White\ Males: \%FM = 1.21\ (triceps + subscapular) - 0.008\ (triceps + subscapular)^2 - 1.7 \quad (1)$$

$$Pubescent\ White\ Males: \%FM = 1.21(triceps + subscapular) - 0.008\ (triceps + subscapular)^2 - 3.4 \quad (2)$$

$$Postpubescent\ White\ Males: \%FM = 1.21(triceps + subscapular) - 0.008\ (triceps + subscapular)^2 - 5.5 \quad (3)$$

For sum of triceps and subscapular greater than 35 mm: $\%FM = 0.783\ (triceps + subscapular) + 1.6$ (4)

Mid-arm muscle circumference (MAMC), mid-arm area (MAA), mid-arm muscle area (MAMA), mid-arm fat area (MAFA), and arm fat index (AFI) were calculated as follows:

$$MAMC = MAC - \left(\pi \times \frac{Triceps\ skinfold}{10}\right) \quad (5)$$

$$MAA = \frac{MAC^2}{4 \times \pi} \quad (6)$$

$$MAMA = \frac{MAMC^2}{4 \times \pi} \quad (7)$$

$$MAFA = MAA - MAMA \quad (8)$$

$$AFI = 100 \times \frac{MAFA}{MAA} \quad (9)$$

Body mass index (BMI) was calculated as weight in kilograms divided by the square of height, expressed in meters. Participants who had a WC >90th percentile, considering McCarthy's waist circumference as a reference [39], were considered to have abdominal obesity, and a cutoff of 0.5 was used to differentiate low waist to height ratio (W/Hr) from high W/Hr [28,40].

2.3. Age and Maturity Status

According to the estimated age at PHV, the maturity status was defined based on the Mirwald et al. equation [4]. Participants were classified into three groups based on their YPHV: pre-PHV (offset <−1 years), circa-PHV (≤±1 years), and post-PHV (offset >+1 years), as a previous study reported [41].

2.4. Statistical Analysis

The Shapiro–Wilk test was performed to check the normality of the data. The analysis of variance (ANOVA) was used to determine the differences between maturity status group (defined as fixed factor) in body composition and anthropometric parameters (defined as dependent variables), and partial eta squared (η^2_p) was calculated to indicate the effect-size (small = 0.01, medium = 0.06, large = 0.14) [42]. When the analysis of variance (ANOVA) showed significant results, a Tukey's post hoc test was used to confirm where the differences occurred. Pearson's correlation coefficient was used to determine the extent of correlation between YPHV and anthropometric measures. Following the appropriate indications [43], the magnitude of correlations was considered as: r = 0.00–0.09, negligible; r = 0.10–0.39, weak; r = 0.40–0.69, moderate; r = 0.70–0.89, strong; r = 0.90–1.00, very strong. Finally, when the necessary conditions were met, the chi-square (χ^2) test for independence was used to check the association between maturity status and the selected categories (BMI, waist circumference, birth quartile, growth velocity, and achievement of peak growth). When data were not normally distributed, the Kruskal–Wallis with Dunn's post-hoc test was used instead of ANOVA and Tukey's post hoc, and Spearman's Rho was used instead of Pearson's r. Descriptive data are presented as mean ± standard deviation, while categorical data as frequency (count and percentage of the group, total count, and percentage of the total). The statistical significance was set at <0.05.

3. Results

3.1. Anthropometric Profile

Table 1 shows the descriptive statistics for the participants' anthropometric and body composition variables divided by maturity offset.

Age, height and weight were significantly different between groups [$p < 0.001$; F (2,39) = 54.732, $p < 0.001$, η^2_p = 0.737; F (2,39) = 23.945, $p < 0.001$, η^2_p = 0.551, respectively], however post hoc analysis did not shows differences between circa-PHV and post-PHV regarding weight (62.66 ± 10.17 vs. 69.29 ± 10.51, p = 0.163). Similarly, statistical difference was found for sitting height [F (2,39) = 54.824, $p < 0.001$, η^2_p = 0.744] and arm span [F (2,39) = 34.722, $p < 0.001$, η^2_p = 0.640]. On the other hand, both arm span to height ratio (AS/Hr) and sitting height to height ratio (SH/Hr) were similar in the three groups (p = 0.522; p = 0.330, respectively).

Regarding skinfolds measurements, a significantly difference was seen for triceps skinfold (p = 0.042) but not for subscapular skinfold, (p = 0.143) with circa-PHV showing the highest values. The mid-arm circumference (MAC) was statistically different [F (2,39) = 7.393, p = 0.002, η^2_p = 0.275] although the Tukey's post hoc demonstrates that such a variable was similar between circa-PHV and post-PHV (26.89 ± 4.31 vs. 28.30 ± 2.03, p = 0.454). Furthermore, the derived mid-arm muscle circumference (MAMC) showed even more significant difference ($p < 0.001$) and in this case the post hoc demonstrates differences also between circa-PHV and post-PHV (21.99 ± 3.70 vs. 25.17 ± 1.57, p = 0.005). Similarly, both the mid-arm area (MAA) and the mid-arm muscle area (MAMA) were significantly different between groups [F (2,39) = 7.610, p = 0.002, η^2_p = 0.281; F (2,39) = 23.213, $p < 0.001$, η^2_p = 0.543], respectively. However the MAA was similar when comparing the circa-PHV with the post-PHV (58.96 ± 17.20 vs. 64.07 ± 9.54, p = 0.527). In addition, also the arm fat index (AFI) showed a significant difference between the three groups of goalkeepers (p = 0.005), but with pre-PHV and circa-PHV participants showing similar results. On the other hand, mid-arm fat area (MAFA) did not showed differences (p = 0.168).

The WC was significantly different between the groups [F (2,39) = 7.782, p = 0.001, η^2_p = 0.285], however the post hoc test showed no difference between circa-PHV and post-PHV (75.21 ± 6.96 vs. 74.09 ± 4.47, p = 0.869). Also waist to height ratio (W/Hr) was different between the groups (p = 0.029). Finally, the percentage of predicted adult height (%PAH) was significantly different ($p < 0.001$), while the predicted adult height (PAH) showed no significant differences [F (2,39) = 0.854, p = 0.434, η^2_p = 0.042].

Table 1. Descriptive data of goalkeepers based on maturity status.

	Pre-PHV (n = 12)		Circa-PHV (n = 14)		Post-PHV (n = 16)			
	M ±SD	Min-Max	M ±SD	Min-Max	M ±SD	Min-Max	p	η^2_p
YPHV [a,b,c]	−2.02 ± 0.93	−4.10–−1.1	−0.26 ± 0.74	−1.0–−1.0	1.99 ± 0.71	1.10–3.60	<0.001	0.822
Age (years) [a,b,c]	11.43 ± 1.37	8.80–13.04	12.86 ± 1.33	10.35–15.0	15.58 ± 0.62	14.30–16.70	<0.001 †	-
Height (cm) [a,b,c]	149.85 ± 7.64	133.30–157.70	166.43 ± 7.61	156.65–179.35	177.00 ± 5.22	171.30–189.30	<0.001	0.737
Weight (kg) [a,b]	44.06 ± 7.88	25.90–54.70	62.66 ± 10.17	47.30–84.55	69.29 ± 10.51	57.80–99.00	<0.001	0.551
Sitting Height (cm) [a,b,c]	77.23 ± 3.55	69.0–81.50	85.94 ± 4.29	82.0–94.0	92.69 ± 3.53	88.0–99.0	<0.001	0.738
Arm Span (cm) [a,b,c]	152.13 ± 10.28	130.60–161.0	169.9 ± 9.11	159.0–185.05	180.13 ± 6.95	169.45–192.0	<0.001	0.640
AS/Hr	1.02 ± 0.03	0.95–1.04	1.02 ± 0.02	0.99–1.05	1.01 ± 0.02	0.98–1.04	0.522 †	-
SH/Hr	0.52 ± 0.01	0.50–0.54	0.52 ± 0.01	0.48–0.54	0.52 ± 0.01	0.50–0.54	0.330 †	-
Triceps Skinfold [c]	13.77 ± 6.44	5.50–23.0	15.61 ± 5.91	5.50–25.0	9.97 ± 3.31	6.0–18.0	0.042 †	-
Subscapular Skinfold	8.31 ± 4.88	3.50–20.75	10.36 ± 4.38	5.0–21.0	7.63 ± 1.99	5.0–12.75	0.143 †	-
MAC (cm) [a]	23.68 ± 2.87	17.50–27.50	26.89 ± 4.31	15.90–33.90	28.30 ± 2.03	25.50–34.0	0.002	0.275
MAMC (cm) [a,b,c]	19.36 ± 1.59	15.62–22.12	21.99 ± 3.70	11.19–26.05	25.17 ± 1.57	22.63–28.35	<0.001†	-
MAA (cm²) [a,b]	45.26 ± 10.51	24.38–60.21	58.96 ± 17.20	20.13–91.50	64.07 ± 9.54	51.77–92.04	0.002	0.281
MAMA (cm²) [a,b,c]	30.02 ± 4.77	19.42–38.94	39.52 ± 11.17	9.97–54.03	50.63 ± 6.39	40.78–63.98	<0.001	0.543
MAFA (cm²)	15.23 ± 7.99	4.97–27.47	19.44 ± 9.03	5.81–37.47	13.45 ± 5.13	7.37–28.06	0.168†	-
AFI [b,c]	31.81 ± 11.26	15.08–45.63	32.79 ± 10.77	15.08–50.47	20.64 ± 5.46	13.00–30.94	0.005†	-
WC (cm) [a,b]	66.59 ± 6.59	54.40–79.50	75.21 ± 6.96	62.0–87.40	74.09 ± 4.47	68.25–87.15	0.001	0.285
W/Hr	0.46 ± 0.05	0.39–0.55	0.45 ± 0.04	0.37–0.53	0.42 ± 0.02	0.38–0.48	0.029†	-
PAH (cm)	180.98 ± 3.26	175.29–186.42	179.23 ± 7.88	166.90–190.61	182.16 ± 6.07	174.39–197.91	0.434	0.042
%PAH [a,b,c]	82.79 ± 3.76	75.28–86.62	92.89 ± 2.87	86.54–95.60	97.22 ± 2.97	87.74–99.86	<0.001 †	-
BMI (kg/m²) [a,b]	19.62 ± 3.38	13.60–26.00	22.57 ± 2.69	18.50–27.60	22.06 ± 2.64	18.90–30.0	0.031	0.163
FM (kg) [a,b]	8.11 ± 1.47	5.27–10.98	10.93 ± 2.22	7.30–14.99	10.33 ± 1.76	8.59–15.50	0.001	0.295
%FM [a,b,c]	18.47 ± 1.25	16.81–20.65	17.36 ± 1.27	15.02–19.47	14.87 ± 0.58	13.86–15.96	<0.001†	-
FMI [c]	3.63 ± 0.75	2.77–5.21	3.94 ± 0.68	2.77–5.37	3.29 ± 0.48	2.64–4.71	0.016†	-
FFMI [a,b]	15.98 ± 2.69	10.85–20.77	18.61 ± 2.06	15.69–22.37	18.77 ± 2.19	16.06–25.33	0.005	0.235

Pre-PHV = pre-peak height velocity; Circa-PHV = circa-peak height velocity; Post-PHV = post-peak height velocity; YPHV = years from peak height velocity; AS/Hr = arm span to height ratio; SH/Hr = sitting height to height ratio; MAC = mid-arm circumference; MAMC = mid-arm muscle circumference; AFI = arm fat index; WC = waist circumference; PAH = predicted adult height; %PAH = percentage of predicted adult height; BMI = body mass index; FM = fat mass; %FM = percentage of fat mass; FMI = fat mass index; FFMI = free fat mass index; W/Hr = waist to height ratio. Data are expressed as mean ± standard deviation. [a] indicates statistical significance for pre-PHV vs. circa-PHV; [b] indicates statistical significance for pre-PHV vs. post-PHV; [c] indicates statistical significance for circa-PHV vs. post-PHV; † indicates Kruskal-Wallis results.

3.2. Body Composition

The three groups of goalkeepers showed a statistically different BMI [F (2,39) = 3.798, p = 0.031, η^2_p = 0.163] although the values between circa-PHV and post-PHV were comparable (22.57 ± 2.69 vs. 22.06 ± 2.64, p = 0.883). Similarly, absolute fat mass was different [F (2,39) = 8.173, p = 0.001, η^2_p = 0.295] while the post hoc revealed that circa-PHV and post-PHV participants fat mass was similar (10.93 ± 2.22 vs. 10.33 ± 1.76, p = 0.649). The %FM was also significantly different (p < 0.001) and showed a decreasing trend from pre-PHV to post-PHV. Likewise, the fat mass index (FMI) and the fat free mass index (FFMI) were different between groups [p = 0.016; F (2,39) = 5.994, p = 0.005, η^2_p = 0.235, respectively], with a significant difference between circa-PHV and post-PHV for FMI (3.94 ± 0.68 vs. 3.29 ± 0.48, p = 0.002) and pre-PHV differing from circa-PHV and post-PHV, regarding FFMI values (15.98 ± 2.69 vs. 18.61 ± 2.06 p = 0.016; 15.98 ± 2.69 vs. 18.77 ± 2.19, p = 0.008, respectively).

3.3. Correlation between Years from Peak Height Velocity (YPHV) and Anthropometric Measures

Correlation analysis showed that YPHV had a significant relationship with weight, height, arm span, sitting height, MAC, MAMC, MAA, MAMA, AFI, WC, W/Hr, %PAH, BMI, FM, %FM, and FFMI. Table 2 contains the complete panel of correlations.

Table 2. This table shows the correlation between YPHV and anthropometric measures.

Selected Variables	Correlation with YPHV (Pearson's r or Spearman's Rho)	p	Lower 95% CI–Upper 95% CI
Weight	0.767	<0.001	0.604–0.869
Height	0.921	<0.001	0.856–0.957
Arm Span	0.875	<0.001	0.778–0.931
AS/Hr	−0.138 †	0.382	−0.424–0.173
Sitting Height	0.941	<0.001	0.892–0.968
SH/Hr	0.289 †	0.064	−0.017–0.545
Triceps Skinfold	−0.284 †	0.069	−0.541–0.022
Subscapular Skinfold	−0.034 †	0.830	−0.335–0.273
MAC	0.550	<0.001	0.295–0.732
MAMC	0.809 †	<0.001	0.670–0.893
MAA	0.541	<0.001	0.284–0.726
MAMA	0.763	<0.001	0.598–0.866
MAFA	−0.087 †	0.584	−0.381–0.223
AFI	−0.437 †	0.004	−0.654–−0.153
WC	0.405	0.008	0.115–0.631
W/Hr	−0.343 †	0.026	−0.586–−0.043
PAH	0.159	0.313	−0.152–0.442
%PAH	0.941 †	<0.001	0.893–0.968
BMI	0.319	0.039	0.017–0.568
FM	0.404	0.008	0.114–0.631
%FM	−0.878 †	<0.001	−0.933–−0.783
FMI	−0.260 †	0.097	−0.522–0.048
FFMI	0.457	0.002	0.178–0.668

YPHV = years from PHV; AS/Hr = arm span to height ratio; SH/Hr = sitting height to height ratio; MAC = mid-arm circumference; MAMC = mid-arm muscle circumference; AFI = arm fat index; WC = waist circumference; PAH = predicted adult height; %PAH = percentage of predicted adult height; BMI = body mass index; FM = fat mass; %FM = percentage of fat mass; FMI = fat mass index; FFMI = free fat mass index; W/Hr = waist to height ratio; † indicates Spearman's Rho.

Specifically, height (r = 0.921), sitting height (r = 0.941), and %PAH (r_s = 0.941) showed a very strong positive correlation. In addition, weight (r = 0.767), arm span (r = 0.875), MAMC (r_s = 0.809) and MAMA (r = 0.763) highlighted a strong direct correlation, while %FM (r_s = −0.878) had strong negative correlation. Also, MAC (r = 0.550), MAA (r = 0.541), WC (r = 0.405), fat mass (r = 0.404), and FFMI (r = 0.457) presented a moderate positive correlation, whereas AFI (r_s = −0.437) showed a moderate negative relationship. Finally, W/Hr (r_s = −0.343) and BMI (r = 0.319) showed weak negative and positive correlations, respectively.

On the other hand, AS/Hr, SH/Hr, subscapular skinfold, MAFA, PAH, FMI, and triceps skinfold did not show a significant correlation with YPHV, although triceps skinfold was close to statistical significance, presenting a weak negative correlation (r = −0.288, p = 0.065).

3.4. Categories for Body Mass Index (BMI), Waist Circumference (WC), Waist to Height Ratio (W/Hr), Birth Quartile, and Achievement of Peak Growth

As stated before, the participants were assigned to the three groups representing the different maturity status (pre-PHV, circa-PHV, and post-PHV), based on their YPHV.

When the data met the required conditions, the χ^2 test of independence was used to check if the association between the groups of goalkeepers and the selected categories were present. Otherwise, the number of subjects and frequencies were calculated (Figure 1).

The selected categories were: BMI (divided into "normal weight" and "overweight/obese"), WC (divided into "not at risk" and "at risk"), birth quartile (divided into "first/second" and "third/fourth"), W/Hr (divided in "normal" and "high"), and achievement in peak growth (divided in "reached" and "not reached").

An association between maturity status and WC categories (χ^2 = 8.956, p = 0.011) was seen (Figure 1a). The circa-PHV group showed the highest number of subjects with a WC >90th percentile and thus was considered at risk regarding this factor (i.e., 10 subjects, representing 71.43% of the circa-PHV group). In the pre-PHV group, 4 subjects (33.33%) were considered at risk, and in the post-PHV, 3 goalkeepers (18.75%) were in the same condition. Taking into account the entire sample of goalkeepers, 17 of them (40.48% of the total) had a WC >90th percentile, while 25 (59.52% of the total) had a normal WC.

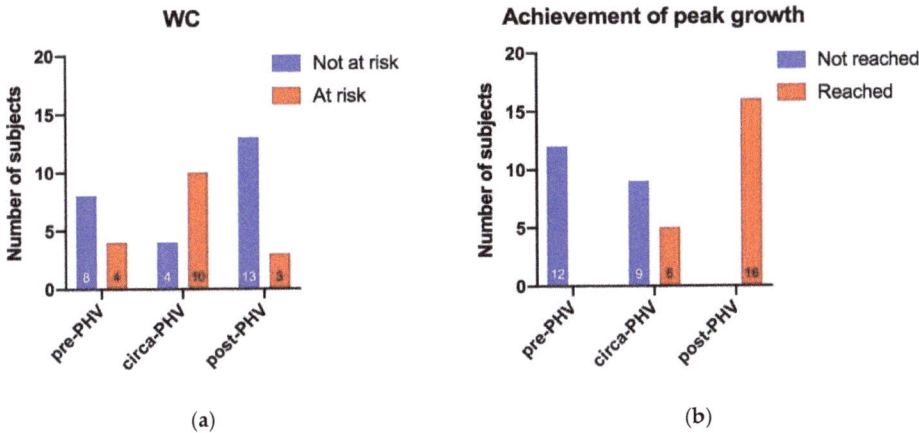

Figure 1. *Cont.*

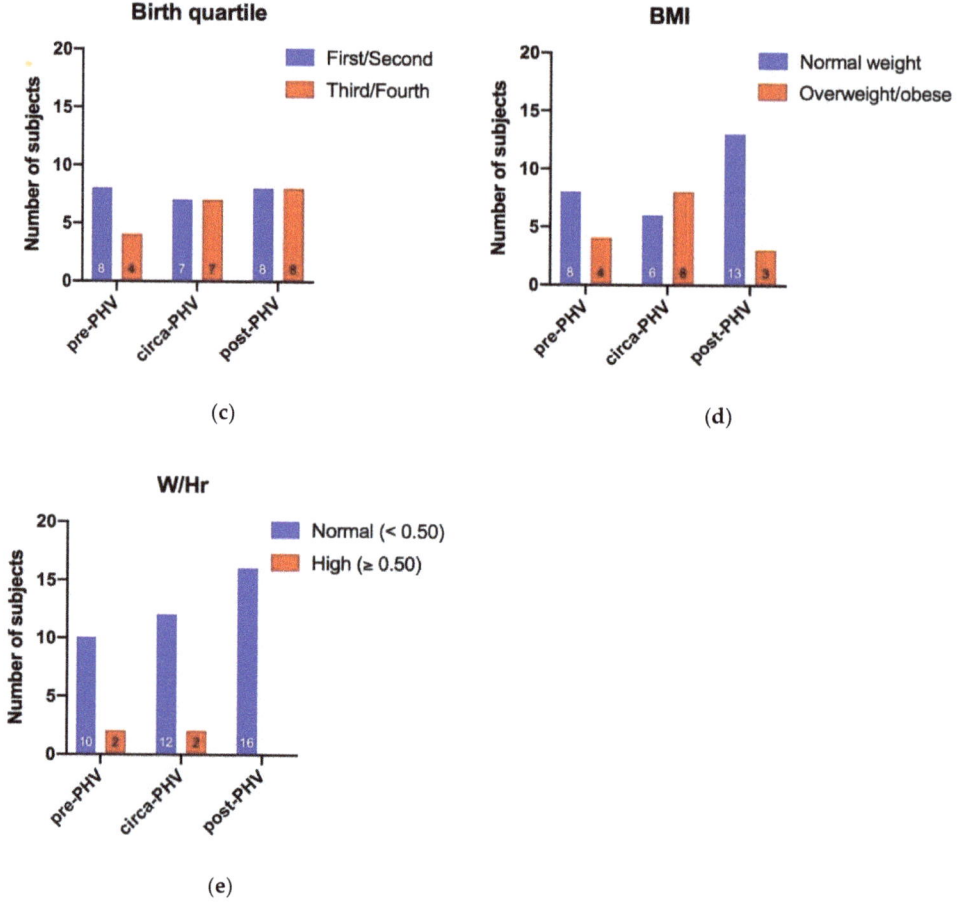

Figure 1. This figure summarizes the association of the three groups of goalkeepers with (**a**) WC, (**b**) achievement of peak growth, (**c**) birth quartile, (**d**) BMI, and (**e**) W/Hr. BMI = body mass index; WC = waist circumference; W/Hr = waist to height ratio.

Moreover, as expected, a strong association between maturity status and peak growth achievement was seen (Figure 1b; $\chi^2 = 29.143$, $p = <0.001$). Indeed, all the participants appertaining at the pre-PHV group ($n = 12$, 100.00%) had not reached the peak growth, whereas all the subjects in the post-PHV group had reached the peak growth ($n = 16$, 100.00%). Regarding the circa-PHV, five subjects (35.71%) had not reached the peak growth, while 9 of them (64.29%) had reached it. Hence, half of the goalkeepers ($n = 21$, 50.00% of the total) had reached the peak growth, and the other half ($n = 21$, 50.00% of the total) had not reached it.

Regarding the birth quartile, the χ^2 test did not showed significance (Figure 1c; $X^2 = 0.961$, $p = 0.618$). The number of subjects born in the first/second quartiles of the year were distributed as follows: pre-PHV, $n = 8$, 66.67%; circa-PHV, $n = 7$, 50.00%; post-PHV, $n = 8$, 50.00%. Overall, 23 participants (54.76%) were born in the first half of the year, while 19 (45.24%) in the second.

BMI and W/Hr data did not meet the required criteria to run the χ^2 test (Figure 1d,e respectively). However, in the pre-PHV group, 4 subjects (33.33%) were overweight/obese, while in the circa-PHV group, 8 subjects (57.14%), and in the post-PHV group 3 (18.75%) subjects were overweight/obese as well. Overall, on the 42 participants, 15 (35.71% of the total) were in overweight/obese condition, and 27 (64.29% of the total) were normal weight.

Finally, two subjects in the pre-PHV group (16.67%) and two subjects in the circa-PHV group (14.29%) presented a high W/Hr.

4. Discussion

In the present study, we investigated the influence of maturity status on the anthropometric profile and body composition of youth goalkeepers from different soccer teams, dividing them considering their somatic maturation state according to their YPHV. In addition, we evaluated whether a RAE was present in the different groups of goalkeepers.

The main results were that, although participating in sport, the group of youth goalkeepers included a high percentage of subjects with unhealthy body composition and that the worst condition was found for the circa-PHV group. Secondly, regarding the RAE, participants in the first and second half of the year were almost equally distributed, and no association was found regarding the number of goalkeepers of the first/second birth quartile and state of maturity. This result agrees with literature reporting that selection based on maturity is more evident in high-level teams [18]. On the other hand, despite the lack of association between goalkeepers' birth quartile and state of maturity, the circa-PHV group was composed mainly of participants who reached the peak growth (64.29%). This result suggests that it is important to pay particular attention to the state of maturity when children are very close to the growth spurt.

As expected, the state of maturity status affected the anthropometric profile and body composition of the goalkeepers. The statistical analysis showed differences in most of the measured variables, indicating an adverse condition regarding body composition for the goalkeepers, mainly in the circa-PHV group compared to the post-PHV group.

For example, although there were differences in age and maturity state, the weight and BMI were similar between circa-PHV and post-PHV, indicating a possible excess in body fat in the younger participants. This aspect was confirmed by comparing body skinfolds and derived body fat measures such as %FM and FMI. We found that triceps skinfold was higher in the circa-PHV, as well as %FM and FMI (Table 1). Although %FM was higher in pre-PHV compared to the others, when fat mass was normalized for height, the circa-PHV group emerged as that with the poorest body composition. Furthermore, the subscapular skinfold was similar among the three groups of goalkeepers but also, in this case, the higher value was found in the circa-PHV.

Considering the entire sample of goalkeepers, 17 (40.48% of the total) showed a high WC that indicated abdominal obesity and increased cardiometabolic risk. A higher number of subjects with abdominal obesity were in the circa-PHV group. Moreover, W/Hr was different between the three states of maturity, and both the pre-PHV and the circa-PHV presented two goalkeepers having the W/Hr higher than 0.5. Waist circumference shows a high correlation with visceral adipose tissue, plasmatic level of lipids, lipoproteins, and the hormone insulin [34], and W/Hr represents a predictor of cardiovascular risk in children and adolescents [28,34].

Assessing anthropometric variables and body composition close to puberty is crucial because it could also predict adult body composition and future health [44]. Typically, in males, there is an increase in FM at 8 years to 14 years, then FM tends to decrease at about 16 years and subsequently tends to reach a plateau [45]. According to this evidence, the subjects appertaining at the circa-PHV group showed increasing adiposity values in our study. However, a major part of them showed pathological conditions and anthropometric values that place them at risk for cardiovascular and metabolic diseases. Furthermore, it is demonstrated that goalkeepers tend to be heavier, taller, and have larger skinfolds than outfielders [13]. However, although it seems that during puberty, FM typically increases and that goalkeepers present higher anthropometric values, in this study, such conditions are exacerbated. Indeed, factors other than normal growth trends could cause such non-optimal condition for circa-PHV.

Overall, an important consideration is that many of the examined youth goalkeepers were in a condition of overweight/obesity and/or presented high WC and W/Hr. In recent years, a worrying increase in pediatric adiposity was observed almost worldwide [46]. Several non-heritable factors contributed to this obesity pandemic among children and adolescents, including nutrition, physical activity, sports participation, sedentary behavior and electronic devices usage, and parental modeling [46–50]. In the present study, a large proportion of participants showed an unfavorable body composition, despite sport participation. In this regard, it is well known that physical exercise and training are potent stimuli that elicit positive adaptation [51–60]. However, a previous study indicated that youth soccer players might fail to reach the recommended physical activity levels during days without sports practice. Furthermore, the less active they were off-training, the less they moved during training practice [21]. Thus, such off-training behaviors could be a major cause of the condition found in our sample [61,62].

In addition, goalkeepers tend to have a lower energy expenditure than outfielders, and such a situation is also reported for high-level professional athletes [63]. Thus, more attention should be paid to youth goalkeepers playing in lower-level teams.

Finally, anthropometry is a valuable tool for monitoring harmful situations associated with adiposity, hormonal status [37], and the extent of cardiovascular risk among children and adolescents [38], as well as avoiding early selection.

Limitations

In this study, we do not measure the levels of physical activity of the participants. However, such an assessment could be useful in future studies investigating anthropometric profile and body composition in youth populations.

5. Conclusions

In conclusion, this study evaluates the anthropometric profile trend of a group of goalkeepers, taking into account the state of maturity. The majority of the variables followed the physiological trend occurring during puberty. However, among the entire examined group, a non-optimal anthropometric situation for many subjects indicated an increased risk of cardiometabolic disease. The results of this study add shreds of evidence that also youth goalkeepers participating in sport could be at health risk, and thus attention should be made to factors known to affect body composition and health (e.g., physical activity, sedentary time, and nutrition habits). Thus, monitoring the anthropometric profile and body composition of children and adolescents participating in sport should be an essential aspect to consider in evaluating possible risk conditions and adopting effective countermeasures.

Author Contributions: Conceptualization, P.I., A.D.C., and A.D.B.; methodology, P.I., A.D.C., and B.G.; formal analysis, P.I., A.D.C..; investigation, P.I., A.D.C., G.G., G.M., R.D.G., and C.P.; data curation, A.D.C., B.G., and G.G.; writing—original draft preparation, A.D.C., P.I., A.D.B., and B.G.; visualization, B.G., G.G., G.M., R.D.G., and C.P.; supervision, P.I., A.D.B., B.G.; funding acquisition, A.D.B. All authors have read and agreed to the published version of the manuscript.

Funding: This research was supported by the Italian Ministry of Education, University and Research (Ministero dell'Istruzione, dell'Università e della Ricerca-MIUR), grant number PRIN 2017ATZ2YK_003.

Conflicts of Interest: The authors declare no conflict of interest.

References

1. WHO. *Physical Status: The Use and Interpretation of Anthropometry. Report of A WHO Expert Committee*; World Health Organization: Geneva, Switzerland, 1995; ISBN 978-92-4-120854-3.
2. Bhattacharya, A.; Pal, B.; Mukherjee, S.; Roy, S.K. Assessment of nutritional status using anthropometric variables by multivariate analysis. *BMC Public Health* **2019**, *19*. [CrossRef] [PubMed]
3. Sherar, L.B.; Mirwald, R.L.; Baxter-Jones, A.D.G.; Thomis, M. Prediction of adult height using maturity-based cumulative height velocity curves. *J. Pediatrics* **2005**, *147*, 508–514. [CrossRef] [PubMed]

4. Mirwald, R.L.; G. Baxter-Jones, A.D.; Bailey, D.A.; Beunen, G.P. An assessment of maturity from anthropometric measurements. *Med. Sci. Sports Exerc.* **2002**, *34*, 689–694. [CrossRef] [PubMed]
5. Rinaldo, N.; Toselli, S.; Gualdi-Russo, E.; Zedda, N.; Zaccagni, L. Effects of Anthropometric Growth and Basketball Experience on Physical Performance in Pre-Adolescent Male Players. *Int. J. Env. Res. Public Health* **2020**, *17*, 2196. [CrossRef] [PubMed]
6. Petri, C.; Campa, F.; Hugo Teixeira, V.; Izzicupo, P.; Galanti, G.; Pizzi, A.; Badicu, G.; Mascherini, G. Body Fat Assessment in International Elite Soccer Referees. *J. Funct. Morphol. Kinesiol.* **2020**, *5*, 38. [CrossRef]
7. Högström, G.M.; Pietilä, T.; Nordström, P.; Nordström, A. Body Composition and Performance: Influence of Sport and Gender Among Adolescents. *J. Strength Cond. Res.* **2012**, *26*, 1799–1804. [CrossRef]
8. Silva, A.M.; Fields, D.A.; Heymsfield, S.B.; Sardinha, L.B. Relationship Between Changes in Total-Body Water and Fluid Distribution With Maximal Forearm Strength in Elite Judo Athletes. *J. Strength Cond. Res.* **2011**, *25*, 2488–2495. [CrossRef]
9. Collings, P.J.; Westgate, K.; Väistö, J.; Wijndaele, K.; Atkin, A.J.; Haapala, E.A.; Lintu, N.; Laitinen, T.; Ekelund, U.; Brage, S.; et al. Cross-Sectional Associations of Objectively-Measured Physical Activity and Sedentary Time with Body Composition and Cardiorespiratory Fitness in Mid-Childhood: The PANIC Study. *Sports Med.* **2017**, *47*, 769–780. [CrossRef]
10. Lago-Peñas, C.; Casais, L.; Dellal, A.; Rey, E.; Domínguez, E. Anthropometric and Physiological Characteristics of Young Soccer Players According to Their Playing Positions: Relevance for Competition Success. *J. Strength Cond. Res.* **2011**, *25*, 3358–3367. [CrossRef]
11. Figueiredo, A.J.; Gonçalves, C.E.; Coelho E Silva, M.J.; Malina, R.M. Youth soccer players, 11–14 years: Maturity, size, function, skill and goal orientation. *Ann. Hum. Biol.* **2009**, *36*, 60–73. [CrossRef] [PubMed]
12. Malina, R.M.; Eisenmann, J.C.; Cumming, S.P.; Ribeiro, B.; Aroso, J. Maturity-associated variation in the growth and functional capacities of youth football (soccer) players 13–15 years. *Eur. J. Appl. Physiol.* **2004**, *91*, 555–562. [CrossRef]
13. Gil, S.M.; Gil, J.; Ruiz, F.; Irazusta, A.; Irazusta, J. Physiological and Anthropometric Characteristics of Young Soccer Players According to Their Playing Position: Relevance for the Selection Process. *J. Strength Cond. Res.* **2007**, *21*, 438. [CrossRef]
14. Gil, S.M.; Zabala-Lili, J.; Bidaurrazaga-Letona, I.; Aduna, B.; Lekue, J.A.; Santos-Concejero, J.; Granados, C. Talent identification and selection process of outfield players and goalkeepers in a professional soccer club. *J. Sports Sci.* **2014**, *32*, 1931–1939. [CrossRef]
15. Carling, C.; Le Gall, F.; Reilly, T.; Williams, A.M. Do anthropometric and fitness characteristics vary according to birth date distribution in elite youth academy soccer players? Relative age effect in elite youth soccer. *Scand. J. Med. Sci. Sports* **2008**, *19*, 3–9. [CrossRef]
16. Musch, J.; Grondin, S. Unequal Competition as an Impediment to Personal Development: A Review of the Relative Age Effect in Sport. *Dev. Rev.* **2001**, *21*, 147–167. [CrossRef]
17. Helsen, W.F.; van Winckel, J.; Williams, A.M. The relative age effect in youth soccer across Europe. *J. Sports Sci.* **2005**, *23*, 629–636. [CrossRef]
18. Cobley, S.; Baker, J.; Wattie, N.; McKenna, J. Annual Age-Grouping and Athlete Development: A Meta-Analytical Review of Relative Age Effects in Sport. *Sports Med.* **2009**, *39*, 235–256. [CrossRef]
19. Singh, G.K.; Kogan, M.D.; Van Dyck, P.C.; Siahpush, M. Racial/Ethnic, Socioeconomic, and Behavioral Determinants of Childhood and Adolescent Obesity in the United States: Analyzing Independent and Joint Associations. *Ann. Epidemiol.* **2008**, *18*, 682–695. [CrossRef]
20. Roberts, J.D.; Rodkey, L.; Ray, R.; Knight, B.; Saelens, B.E. Electronic media time and sedentary behaviors in children: Findings from the Built Environment and Active Play Study in the Washington DC area. *Prev. Med. Rep.* **2017**, *6*, 149–156. [CrossRef]
21. Ala-Kitula, A.; Peltonen, J.; Finni, T.; Linnamo, V. Physical activity on days with and without soccer practice in 12–13 year-old boys. *Sci. Med. Footb.* **2019**, *3*, 245–250. [CrossRef]
22. Izzicupo, P.; Di Blasio, A.; Di Credico, A.; Gaggi, G.; Vamvakis, A.; Napolitano, G.; Ricci, F.; Gallina, S.; Ghinassi, B.; Di Baldassarre, A. The Length and Number of Sedentary Bouts Predict Fibrinogen Levels in Postmenopausal Women. *Int. J. Environ. Res. Public Health* **2020**, *17*, 3051. [CrossRef] [PubMed]

23. Kokkinos, P.; Sheriff, H.; Kheirbek, R. Physical Inactivity and Mortality Risk. *Cardiol. Res. Pract.* **2011**, *2011*, 1–10. [CrossRef]
24. Ricci, F.; Izzicupo, P.; Moscucci, F.; Sciomer, S.; Maffei, S.; Di Baldassarre, A.; Mattioli, A.V.; Gallina, S. Recommendations for Physical Inactivity and Sedentary Behavior During the Coronavirus Disease (COVID-19) Pandemic. *Front. Public Health* **2020**, *8*. [CrossRef]
25. Ceschia, A.; Giacomini, S.; Santarossa, S.; Rugo, M.; Salvadego, D.; Da Ponte, A.; Driussi, C.; Mihaleje, M.; Poser, S.; Lazzer, S. Deleterious effects of obesity on physical fitness in pre-pubertal children. *Eur. J. Sport Sci.* **2016**, *16*, 271–278. [CrossRef] [PubMed]
26. Must, A.; Anderson, S.E. Body mass index in children and adolescents: Considerations for population-based applications. *Int. J. Obes.* **2006**, *30*, 590–594. [CrossRef]
27. Nevill, A.M.; Stewart, A.D.; Olds, T.; Holder, R. Relationship between adiposity and body size reveals limitations of BMI. *Am. J. Phys. Anthropol.* **2006**, *129*, 151–156. [CrossRef]
28. Maffeis, C.; Banzato, C.; Talamini, G. Waist-to-Height Ratio, a Useful Index to Identify High Metabolic Risk in Overweight Children. *J. Pediatrics* **2008**, *152*, 207–213.e2. [CrossRef]
29. Wells, J.C.K. Measurement: A critique of the expression of paediatric body composition data. *Arch. Dis. Child.* **2001**, *85*, 67–72. [CrossRef]
30. Shypailo, R.J.; Wong, W.W. Fat and fat-free mass index references in children and young adults: Assessments along racial and ethnic lines. *Am. J. Clin. Nutr.* **2020**. [CrossRef]
31. Addo, O.Y.; Himes, J.H. Reference curves for triceps and subscapular skinfold thicknesses in US children and adolescents. *Am. J. Clin. Nutr.* **2010**, *91*, 635–642. [CrossRef] [PubMed]
32. de Arriba Muñoz, A.; Domínguez Cajal, M.; Rueda Caballero, C.; Labarta Aizpún, J.I.; Mayayo Dehesa, E.; Ferrández Longás, Á. Sitting height/standing height ratio in a Spanish population from birth to adulthood. *Arch Argent Pediatr* **2013**, *111*, 309–314. [CrossRef] [PubMed]
33. Bedogni, G.; Iughetti, L.; Ferrari, M.; Malavolti, M.; Poli, M.; Bernasconi, S.; Battistini, N. Sensitivity and specificity of body mass index and skinfold thicknesses in detecting excess adiposity in children aged 8–12 years. *Ann. Hum. Biol.* **2003**, *30*, 132–139. [CrossRef]
34. Savva, S.; Tornaritis, M.; Savva, M.; Kourides, Y.; Panagi, A.; Silikiotou, N.; Georgiou, C.; Kafatos, A. Waist circumference and waist-to-height ratio are better predictors of cardiovascular disease risk factors in children than body mass index. *Int. J. Obes.* **2000**, *24*, 1453–1458. [CrossRef]
35. Ashwell, M.; Gibson, S. Waist-to-height ratio as an indicator of 'early health risk': Simpler and more predictive than using a 'matrix' based on BMI and waist circumference. *BMJ Open* **2016**, *6*, e010159. [CrossRef] [PubMed]
36. Cacciari, E.; Milani, S.; Balsamo, A.; Spada, E.; Bona, G.; Cavallo, L.; Cerutti, F.; Gargantini, L.; Greggio, N.; Tonini, G.; et al. Italian cross-sectional growth charts for height, weight and BMI (2 to 20 yr). *J. Endocrinol. Investig.* **2006**, *29*, 581–593. [CrossRef]
37. Opstoel, K.; Pion, J.; Elferink-Gemser, M.; Hartman, E.; Willemse, B.; Philippaerts, R.; Visscher, C.; Lenoir, M. Anthropometric Characteristics, Physical Fitness and Motor Coordination of 9 to 11 Year Old Children Participating in a Wide Range of Sports. *PLoS ONE* **2015**, *10*, e0126282. [CrossRef]
38. Slaughter, M.H.; Lohman, T.G.; Boileau, R.A.; Horswill, C.A.; Stillman, R.J.; Van Loan, M.D.; Bemben, D.A. Skinfold equations for estimation of body fatness in children and youth. *Hum. Biol.* **1988**, *60*, 709–723.
39. McCarthy, H.; Jarrett, K.; Crawley, H. The development of waist circumference percentiles in British children aged 5.0–16.9 y. *Eur. J. Clin. Nutr.* **2001**, *55*, 902–907. [CrossRef]
40. McCarthy, H.D.; Ashwell, M. A study of central fatness using waist-to-height ratios in UK children and adolescents over two decades supports the simple message—'Keep your waist circumference to less than half your height'. *Int. J. Obes.* **2006**, *30*, 988–992. [CrossRef]
41. Emmonds, S.; Morris, R.; Murray, E.; Robinson, C.; Turner, L.; Jones, B. The influence of age and maturity status on the maximum and explosive strength characteristics of elite youth female soccer players. *Sci. Med. Footb.* **2017**, *1*, 209–215. [CrossRef]
42. Cohen, J. *Statistical Power Analysis for the Behavioral Sciences*, 2nd ed.; Routledge: New York, NY, USA, 2013; ISBN 978-0-203-77158-7.

43. Schober, P.; Boer, C.; Schwarte, L.A. Correlation Coefficients: Appropriate Use and Interpretation. *Anesth. Analg.* **2018**, *126*, 1763–1768. [CrossRef]
44. Loomba-Albrecht, L.A.; Styne, D.M. Effect of puberty on body composition. *Curr. Opin. Endocrinol. Diabetes Obes.* **2009**, *16*, 10–15. [CrossRef] [PubMed]
45. Siervogel, R.M.; Demerath, E.W.; Schubert, C.; Remsberg, K.E.; Chumlea, W.C.; Sun, S.; Czerwinski, S.A.; Towne, B. Puberty and Body Composition. *Horm. Res. Paediatr.* **2003**, *60*, 36–45. [CrossRef]
46. Xu, S.; Xue, Y. Pediatric obesity: Causes, symptoms, prevention and treatment. *Exp. Ther. Med.* **2016**, *11*, 15–20. [CrossRef]
47. Kim, J.; Lim, H. Nutritional Management in Childhood Obesity. *J. Obes. Metab. Syndr.* **2019**, *28*, 225–235. [CrossRef]
48. Scarafile, G. Childhood obesity in Italian primary schools: Eating habits, physical activity and perception of weight by parents. *Rev. Health Care* **2015**, *6*, 129–139. [CrossRef]
49. Robinson, T.N.; Banda, J.A.; Hale, L.; Lu, A.S.; Fleming-Milici, F.; Calvert, S.L.; Wartella, E. Screen Media Exposure and Obesity in Children and Adolescents. *Pediatrics* **2017**, *140*, S97–S101. [CrossRef]
50. Huang, H.; Wan Mohamed Radzi, C.; Salarzadeh Jenatabadi, H. Family Environment and Childhood Obesity: A New Framework with Structural Equation Modeling. *Int. J. Environ. Res. Public Health* **2017**, *14*, 181. [CrossRef]
51. Egan, B.; Zierath, J.R. Exercise Metabolism and the Molecular Regulation of Skeletal Muscle Adaptation. *Cell Metab.* **2013**, *17*, 162–184. [CrossRef]
52. Di Credico, A.; Izzicupo, P.; Gaggi, G.; Di Baldassarre, A.; Ghinassi, B. Effect of Physical Exercise on the Release of Microparticles with Angiogenic Potential. *Appl. Sci.* **2020**, *10*, 4871. [CrossRef]
53. Camera, D.M.; Smiles, W.J.; Hawley, J.A. Exercise-induced skeletal muscle signaling pathways and human athletic performance. *Free Radic. Biol. Med.* **2016**, *98*, 131–143. [CrossRef]
54. Izzicupo, P.; Ghinassi, B.; D'Amico, M.A.; Di Blasio, A.; Gesi, M.; Napolitano, G.; Gallina, S.; Di Baldassarre, A. Effects of ACE I/D Polymorphism and Aerobic Training on the Immune–Endocrine Network and Cardiovascular Parameters of Postmenopausal Women. *J. Clin. Endocrinol. Metab.* **2013**, *98*, 4187–4194. [CrossRef]
55. Izzicupo, P.; D'Amico, M.A.; Bascelli, A.; Di Fonso, A.; D'Angelo, E.; Di Blasio, A.; Bucci, I.; Napolitano, G.; Gallina, S.; Di Baldassarre, A. Walking training affects dehydroepiandrosterone sulfate and inflammation independent of changes in spontaneous physical activity. *Menopause J. North Am. Menopause Soc.* **2012**, *1*. [CrossRef] [PubMed]
56. Gaggi, G.; Di Credico, A.; Izzicupo, P.; Antonucci, I.; Crescioli, C.; Di Giacomo, V.; Di Ruscio, A.; Amabile, G.; Alviano, F.; Di Baldassarre, A.; et al. Epigenetic Features of Human Perinatal Stem Cells Redefine Their Stemness Potential. *Cells* **2020**, *9*, 1304. [CrossRef] [PubMed]
57. Falone, S.; Mirabilio, A.; Passerini, A.; Izzicupo, P.; Cacchio, M.; Gallina, S.; Baldassarre, A.D.; Amicarelli, F. Aerobic Performance and Antioxidant Protection in Runners. *Int. J. Sports Med.* **2009**, *30*, 782–788. [CrossRef] [PubMed]
58. Izzicupo, P.; Di Valerio, V.; D'Amico, M.A.; Di Mauro, M.; Pennelli, A.; Falone, S.; Alberti, G.; Amicarelli, F.; Miscia, S.; Gallina, S.; et al. Nad(P)H Oxidase and Pro-Inflammatory Response during Maximal Exercise: Role of C242T Polymorphism of the P22PHOX Subunit. *Int. J. Immunopathol. Pharmacol.* **2010**, *23*, 203–211. [CrossRef]
59. Filardi, T.; Ghinassi, B.; Di Baldassarre, A.; Tanzilli, G.; Morano, S.; Lenzi, A.; Basili, S.; Crescioli, C. Cardiomyopathy Associated with Diabetes: The Central Role of the Cardiomyocyte. *Int. J. Mol. Sci.* **2019**, *20*, 3299. [CrossRef]
60. D'amico, M.A.; Ghinassi, B.; Izzicupo, P.; Di Ruscio, A.; Di Baldassarre, A. IL-6 Activates PI3K and PKCζ Signaling and Determines Cardiac Differentiation in Rat Embryonic H9c2 Cells: IL-6 and cardiac differentiation of H9C2 cells. *J. Cell. Physiol.* **2016**, *231*, 576–586. [CrossRef]
61. Exel, J.; Mateus, N.; Travassos, B.; Gonçalves, B.; Gomes, I.; Leite, N.; Sampaio, J. Off-Training Levels of Physical Activity and Sedentary Behavior in Young Athletes: Preliminary Results during a Typical Week. *Sports* **2018**, *6*, 141. [CrossRef]

62. Izzicupo, P.; Di Baldassarre, A.; Ghinassi, B.; Reichert, F.F.; Kokubun, E.; Nakamura, F.Y. Can Off-Training Physical Behaviors Influence Recovery in Athletes? A Scoping Review. *Front. Physiol.* **2019**, *10*. [CrossRef]
63. Anderson, L.; Close, G.L.; Morgans, R.; Hambly, C.; Speakman, J.R.; Drust, B.; Morton, J.P. Assessment of Energy Expenditure of a Professional Goalkeeper From the English Premier League Using the Doubly Labeled Water Method. *Int. J. Sports Physiol. Perform.* **2019**, *14*, 681–684. [CrossRef]

Publisher's Note: MDPI stays neutral with regard to jurisdictional claims in published maps and institutional affiliations.

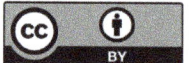

© 2020 by the authors. Licensee MDPI, Basel, Switzerland. This article is an open access article distributed under the terms and conditions of the Creative Commons Attribution (CC BY) license (http://creativecommons.org/licenses/by/4.0/).

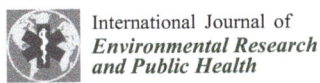

Article

Differences in Fat Mass Estimation Formulas in Physically Active Adult Population and Relationship with Sums of Skinfolds

Raquel Vaquero-Cristóbal [1,2], Mario Albaladejo-Saura [2], Ana E. Luna-Badachi [2] and Francisco Esparza-Ros [2,*]

1. Faculty of Sport, Catholic University San Antonio of Murcia (UCAM), Av. de los Jerónimos 135, 30107 Murcia, Spain; rvaquero@ucam.edu
2. Kinanthropometry International Chair, Catholic University San Antonio of Murcia (UCAM), Av. de los Jerónimos 135, 30107 Murcia, Spain; mdalbaladejosaura@ucam.edu (M.A.-S.); anaelenalunab@gmail.com (A.E.L.-B.)
* Correspondence: fesparza@ucam.edu; Tel.: +34-9-6827-8655

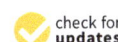

Received: 22 September 2020; Accepted: 22 October 2020; Published: 23 October 2020

Abstract: Changes in body composition and specifically fat mass, has traditionally been used as a way to monitor the changes produced by nutrition and training. The objective of the present study was to analyse the differences between the formulas used to estimate fat mass and to establish the existing relationship with the body mass index and sums of skinfolds measurement in kinanthropometry. A total of 2458 active adults participated in the study. Body mass index (BMI) and skinfolds were measured, and the Kerr, Durnin-Womersley, Faulkner and Carter equations were used to assess fat mass. Significant differences were found between all the formulas for the percentage of fat mass, ranging from 10.70 ± 2.48 to 28.43 ± 5.99% ($p < 0.001$) and fat mass from 7.56 ± 2.13 to 19.89 ± 4.24 kg ($p < 0.001$). The correlations among sums of skinfolds and the different equations were positive, high and significant in all the cases (r from 0.705 to 0.926 $p < 0.001$), unlike in the case of BMI, were the correlation was lower and both positive or negative (r from −0.271 to 0.719; $p < 0.001$). In conclusion, there were differences between all the formulas used to estimate fat mass; thus, for the evaluation of fat mass with kinanthropometry of an active adult, the use of the same formula is recommended on all occasions when the results are going to be compared or when an athlete is compared with a reference.

Keywords: kinanthropometry; physical performance; body weight; health

1. Introduction

The changes in body composition, and specifically the percentage of fat mass, have traditionally been used as a way to monitor the effects produced by training and nutrition in athletes and non-athlete population [1–4]. Nutritional interventions and training programs aimed at improving the performance of athletes have also been shown to be effective in reducing fat mass [5,6]. In fact, there is a relationship between fat mass and sports performance [7,8], because an excess of fat mass reduces sports performance in most sport modalities such as aesthetic and endurance sports [9,10]. Athletes can be characterized according to the type of sport and the specific field position according to fat mass [11].

However, there is also a relationship between fat mass and health indicators of different groups of non-athlete populations [12]. Fat mass can play an important role in the current obesity epidemic, which has become a major public health problem [13,14]. In fact, obesity is defined as the accumulation of excess body fat to the extent that it may have adverse effects on health [15]. Furthermore, excessive fat mass is associated with other health risk factors such as elevated plasma cholesterol, plasma glucose, and resting blood pressure, which contribute to the development of cardiovascular disease and type 2 diabetes, among other diseases [14,16–18].

In the scientific literature, a multitude of methods for assessing body composition can be found [19,20]. The most common methods for performing an in vivo assessment of body composition are bioimpedance (BIA), dual-energy X-ray absorptiometry (DXA) and kinanthropometry, among others, and all of them have positive and negative aspects [21]. BIA is a method based on the electrical conductivity properties of the human body, and its main advantages are that it is a safe, observer-independent, inexpensive field test and it is easy to perform [14]. However, some limitations have been showed by this method, such as its low sensitivity in the evaluation of the trunk; the influence of previous exercise, body position, skin temperature or dietary intake; the need of the examined subject to match the reference population from which the regression equation was obtained, to utilize a valid method because conductivity depends on age, ethnicity, hydration, health status, etc.; or a controversial assessment of longitudinal changes in fat mass when significant weight loss occurs due to concurrent changes in volume and composition of the conducting tissue. In addition, the portability of the most valid models is limited [14,22–25].

DXA is based on the attenuation of calibrated X-ray beams with dual photon energy so each atomic element has a characteristic mass attenuation coefficients for a given photon energy [14]. The advantages of DXA as a method of body composition measurement include observer independence, excellent precision for whole-body measurements, modest demands for the cooperation of the patient [14]. However, there are some negative aspects in the body composition evaluation with this method as well. For example, the equipment is expensive, the influence of the inaccurate positioning of the subjects on the final result; presence of metal implants; administration of radioactive substances to the subject; bias in determination of body fat from 38% to 28%; underestimation of fat mass in lean individuals; a variability from 0.8% to 27% in sequential measurements; or that it is not a portable method [14,26].

Alternatively, kinanthropometry uses the measurement of certain skinfolds to establish a percentage of fat mass through the use of different equations [19,20]. The use of skinfold thickness to estimate body fat is based on the relationship between subcutaneous adipose tissue and total body fat [14]. Its principal advantages are that it is easy, inexpensive, easy to transport and quick to apply [19,27]. Furthermore, kinanthropometry has been shown to have sufficient validity and reliability to be considered a useful tool in the assessment of fat percentage in the athlete population [28]. However, reliability can be affected by the error introduced by the researcher [29]. In fact, the error introduced by a non-expert researcher can vary between 3% and 11% [19,20,29].

If all the methods to estimate body composition have advantages and defects, there is a clear trend among professionals interested in body composition to choose methods with a better benefit to cost ratio, and the kinanthropometric method as a field test is one of the most widely used in the assessment of body composition of athletes [20]. However, the despite different methods for assessing body composition demonstrating reliability and validity in samples of the general population and athletes, it has been shown that it is not possible to compare between the body composition results obtained with different methods [28,30]. Furthermore, many formulas have been validated to estimate fat mass through kinanthropometry [29], and no studies have been found that compare the variety of fat masses depending on the formula used to estimate it with kinanthropometry. This comparison is needed in order to verify if references and measurements with different formulas can be compared, even when these formulas have been validated in similar populations. In addition, it is common to find that when fat mass is estimated in athletes with kinanthropometry, most of the attention is placed on the result (percentage or kg), without any importance attached to the formula chosen for the calculation, despite the importance it could have on the final result.

Therefore, the objective of the present study was to analyze the differences between the formulas used to estimate fat mass with kinanthropometry and to establish the existing relationship with the body mass index and sums of skinfolds in kinanthropometry.

2. Materials and Methods

2.1. Participants

The calculations for establishing the sample size were performed using Rstudio 3.15.0 software (Rstudio Inc., Boston, MA, USA). The significance level was set at $\alpha = 0.05$. The standard deviation (SD) was established based on previous studies of fat mass (mean SD = 1.7) [10], the percentage of fat mass (mean SD = 2.3), sum of six skinfolds (mean SD = 8.4) and sum of eight skinfolds in kinanthropometry (mean SD = 9.7) [31]. With an estimated error (d) of 0.067 kg of fat mass, of 0.092% in the percentage of fat mass, 0.33 mm in the sum of six skinfolds and 0.38 mm in the sum of eight skinfolds in kinanthropometry. The sample needed was 2458 subjects.

Participants were volunteers from the Region of Murcia (Spain) and the selection of the participants was non-probabilistic for convenience. The inclusion criteria were (1) to be aged between 18 and 50 years old and (2) to practice any sport or exercise on a regular basis. To determine if the participants could be considered physically active, the IPAQ questionnaire was utilized [32], and the Global Recommendations on Physical Activity for Health of the World Health Organization were set as the criteria [33].

2.2. Procedure

The Institutional Ethical Committee reviewed and authorized the protocol designed for data collection according to the Code of the World Medical Association (number 23/02/2013). The statements of the Declaration of Helsinki were followed during the entire process. All the participants were informed about the procedures and signed an informed consent form before the start of the study. The protocol was registered (ClinicalTrials.gov Identifier: NCT04429581).

Kinanthropometric variables were measured following the guidelines of the International Society for the Advancement in Kinanthropometry (ISAK) [34] between 2013 and 2018. Basic measurements of body mass and stretch stature; and the triceps, subscapular, biceps, iliac crest, supraspinale, abdominal, thigh and calf skinfolds were measured by level 2, 3 and 4 anthropometrists accredited by the ISAK. The intra- and inter-evaluator technical error of measurement (TEM) were calculated in a sub-sample. The intra-evaluator TEM was 0.01% in basic measures and 1.13% in skinfolds; and the inter-evaluator TEM was 0.03% in basic measures and 2.97% in skinfolds.

A SECA 862 scale (SECA, Hambourg, Germany) with 100 g precision was used to measure body mass; a SECA stadiometer (SECA, Hambourg, Germany) with 0.1 mm precision was used for the assessment of stretch stature, while skinfolds were measured with a Harpenden caliper (Harpenden, London, UK), with a precision of 0.2 mm.

Each measurement was performed twice. In case the differences between measurements was higher than 1% in basic measurements or 5% in skinfolds, the measurement was performed a third time. The final value for the data analysis was the mean if two measurement were taken or the median if three measurements were taken. The participants were told to avoid heavy foods and physical activity starting from the day before the measurement session. All the measurements were performed in a room with a standardized temperature of 24 °C, from 9:00 to 14:00.

The BMI, sum of six skinfolds (triceps, subscapular, supraespinale, abdominal, thigh and calf) and sum of eight skinfolds (triceps, subscapular, biceps, iliac crest, supraspinale, abdominal, thigh and calf) were calculated. The equations used to estimate fat mass and the percentage of fat mass were those proposed by Kerr [35], Durning-Womersley [7], Faulkner [36] and Carter [37]. All of them had been validated in the measurement of athletes.

2.3. Statistical Analysis

The normality of the distribution was checked with the Kolmogorov-Smirnov test. The kurtosis analysis showed a platikurtic distribution for all the variables. All the variables included in the analysis followed a normal distribution, so a parametric statistics test was performed. A descriptive statistics test was performed for all the variables. The differences between fat mass equations were analysed with a one-way analysis of variance (ANOVA) for repeated measurements. The confidence interval (CI) of the differences (CI of 95%) was included and effect size (Cohen´s D) was calculated [38]. Threshold values for effect size were set as ≥ 0.2 (small), ≥ 0.5 (moderate) and ≥ 0.8 (large). Pearson's correlation was performed between BMI, sums of six and eight skinfolds and fat mass equations. Percentiles relating all the variables were included in the analysis. The level of significance was set at $p \leq 0.05$. The software used to perform the statistical analysis was SPSS (v.23, IBM, Endicott, NY, USA).

3. Results

The present study was conducted with a sample of 2458 active subjects (mean age: 27.98 ± 7.43 years-old; mean metabolic equivalents (MET)—minute/week: 3728.63 ± 132,815), of which 1775 were men (mean age: 27.99 ± 7.46 years) and 681 was women (mean age: 27.94 ± 7.37 years). The descriptive analysis of body mass index (BMI), sums of skinfolds and fat masses and percentages estimated are shown in Table 1.

Table 1. Descriptive analysis of kinanthropometry variables and fat masses and percentages.

Variable	Mean ± SD	Max.	Min.
Height (cm)	173.52 ± 8.58	200.00	148.00
Weight (kg)	70.74 ± 10.89	108.45	43.40
BMI	23.38 ± 2.28	29.98	18.50
Sum of 6 skinfolds (mm)	77.32 ± 23.67	144.80	37.30
Sum of 8 skinfolds (mm)	98.02 ± 29.68	171.00	49.60
FM Kerr (kg)	19.89 ± 4.24	36.37	10.28
FM Durnin-Womersley (kg)	13.55 ± 3.87	28.37	4.96
FM Faulkner (kg)	9.56 ± 2.47	21.08	4.40
FM Carter (kg)	7.56 ± 2.13	15.63	3.18
% Kerr	28.43 ± 5.99	49.49	15.79
% Durnin-Womersley	19.43 ± 5.81	35.30	7.37
% Faulkner	13.46 ± 2.36	22.31	8.98
% Carter	10.70 ± 2.48	17.79	6.50

BMI: Body mass index; FM: fat mass weight; %: percentage of fat mass.

3.1. Differences Between Fat Mass Prediction Equations

The analysis of the differences between fat mass equations can be observed in Tables 2 and 3. All the equations used to estimate fat mass and the percentage of fat mass showed statistical differences ($p < 0.001$). The effect side observed was high in all the cases (D from 0.87 to 3.86) (Tables 2 and 3).

3.2. Correlations Among Fat Mass Equations, Sum of Skinfolds and BMI

The Pearson's correlation analysis between BMI, sums of skinfolds and fat masses and fat percentages are shown in Tables 4 and 5, respectively. The correlations of the different equations were positive, high and significant between themselves (r from 0.732 to 0.940; $p < 0.001$). The correlations between BMI and six and eight sums of skinfolds was significant, but low in both cases ($r = 0.187$ and 0.218, respectively; $p < 0.001$) (Tables 4 and 5).

Table 2. Differences between fat mass equations in kg.

	FM Kerr	FM Durnin-Womersley	FM Faulkner	FM Carter
FM Kerr	-	Mean differences ± SD: 6.33 ± 0.05 95% CI: 6.20–6.48 $p < 0.001$ Cohen's D: 1.56	Mean differences ± SD: 10.32 ± 0.05 95% CI: 10.19–10.46 $p < 0.001$ Cohen's D: 2.97	Mean differences ± SD: 12.32 ± 0.05 95% CI: 12.20–12.44 $p < 0.001$ Cohen's D: 3.67
FM Durnin-Womersley	Mean differences ± SD: 6.33 ± 0.05 95% CI: 6.20–6.48 $p < 0.001$ Cohen's D: 1.56	-	Mean differences ± SD: 3.98 ± 0.05 95% CI: 3.84–4.12 $p < 0.001$ Cohen's D: 1.23	Mean differences ± SD: 5.98 ± 0.05 95% CI: 5.85–6.11 $p < 0.001$ Cohen's D: 1.91
FM Faulkner	Mean differences ± SD: 10.32 ± 0.05 95% CI: 10.19–10.46 $p < 0.001$ Cohen's D: 2.97	Mean differences ± SD: 3.98 ± 0.05 95% CI: 3.84–4.12 $p < 0.001$ Cohen's D: 1.23	-	Mean differences ± SD: 1.99 ± 0.02 95% CI: 1.95–2.04 $p < 0.001$ Cohen's D: 0.87
FM Carter	Mean differences ± SD: 12.32 ± 0.05 95% CI: 12.20–12.44 $p < 0.001$ Cohen's D: 3.67	Mean differences ± SD: 5.98 ± 0.05 95% CI: 5.85–6.11 $p < 0.001$ Cohen's D: 1.91	Mean differences ± SD: 1.99 ± 0.02 95% CI: 1.95–2.04 $p < 0.001$ Cohen's D: 0.87	-

FM: fat mass weight.

Table 3. Differences between fat mass equations in percentages.

	% Kerr	% Durnin-Womersley	% Faulkner	% Carter
% Kerr	-	Mean differences ± SD: 8.99 ± 0.07 95% CI: 8.80–9.19 $p < 0.001$ Cohen's D: 1.52	Mean differences ± SD: 14.97 ± 0.09 95% CI: 14.72–15.21 $p < 0.001$ Cohen's D: 3.28	Mean differences ± SD: 17.72 ± 0.08 95% CI: 17.51–17.93 $p < 0.001$ Cohen's D: 3.86
% Durnin-Womersley	Mean differences ± SD: 8.99 ± 0.07 95% CI: 8.80–9.19 $p < 0.001$ Cohen's D: 1.52	-	Mean differences ± SD: 5.97 ± 0.09 95% CI: 5.73–6.21 $p < 0.001$ Cohen's D: 1.35	Mean differences ± SD: 8.72 ± 0.08 95% CI: 8.51–8.84 $p < 0.001$ Cohen's D: 1.95
% Faulkner	Mean differences ± SD: 14.97 ± 0.09 95% CI: 14.72–15.21 $p < 0.001$ Cohen's D: 3.28	Mean differences ± SD: 5.97 ± 0.09 95% CI: 5.73–6.21 $p < 0.001$ Cohen's D: 1.35	-	Mean differences ± SD: 2.76 ± 0.02 95% CI: 2.70–2.81 $p < 0.001$ Cohen's D: 1.14
% Carter	Mean differences ± SD: 17.72 ± 0.08 95% CI: 17.51–17.93 $p < 0.001$ Cohen's D: 3.86	Mean differences ± SD: 8.72 ± 0.08 95% CI: 8.51–8.84 $p < 0.001$ Cohen's D: 1.95	Mean differences ± SD: 2.76 ± 0.02 95% CI: 2.70–2.81 $p < 0.001$ Cohen's D: 1.14	-

%: percentage of fat mass.

Table 4. Correlation between BMI; sums of skinfolds and fat mass.

	Sum of 6 Skinfolds	Sum of 8 Skinfolds	FM Kerr	FM Durnin-Womersley	FM Faulkner	FM Carter
BMI	$r = 0.187$ $p < 0.001$	$r = 0.218$ $p < 0.001$	$r = 0.331$ $p < 0.001$	$r = 0.411$ $p < 0.001$	$r = 0.719$ $p < 0.001$	$r = 0.613$ $p < 0.001$
Sum of 6 skinfolds	-	$r = 0.989$ $p < 0.001$	$r = 0.841$ $p < 0.001$	$r = 0.816$ $p < 0.001$	$r = 0.613$ $p < 0.001$	$r = 0.806$ $p < 0.001$
Sum of 8 skinfolds		-	$r = 0.847$ $p < 0.001$	$r = 0.849$ $p < 0.001$	$r = 0.645$ $p < 0.001$	$r = 0.820$ $p < 0.001$
FM Kerr			-	$r = 0.793$ $p < 0.001$	$r = 0.840$ $p < 0.001$	$r = 0.939$ $p < 0.001$
FM Durnin-Womersley				-	$r = 0.732$ $p < 0.001$	$r = 0.824$ $p < 0.001$
FM Faulkner					-	$r = 0.940$ $p < 0.001$

Table 5. Correlation between BMI, sums of skinfolds and fat mass percentage.

	Sum of 6 Skinfolds	Sum of 8 Skinfolds	% Kerr	% Durnin-Womersley	% Faulkner	% Carter
BMI	r = 0.187 p < 0.001	r = 0.218 p < 0.001	r = −0.271 p < 0.001	r = −0.055 p < 0.001	r = 0.338 p < 0.001	r = 0.187 p < 0.001
Sum of 6 skinfolds	-	r = 0.989 p < 0.001	r = 0.889 p < 0.001	r = 0.812 p < 0.001	r = 0.916 p < 0.001	r = 0.999 p < 0.001
Sum of 8 skinfolds		-	r = 0.865 p < 0.001	r = 0.821 p < 0.001	r = 0.929 p < 0.001	r = 0.989 p < 0.001
% Kerr			-	r = 0.812 p < 0.001	r = 0.739 p < 0.001	r = 0.889 p < 0.001
% Durnin-Womersley				-	r = 0.705 p < 0.001	r = 0.812 p < 0.001
% Faulkner					-	r = 0.916 p < 0.001

BMI: Body mass index; %: percentage of fat mass.

A positive low to high positive correlation was found between BMI and most of the fat mass and percentage equations (r from 0.187 to 0.719; $p < 0.001$); although a negative low correlation was found with fat percentages estimated by Kerr and Durnin-Womersley ($r = -0.271$ and -0.055, respectively; $p < 0.001$). A positive moderate to high correlation was found among fat mass equations and the sums of six and eight skinfolds (r from 0.613 to 0.849; $p < 0.001$).

The percentile analysis relating the measurements included in the study can be observed in Table 6.

Table 6. Percentile relationship of the sums of skinfolds and the kilograms and percentage calculated.

Percentile	BMI (kg/m²)	Sum of 6 Skinfolds (mm)	Sum of 8 Skinfolds (mm)	FM Kerr (kg)	FM Durnin-Womersley (kg)	FM Faulkner (kg)	FM Carter (kg)	% Kerr	% Durnin-Womersley	% Faulkner	% Carter
5	19.73	44.00	56.20	13.77	7.68	6.24	4.69	20.16	11.30	10.19	7.20
10	20.48	47.60	60.75	14.71	8.71	6.81	5.07	21.43	12.49	10.60	7.58
15	20.97	51.45	65.99	15.40	9.37	7.12	5.41	22.30	13.42	10.91	7.99
20	21.36	54.90	69.85	16.06	10.00	7.48	5.65	23.12	14.22	11.28	8.35
25	21.72	58.74	74.24	16.70	10.61	7.76	5.95	23.80	14.90	11.60	8.75
30	22.05	61.50	78.50	17.22	11.17	8.06	6.25	24.52	15.61	11.90	9.04
35	22.40	64.50	82.50	17.84	11.69	8.33	6.49	25.24	16.36	12.21	9.36
40	22.67	67.78	85.75	18.42	12.27	8.63	6.75	25.89	17.07	12.52	9.70
45	22.98	71.00	89.50	18.89	12.76	8.90	7.01	26.57	17.77	12.82	10.04
50	23.29	74.20	93.90	19.48	13.25	9.20	7.26	27.41	18.55	13.13	10.38
55	23.60	77.30	98.25	19.96	13.78	9.48	7.54	28.47	19.25	13.45	10.70
60	23.90	81.20	103.00	20.52	14.34	9.79	7.83	29.28	20.18	13.82	11.11
65	24.21	85.50	108.00	21.30	14.97	10.14	8.16	30.21	21.18	14.20	11.57
70	24.54	89.00	112.93	21.99	15.48	10.50	8.46	31.14	22.23	14.60	11.93
75	24.87	94.30	119.43	22.67	16.21	10.91	8.81	32.28	23.31	15.04	12.49
80	25.25	99.00	125.20	23.52	16.86	11.37	9.20	33.59	24.50	15.54	12.98
85	25.78	104.52	132.77	24.33	17.73	12.00	9.73	35.17	26.10	16.19	13.56
90	26.40	112.00	142.02	25.73	18.88	12.94	10.49	37.18	28.16	16.80	14.35
95	27.42	120.85	153.72	27.63	20.37	14.31	11.67	39.48	30.62	17.81	15.28

BMI: Body mass index; FM: fat mass weight; %: percentage of fat mass.

4. Discussion

The objective of the present study was to analyze the differences between the formulas used to estimate fat mass with kinanthropometry and to establish the existing relationship with sums of skinfolds. It has been observed that even when using the same method to estimate fat mass, problems can occur when comparing results. In widely-used methods for body estimation, such as BIA, it has been observed that various factors can produce inaccuracies between measurements [39]. Among these factors, those related to the placement of the electrodes and the equations used stand out, making the results obtained vary by around 4% between instruments [39]. The same occurs with DXA, and significant differences in body composition have been shown when comparing machines from different manufacturers, different models from the same manufacturer or the same scanner model [40–43], or the version of the software. However, previous studies focused on the use of kinanthropometry have not been found. The main finding was that there are significant differences between all the formulas. In fact, differences found between the fat mass formulas ranged from $10.70 \pm 2.48\%$ to $28.43 \pm 5.99\%$ and from 7.56 ± 2.13 kg to 19.89 ± 4.24 kg although all the formulas had been validated with active adults [7,35–37]. These data agree with what was found in the previous literature, supporting the idea that there are significant intra-method differences when using various formulas to estimate fat mass [44,45].

The differences found may be due to the method used in the validation of the formula, as Kerr used cadaver dissection as a method to compare the results [35], while Durnin-Womersley, Faulkner and Carter used hydrostatic weighing [7,36,37]. The hydrostatic weighing assumes certain sources of error. The body density is obtained by weighing the subject in air and fully submerged [20]. The air found in the lungs and in the gastrointestinal (GI) tract is one of the factors that can affect body density [20]. There is a consensus about the value given to the GI tract air, set as 100 mL [46], but the residual volume of the lungs generates uncertainty [47], perhaps affecting the final result. Once the body density value is obtained, estimation equations are used to estimate the fat percentage [20]. These equations use a constant value for the density of fat mass and free fat mass [20]. While the use of a constant value for fat mass is well accepted, free fat mass has been demonstrated to be affected by age, gender and race [48–50], thereby being another aspect of bias. Thus, Kerr [35] is the only formula that was validated with a direct method, while the other formulas were validated with indirect methods. Therefore, an error in the estimation of fat mass with these methods has to be assumed [29].

Another reason why these differences may occur is due to the diversity of the target population [45]. Although all of participants were adults, the Kerr [35] and Durnin-Womersley [7] formulas were validated in the general population. Instead, the equations proposed by Faulkner and Carter were validated in elite athlete populations, specifically in swimmers and Olympic athletes, respectively [36,37]. Other factors that may introduce differences in the calculation of body composition are gender and age [39]. In this way, Kerr's proposed a unique fat mass prediction formula [35]; Durnin-Womersley proposed different equations according to the age group [7]; while Faulkner and Carter established a formula for men and another for women [36,37].

However, statistically significant and positive correlations were observed between all fat mass formulas (r from 0.705 to 0.926; $p < 0.001$). This can be attributed to all of these formulas using skinfolds, as Carter and Kerr proposed the use of the sum of six skinfolds [35,37], Durnin-Womersley used four skinfolds (triceps, biceps, subscapular and iliac crest) [7] and Faulkner used another four skinfolds (triceps, subscapular, supraspinale and abdominal) [36]. In fact, a high correlation was found between fat mass formulas with sums of six and eight skinfolds (r from 0.613 to 0.849; $p < 0.001$). The skinfolds represent the subcutaneous fat, 40%-60% of the total body fat [29,51]. Due to the lack of uniformity in the distribution of the thickness of the subcutaneous fat tissue, skinfolds in different locations of the body have to be measured, including trunk, upper and lower limbs, to ensure the correct assessment of fat mass [29,51]. The skinfold measurements from different locations used in the equations analysed could explain the high correlation found between them and the sums of six and eight skinfolds.

Furthermore, in this study, a low correlation was also observed between BMI and sums of skinfolds and the formulas for estimating fat mass (r from 0.055 to 0.338; $p < 0.001$). Despite BMI being a variable that has been traditionally used for weight control, and related with health [52], in an athlete population, it has been shown not to have a sufficient precision to assess the adiposity of the subjects [53]. This may be due to the fact that BMI does not discriminate between the contribution of fatty tissue and muscle tissue to the total weight [54]. The practice of sports can produce lean muscle mass gain [55], and as the muscle is denser than the fat tissue, BMI could not be a valid instrument to assess changes in a physically-active population [20,56]. Furthermore, systematic exercise practice can reduce the sums of skinfolds, as a consequence of the loss of subcutaneous fat, with no changes in BMI because the decrease of fat mass is compensated by the increase in muscle mass [57], which can explain why the correlation between BMI and sums of skinfolds in the present study was also low.

For all the aforementioned reasons, the same method should always be used to assess fat mass using kinanthropometry and estimation formulas, to reduce the bias introduced by the formula. In fact, fat mass estimation with different formulas cannot be compared, so it is necessary to have a percentile table as it is included in the current study to know the equivalences between methods. However, to avoid this kind of challenges, the sums of six and eight skinfolds are proposed as the measurement of the changes of subcutaneous fat. If the measurements are taken by an experienced researcher and with a calibrated calliper, the error can be reduced with respect to the use of formulas [19,20,29].

Some limitations should be acknowledged. The main limitation was that the assessment of fat mass did not include a comparison between a gold standard and the estimation formulas, so this study is not able to check on the most accurate formula. A comparison with a reference method (e.g., DXA) would have been useful in order to determine the accuracy of each equation. This is an important issue for future research. Other research designs that could be utilized after this study include longitudinal studies to analyse the reliability of body composition measurement with formulas and skinfold sums to find the most appropriate measurement for monitoring changes in body composition.

5. Conclusions

There were differences between all the formulas used to estimate fat mass with kinanthropometry. Thus, for the evaluation of fat mass of active adults, the use of the same formula is recommended on all occasions when the results are going to be compared, both to analyse the changes in the athlete or because the athlete's results are going to be compared with a reference. Furthermore, sums of skinfolds are related with fat mass, thus this method could be an alternative option when a comparison with the same formula is not possible. However, BMI seems not to be a reliable indicator of fat mass in a physically-active population.

Author Contributions: Conceptualization, R.V.-C. and F.E.-R.; methodology, R.V.-C. and F.E.-R.; formal analysis, R.V.-C. and M.A.-S.; investigation, R.V.-C., M.A.-S., A.E.L.-B. and F.E.-R.; data curation, R.V.-C., M.A.-S. and A.E.L.-B.; writing—original draft preparation, R.V.-C. and M.A.-S.; writing—review and editing, R.V.-C., M.A.-S. and F.E.-R. All authors have read and agreed to the published version of the manuscript.

Funding: This research received no external funding.

Conflicts of Interest: The authors declare no conflict of interest.

References

1. Tanda, G.; Knechtle, B. Effects of training and anthropometric factors on marathon and 100 km ultramarathon race performance. *Open Access J. Sports Med.* **2015**, *6*, 129–136. [CrossRef] [PubMed]
2. Albaladejo, M.; Vaquero-Cristóbal, R.; Esparza-Ros, F. Effect of preseason trainning on anthtopometric and derived variables in professional basketball players. *Retos: Nuevas Tendencias en Educación Física Deportes y Recreación* **2019**, *36*, 474–479. [CrossRef]
3. Fernández-García, J.C.; Gálvez-Fernández, I.; Mercadé-Melé, P.; Gavala-González, J. Longitudinal Study of Body Composition and Energy Expenditure in Overweight or Obese Young Adults. *Sci. Rep.* **2020**, *10*, 5305. [CrossRef] [PubMed]

4. Cordellat, A.; Padilla, B.; Grattarola, P.; García-Lucerga, C.; Crehuá-Gaudiza, E.; Núñez, F.; Martínez-Costa, C.; Blasco-Lafarga, C. Multicomponent exercise training Combined with nutritional counselling improves physical function, biochemical and anthropometric profiles in obese children: A pilot study. *Nutrients* **2020**, *12*, 2723. [CrossRef]
5. Garthe, I.; Raastad, T.; Refsnes, P.E.; Sundgot-Borgen, J. Effect of nutritional intervention on body composition and performance in elite athletes. *Eur. J. Sport Sci.* **2013**, *13*, 295–303. [CrossRef]
6. Hector, A.J.; Phillips, S.M. Protein Recommendations for Weight Loss in Elite Athletes: A Focus on Body Composition and Performance. *Int. J. Sport Nutr. Exerc. Metab.* **2018**, *28*, 170–177. [CrossRef]
7. Durnin, J.V.; Womersley, J. Body fat assessed from total body density and its estimation from skinfold thickness: Measurements on 481 men and women aged from 16 to 72 years. *Br. J. Nutr.* **1974**, *32*, 77–97. [CrossRef]
8. Moon, J.R. Body composition in athletes and sports nutrition: An examination of the bioimpedance analysis technique. *Eur. J. Clin. Nutr.* **2013**, *67*, S54–S59. [CrossRef]
9. Bridge, C.A.; Ferreira da Silva Santos, J.; Chaabène, H.; Pieter, W.; Franchini, E. Physical and physiological profiles of taekwondo athletes. *Sports Med.* **2014**, *44*, 713–733. [CrossRef]
10. Genton, L.; Mareschal, J.; Karsegard, V.L.; Achamrah, N.; Delsoglio, M.; Pichard, C.; Graf, C.; Herrmann, F.R. An Increase in Fat Mass Index Predicts a Deterioration of Running Speed. *Nutrients* **2019**, *11*, 701. [CrossRef]
11. Santos, D.A.; Dawson, J.A.; Matias, C.N.; Rocha, P.M.; Minderico, C.S.; Allison, D.B.; Sardinha, L.B.; Silva, A.M. Reference values for body composition and anthropometric measurements in athletes. *PLoS ONE* **2014**, *9*, e97846. [CrossRef] [PubMed]
12. Marcos-Pardo, P.J.; Orquin-Castrillón, F.J.; Gea-García, G.M.; Menayo-Antúnez, R.; González-Gálvez, N.; Vale, R.G.S.; Martínez-Rodríguez, A. Effects of a moderate-to-high intensity resistance circuit training on fat mass, functional capacity, muscular strength, and quality of life in elderly: A randomized controlled trial. *Sci. Rep.* **2019**, *9*, 7830. [CrossRef] [PubMed]
13. Kelly, T.; Yang, W.; Chen, C.S.; Reynolds, K.; He, J. Global burden of obesity in 2005 and projections to 2030. *Int. J. Obes. (Lond.)* **2008**, *32*, 1431–1437. [CrossRef] [PubMed]
14. Goossens, G.H. The Metabolic Phenotype in Obesity: Fat Mass, Body Fat Distribution, and Adipose Tissue Function. *Obes. Facts* **2017**, *10*, 207–215. [CrossRef]
15. Ho-Pham, L.T.; Lai, T.Q.; Nguyen, M.T.; Nguyen, T.V. Relationship between Body Mass Index and Percent Body Fat in Vietnamese: Implications for the Diagnosis of Obesity. *PLoS ONE* **2015**, *10*, e0127198. [CrossRef]
16. Abdullah, A.; Peeters, A.; de Courten, M.; Stoelwinder, J. The magnitude of association between overweight and obesity and the risk of diabetes: A meta-analysis of prospective cohort studies. *Diabetes Res. Clin. Pract.* **2010**, *89*, 309–319. [CrossRef]
17. Maggio, C.A.; Pi-Sunyer, F.X. Obesity and type 2 diabetes. *Endocrinol. Metab. Clin. N. Am.* **2003**, *32*, 805–822. [CrossRef]
18. Strasser, B.; Schobersberger, W. Evidence for resistance training as a treatment therapy in obesity. *J. Obes.* **2011**, *2011*. [CrossRef]
19. Ayvaz, G.; Çimen, A.R. Methods dor body composition analysis in adults. *Open Obes. J.* **2011**, *3*, 62–69. [CrossRef]
20. Mattsson, S.; Thomas, B.J. Development of methods for body composition studies. *Phys. Med. Biol.* **2006**, *51*, 203–228. [CrossRef]
21. Fosbøl, M.; Zerahn, B. Contemporary methods of body composition measurement. *Clin. Physiol. Funct. Imaging* **2015**, *35*, 81–97. [CrossRef] [PubMed]
22. Swan, P.D.; McConnell, K.E. Anthropometry and bioelectrical impedance inconsistently predicts fatness in women with regional adiposity. *Med. Sci. Sports Exerc.* **1999**, *31*, 1068–1075. [CrossRef] [PubMed]
23. Kushner, R.F.; Gudivaka, R.; Schoeller, D.A. Clinical characteristics influencing bioelectrical impedance analysis measurements. *Am. J. Clin. Nutr.* **1996**, *64*, 423S–427S. [CrossRef] [PubMed]
24. Gudivaka, R.; Schoeller, D.; Kushner, R.F. Effect of skin temperature on multifrequency bioelectrical impedance analysis. *J. Appl. Physiol. (1985)* **1996**, *81*, 838–845. [CrossRef] [PubMed]
25. Buchholz, A.C.; Bartok, C.; Schoeller, D.A. The validity of bioelectrical impedance models in clinical populations. *Nutr. Clin. Pract.* **2004**, *19*, 433–446. [CrossRef]
26. Hind, K.; Oldroyd, B.; Truscott, J.G. In vivo precision of the GE Lunar iDXA densitometer for the measurement of total body composition and fat distribution in adults. *Eur. J. Clin. Nutr.* **2011**, *65*, 140–142. [CrossRef]

27. Tellez, M.J.A.; Silva, A.M.; Ruiz, J.R.; Martins, S.S.; Palmeira, A.L.; Branco, T.L.; Minderico, C.S.; Rocha, P.M.; Themudo-Barata, J.; Teixeira, P.J.; et al. Neck circumference is associated with adipose tissue content in thigh skeletal muscle in overweight and obese premenopausal women. *Sci. Rep.* **2020**, *10*, 8324. [CrossRef]
28. Arias Téllez, M.J.; Carrasco, F.; España Romero, V.; Inostroza, J.; Bustamante, A.; Solar Altamirano, I. A comparison of body composition assessment methods in climbers: Which is better? *PLoS ONE* **2019**, *14*, e0224291. [CrossRef]
29. Costa-Moreira, O.; Alonso-Aubin, D.A.; Patrocinio de Oliveira, C.E.; Candia-Luján, R.; de Paz, J.A. Methods of assessment of body composition: An updated review of description, application, advanteges and disadvantages. *AMD* **2015**, *32*, 387–394.
30. Lozano Berges, G.; Matute Llorente, Á.; Gómez Bruton, A.; González Agüero, A.; Vicente Rodríguez, G.; Casajús, J.A. Body fat percentage comparisons between four methods in young football players: Are they comparable? *Nutr. Hosp.* **2017**, *34*, 1119–1124. [CrossRef]
31. Sánchez Muñoz, C.; Muros, J.J.; López Belmonte, Ó.; Zabala, M. Anthropometric Characteristics, Body Composition and Somatotype of Elite Male Young Runners. *Int. J. Environ. Res. Public Health* **2020**, *17*, 674. [CrossRef]
32. Craig, C.L.; Marshall, A.L.; Sjöström, M.; Bauman, A.E.; Booth, M.L.; Ainsworth, B.E.; Pratt, M.; Ekelund, U.; Yngve, A.; Sallis, J.F.; et al. International physical activity questionnaire: 12-country reliability and validity. *Med. Sci. Sports Exerc.* **2003**, *35*, 1381–1395. [CrossRef] [PubMed]
33. World Health Organization. *Global Recommendations on Physical Activity for Health*; WHO: Geneva, Switzerland, 2010.
34. Stewart, A.; Marfell-Jones, M.; Olds, T.; de Ridder, H. *International Protocol for the Anthropometric Assessement*; International Society for the Advancement in Kinanthropometry: Portsmouth, Australia, 2011.
35. Ross, W.D.; Kerr, D.A. Fraccionamiento de la masa corporal: Un nuevo método para utilizar en nutrición clínica y medicina deportiva. *Apunts Med. Sport* **1991**, *18*, 175–187.
36. Faulkner, J. Physiology of swimming and diving. In *Exercise Physiology*; Falls, H., Ed.; Academic Press: Baltimore, MD, USA, 1968.
37. Carter, J. Body composition of Montreal Olympic athletes. In *Physical Structure of Olympic Athletes Part I: The Montreal Olympic Games Anthropological Project*; Carter, J., Ed.; Karger: Basel, Switzerland, 1982.
38. Hopkins, W.G.; Marshall, S.W.; Batterham, A.M.; Hanin, J. Progressive statistics for studies in sports medicine and exercise science. *Med. Sci. Sports Exerc.* **2009**, *41*, 3–13. [CrossRef] [PubMed]
39. Khalil, S.F.; Mohktar, M.S.; Ibrahim, F. The theory and fundamentals of bioimpedance analysis in clinical status monitoring and diagnosis of diseases. *Sensors* **2014**, *14*, 10895–10928. [CrossRef] [PubMed]
40. Soriano, J.M.; Ioannidou, E.; Wang, J.; Thornton, J.C.; Horlick, M.N.; Gallagher, D.; Heymsfield, S.B.; Pierson, R.N. Pencil-beam vs fan-beam dual-energy X-ray absorptiometry comparisons across four systems: Body composition and bone mineral. *J. Clin. Densitom.* **2004**, *7*, 281–289. [CrossRef]
41. Malouf, J.; DiGregorio, S.; Del Rio, L.; Torres, F.; Marin, A.M.; Farrerons, J.; Herrera, S.; Domingo, P. Fat tissue measurements by dual-energy x-ray absorptiometry: Cross-calibration of 3 different fan-beam instruments. *J. Clin. Densitom.* **2013**, *16*, 212–222. [CrossRef] [PubMed]
42. Hull, H.; He, Q.; Thornton, J.; Javed, F.; Allen, L.; Wang, J.; Pierson, R.N.; Gallagher, D. iDXA, Prodigy, and DPXL dual-energy X-ray absorptiometry whole-body scans: A cross-calibration study. *J. Clin. Densitom.* **2009**, *12*, 95–102. [CrossRef]
43. Van, L.; Keim, N.L.; Berg, K.; Mayclin, P. Evaluation of body composition by dual energy xray absorptiometry and two different software packages. *Med. Sci. Sport Exerc.* **1995**, *27*, 587–591.
44. Knechtle, B.; Wirth, A.; Knechtle, P.; Rosemann, T.; Rüst, C.A.; Bescós, R. A comparison of fat mass and skeletal muscle mass estimation in male ultra-endurance athletes using bioelectrical impedance analysis and different anthropometric methods. *Nutr. Hosp.* **2011**, *26*, 1420–1427. [CrossRef]
45. Espana Romero, V.; Ruiz, J.R.; Ortega, F.B.; Artero, E.G.; Vicente-Rodriguez, G.; Moreno, L.A.; Castillo, M.J.; Gutierrez, A. Body fat measurement in elite sport climbers: Comparison of skinfold thickness equations with dual energy X-ray absorptiometry. *J. Sports Sci.* **2009**, *27*, 469–477. [CrossRef] [PubMed]
46. Buskirk, E.R. Underwater weighing and body density: A review of procedures. In *Techniques for Measuring Body Composition*; Henschel, J.B.a.A., Ed.; National Academy od Sciences: Washington, DC, USA, 1961.
47. Hackney, A.C.; Deutsch, D.T. Accuracy of residual volume prediction–Effects on body composition estimation in pulmonary dysfunction. *Can. J. Appl. Sport Sci.* **1985**, *10*, 88–93.
48. Lohman, T.G. Assessment of body composition in children. *Pediatr. Exer. Sci.* **1989**, *1*, 9–30. [CrossRef]

49. Millard-Stafford, M.L.; Collins, M.A.; Modlesky, C.M.; Snow, T.K.; Rosskopf, L.B. Effect of race and resistance training status on the density of fat-free mass and percent fat estimates. *J. Appl. Physiol. (1985)* **2001**, *91*, 1259–1268. [CrossRef] [PubMed]
50. Werkman, A.; Deurenberg-Yap, M.; Schmidt, G.; Deurenberg, P. A Comparison between Composition and Density of the Fat-Free Mass of Young Adult Singaporean Chinese and Dutch Caucasians. *Ann. Nutr. Metab.* **2000**, *44*, 235–242. [CrossRef] [PubMed]
51. Wang, J.; Thornton, J.C.; Kolesnik, S.; Pierson, R.N. Anthropometry in body composition. An overview. *Ann. N. Y. Acad. Sci.* **2000**, *904*, 317–326. [CrossRef] [PubMed]
52. Oviedo, G.; Marcano, M.; Morón de Salim, A.; Solano, L. Exceso de peso y patologías en mujeres adultas. *Nutr. Hosp.* **2007**, *22*, 358–362.
53. Ode, J.J.; Pivarnik, J.M.; Reeves, M.J.; Knous, J.L. Body mass index as a predictor of percent fat in college athletes and nonathletes. *Med. Sci. Sports Exerc.* **2007**, *39*, 403–409. [CrossRef]
54. Kruschitz, R.; Wallner-Liebmann, S.J.; Hamlin, M.J.; Moser, M.; Ludvik, B.; Schnedl, W.J.; Tafeit, E. Detecting body fat-A weighty problem BMI versus subcutaneous fat patterns in athletes and non-athletes. *PLoS ONE* **2013**, *8*, e72002. [CrossRef]
55. Westcott, W.L. Resistance training is medicine: Effects of strength training on health. *Curr. Sports Med. Rep.* **2012**, *11*, 209–216. [CrossRef]
56. Klungland Torstveit, M.; Sundgot-Borgen, J. Are under- and overweight female elite athletes thin and fat? A controlled study. *Med. Sci. Sports Exerc.* **2012**, *44*, 949–957. [CrossRef] [PubMed]
57. Vaquero-Cristóbal, R.; Alacid, F.; Esparza-Ros, F.; López-Plaza, D.; Muyor, J.M.; López-Miñarro, P.A. The effects of a reformer Pilates program on body composition and morphological characteristics in active women after a detraining period. *Women Health* **2016**, *56*, 784–806. [CrossRef]

Publisher's Note: MDPI stays neutral with regard to jurisdictional claims in published maps and institutional affiliations.

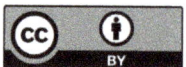

© 2020 by the authors. Licensee MDPI, Basel, Switzerland. This article is an open access article distributed under the terms and conditions of the Creative Commons Attribution (CC BY) license (http://creativecommons.org/licenses/by/4.0/).

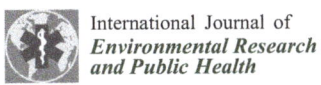

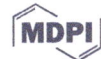

Article

Maximal Oxygen Uptake Adjusted for Skeletal Muscle Mass in Competitive Speed-Power and Endurance Male Athletes: Changes in a One-Year Training Cycle

Jacek Trinschek, Jacek Zieliński and Krzysztof Kusy *

Department of Athletics, Strength and Conditioning, Faculty of Sport Sciences, Poznan University of Physical Education, ul. Królowej Jadwigi 27/39, 61-871 Poznań, Poland; jactri@wp.pl (J.T.); jacekzielinski@wp.pl (J.Z.)
* Correspondence: kusy@awf.poznan.pl; Tel.: +48-61-8355270

Received: 31 July 2020; Accepted: 25 August 2020; Published: 27 August 2020

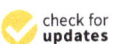

Abstract: We compared the changes in maximum oxygen uptake ($\dot{V}O_2$max) calculated per skeletal muscle mass (SMM) with conventional $\dot{V}O_2$max measures in a 1-year training cycle. We hypothesized that the pattern of changes would differ between SMM-adjusted and absolute or weight-adjusted values, and the differences between groups of distinct training specialization and status will depend on the measure used. Twelve sprinters (24.7 ± 3.3 years), 10 endurance runners (25.3 ± 5.3 years), and 10 recreationally trained controls (29 ± 4.5 years) performed a treadmill test until exhaustion to determine $\dot{V}O_2$max. Their SMM was estimated based on the dual X-ray absorptiometry method and a regression equation. The significance of differences was assessed using analysis of variance ($p \leq 0.05$). The pattern of the longitudinal change was not different between $\dot{V}O_2$max/SMM and standard measures. Also, the significance of differences between sprinters and endurance athletes remained similar regardless of the $\dot{V}O_2$max measure. Sprinters and controls had similar absolute (~4.3 L·min^{-1}) and total weight-adjusted (~52 vs. ~56 mL·min^{-1}·kg) $\dot{V}O_2$max, but they significantly differed in SMM-adjusted $\dot{V}O_2$max (~110 vs. ~130 mL·min^{-1}·kg SMM^{-1}). In summary, SMM-adjusted $\dot{V}O_2$max is not more useful than standard measures to track longitudinal changes in competitive athletes. However, it allows to better distinguish between groups or individuals differing in training status. The results of our study are limited to male athletes.

Keywords: maximum aerobic capacity; total weight; lean body mass; fat mass; DXA method

1. Introduction

Maximal oxygen uptake ($\dot{V}O_2$max) is a widely used indicator of human aerobic capacity defined as the maximum rate of oxygen consumption. Conventionally, $\dot{V}O_2$max is expressed as an absolute rate of oxygen uptake per unit of time (mL·min^{-1}) or as a weight-adjusted rate (mL·min^{-1}·kg^{-1}) [1–4]. The latter is a standard measure in athletes of various sports disciplines. Skeletal muscle mass (SMM) is the largest component of the adipose tissue-free body mass in humans [5], essential for athletic performance. Despite many differences in training and competition specificity, available research indicates that SMM content in athletes ranges from 40% to 48% of total body mass [6–11].

The body of literature on $\dot{V}O_2$max in competitive athletes in the context of SMM is very scarce (unlike the relationships with total body mass). This can be due to problems with accurate SMM estimation. Of particular interest are, therefore, studies where authors used most advanced methods, e.g., magnetic resonance imaging or dual-energy X-ray absorptiometry (DXA) to estimate SMM. Proctor & Joyner [11] demonstrated that reduced aerobic capacity per kilogram of appendicular SMM in highly trained older men and women contributed to reduced whole body $\dot{V}O_2$max. Sanada et al. [12]

revealed that absolute peak $\dot{V}O_2$ was closely associated with total and regional SMM regardless of the whole body or fat-free mass. Similarly, Beekley et al. [13] indicated a strong relationship between SMM (kg) and absolute $\dot{V}O_2$max (L·min^{-1}) in high-performance athletes. However, they also noticed that above a certain SMM level (~45 kg), the relationship between $\dot{V}O_2$ uptake and SMM was weakening and aerobic abilities of athletes reached a "plateau".

It is suggested that in highly trained athletes, not only standard measures of $\dot{V}O_2$ (per kg of total body mass) but also SMM-adjusted $\dot{V}O_2$max, called "aerobic muscle quality", should be taken into account to obtain more accurate and reliable information on the changes in the training status [13]. To our best knowledge, there are no scientific reports that have compared the changes in SMM-adjusted $\dot{V}O_2$max in high-performance athletes of different specializations over a long period. This study aimed to evaluate the changes in SMM-adjusted $\dot{V}O_2$max in competitive highly trained speed-power and endurance athletes in a 1-year training cycle. We hypothesized that (i) the profile of changes in $\dot{V}O_2$max per kg SMM would differ from that per kg total body mass and (ii) the size of the differences in $\dot{V}O_2$max between speed-power, endurance, and amateur male athletes would depend on the measure of $\dot{V}O_2$max used (SMM- vs. total weight-adjusted).

2. Materials and Methods

2.1. Subjects

The study included 22 highly trained male athletes divided into two groups differing in sport specialization. Sprinters ($n = 12$) specialized in the distances of 100 and 200 m, were 24.7 ± 3.3 (range 21–31) years old with a training history of 7.42 ± 2.5 years. Endurance athletes were long-distance runners and triathletes ($n = 10$) aged 25.3 ± 5.3 (range 15–35) years with a competitive sport history of 8.0 ± 2.4 years. Some athletes were members of the Polish national team. The control group consisted of 10 healthy recreationally active men aged 29 ± 4.5 (range 23–35) years without previous and current professional sports experience, representing the model of regular but not competitive physical activity. The controls were invited to participate in the study through announcements in local mass media. The project was approved by the Ethics Committee at the Poznan University of Medical Sciences (decision No 1252/18 issued on 6 December 2018) and has been performed according to the ethical standards laid down in the Declaration of Helsinki. The participants were fully informed of the purpose and risks of the study and gave their written consent to participate. Basic characteristics of the participants at the start of the study are presented in Table 1. Controls were older than athletes. Sprinters were taller and had higher relative skeletal muscle mass index than endurance athletes and controls.

Table 1. Basic characteristics of the athletic groups and controls.

	Sprint	Endurance	Controls	ANOVA p-Value	Effect Size η^2
Age (yars)	24.7 ± 3.3 (22.1–26.2) *	25.3 ± 5.3 (22.3–28.2) *	29 ± 4.5 (26–32)	<0.001	0.22
Sports history (years)	7.4 ± 2.5 (5.8–9.0)	8.0 ± 2.4 (6.3–9.7)	–	0.120	0.30
Height (cm)	185.8 ± 5.0 (182.1–188.2) *	181.6 ± 6.1 (178.2–185)	178.1 ± 5.6 (174.3–181.9)	0.029	0.33
BMI (kg·m^{-2})	23.6 ± 1.0 (22.8–24.3)	22.8 ± 1.9 (21.8–23.9)	24.8 ± 2.0 (23.4–26.1)	0.080	0.24
RSMI (kg)	9.6 ± 0.6 # (9.1–10.0) #	8.5 ± 0.6 (8.1–8.9)	9.0 ± 0.6 (8.6–9.4)	0.007	0.42

Values are expressed as mean ± SD (95% CI). Abbreviations: BMI = body mass index; RSMI = relative skeletal muscle mass index. * $p < 0.05$—significantly different from the control group; # $p < 0.01$—significantly different from endurance athletes.

2.2. Study Design

A repeated-measures design was used to follow the changes in $\dot{V}O_2$max and body composition across a 1-year training cycle. We aimed to find patterns of the longitudinal change and between-group differences depending on the $\dot{V}O_2$max measure, i.e., absolute, weight-, LBM-, and SMM-adjusted values. All measurements were repeated four times in the following training phases of the annual training cycle: (1) beginning of the general preparation period, (2) beginning of the specific preparation period, (3) beginning of the pre-competition period, and (4) beginning of the competition period. Training units and workloads used in the training process were strictly planned by the national team coaches. The 12-week general preparation aimed to develop physiological foundation for performance. Training volume was high and the intensity was low but slowly increasing (the number of training sessions in triathletes, long-distance runners, and sprinters was 181, 122, and 80, respectively). During the specific preparation period, also lasting 12 weeks, training volume decreased, whereas the intensity increased substantially (the number of training sessions: 132, 96, and 61, respectively). In the pre-competition period (10 weeks), training volume further decreased and the intensity increased (the number of training sessions: 179, 120, and 87, respectively). The competition period was characterized by reduced training volume and emphasis was placed on increasing intensity and quality of work to achieve peak performance before upcoming competitions. Sprinters were examined three times, i.e., they did not perform the exercise test until exhaustion in the competition phase to avoid any adverse effect on sprint ability. The control group did not periodize their training during the year analyzed. During the whole study period, they did workouts three to seven times a week at relatively constant training volume and intensity.

2.3. Methodology

Participants were recommended to avoid high-intensity and long-duration training sessions 24–48 h before each examination. All tests were conducted at the Human Movement Laboratory "LaBthletics" of the Poznan University of Physical Education. The measurements were performed in the morning, 2 h after a light breakfast (bread and butter, water, without coffee or tea). Before each exercise test, body composition was assessed. Then, subjects performed an incremental treadmill test until exhaustion. During all examinations, the ambient temperature was kept at 20–21 °C.

2.3.1. Body Composition and Skeletal Muscle Mass

Weight and height were measured using the SECA 285 measuring station (SECA GmbH, Hamburg, Germany) with an accuracy of 0.05 kg and 1 mm, respectively. To evaluate body composition, the DXA method (Lunar Prodigy device, GE Healthcare, Chicago, IL, USA) was used. Before each measurement session, the device was calibrated using a phantom, according to the manufacturer guidelines. During the examination, subjects only wore their underwear without jewelry or other metal objects, to minimize measurement error. All DXA scans were performed and analyzed by the same trained technician using enCORE 16 SP1 software (GE Healthcare, Chicago, IL, USA). All measurements were done following the standardized protocol proposed by Nana et al. [14] and manufacturer's instructions. Three main components of the total-body model were measured: lean body mass (LBM), fat mass, and bone mineral content (the latter not analyzed in this study). In the literature, the DXA technical errors of measurement (expressed as intra-assay coefficients of variation or %CV) have been reported to be 0.1% for total body mass, 0.4% for LBM, 1.9% for fat mass, and 0.7% for BMC (21). In our laboratory, %CV values in young athletic individuals aged 23 ± 2.1 years were 0.2%, 0.4%, 1.0%, and 0.5%, respectively. Also, we calculated %CV for appendicular lean soft tissue (ALST; the sum of upper and lower limb LBM) and obtained a value of 0.8%. The regression model proposed by Kim et al. [5] was used to calculate SMM (kg) = 1.13ALST − 0.02Age + 0.61Sex + 0.97, where 0 and 1 denoted women or men, respectively. Also, the relative skeletal muscle mass index was calculated according to the formula: RSMI = ALST/Height^2 (kg·m^{-2}).

2.3.2. Maximum Oxygen Uptake

All athletes underwent incremental running tests (h/p Cosmos Pulsar treadmill, Sports & Medical GmbH, Nussdorf-Traunstein, Germany) to determine $\dot{V}O_2$max. The initial speed was set at 4 km·h^{-1} and after 3 min increased to 8 km·h^{-1}. After that point, the speed of the moving strip was progressively increasing by 2 km·h^{-1} every 3 min until voluntary exhaustion. Main cardiorespiratory variables (minute ventilation, $\dot{V}E$; oxygen uptake, $\dot{V}O_2$; carbon dioxide output, $\dot{V}CO_2$) were measured constantly (breath by breath) using the MetaLyzer 3B ergospirometer and analyzed using the MetaSoft Studio 5.1.0 software package (Cortex Biophysik GmbH, Leipzig, Germany). Before each test, the system was calibrated according to the manufacturer's instructions. Maximal oxygen uptake was considered achieved if at least three of the following criteria were met: (i) a plateau in $\dot{V}O_2$ despite an increase in speed and minute ventilation; (ii) blood lactate concentration ≥ 9 mmol·L^{-1}; (iii) respiratory exchange ratio ≥ 1.10; and (iv) heart rate $\geq 95\%$ of the age-predicted maximum heart rate [15]. Heart rate was measured continuously with the Polar Bluetooth Smart H6 monitor (Polar Electro Oy, Kempele, Finland).

2.3.3. Statistical Analysis

Data were presented as means and standard deviations (SD), and confidence intervals of the mean (95% CI). The Shapiro–Wilk test was used to check the data for normality of distribution. The assumption on sphericity was tested using the Mauchley's test, verifying if variances of certain variables were identical and equal to respective co-variances. The one-way analysis of variance (ANOVA) with repeated measures was used to compare the change between three (sprinters) or four (endurance athletes and controls) examinations across the annual training cycle. The one-way ANOVA was used to compare differences between the groups at each single training phase. The post hoc Scheffe's test was applied to indicate between which particular examinations or groups there were significant differences. The effect size for ANOVA was expressed as η^2 and defined as small (0.01), medium (0.06), or large (0.14). The statistical significance was set at $p < 0.05$. All analyses were performed using the Statistica 13.0 software package (Tibco Software Inc., Palo Alto, CA, USA).

3. Results

3.1. Body Composition

Sprinters had significantly higher total body mass than endurance athletes in three training periods (general, specific and pre-competition) (Table A1). In sprinters, total mass increased from general to specific and pre-competition phases, whereas no significant longitudinal changes were revealed in endurance athletes and controls.

Absolute and percentage fat mass was similar in sprinters and endurance athletes in all examinations, although slightly lower values were noted in sprinters (insignificant differences) (Figure 1A,B; Table A1). Both sprint and endurance groups had significantly lower absolute and percentage fat mass than controls in almost all examinations, except for the general phase (a non-significant difference between endurance athletes and controls). In sprinters and endurance athletes, absolute and percentage fat mass was significantly higher in the general phase than in the subsequent training phases. No significant change was detected in controls, even though there was a certain trend towards lower values in the competition phase, however, accompanied by large standard deviation.

Sprinters had significantly higher absolute LBM than endurance athletes and controls in the general, specific, and pre-competition phases (Figure 1C; Table A1). Endurance athletes had higher percentage LBM than controls in all training phases, except for the general phase (Figure 1D). Absolute LBM in sprinters and percentage LBM in both sprinters and endurance runners significantly increased between the general and the subsequent training phases (Figure 1C,D). No significant change in LBM was shown in the control group, in spite of slightly increasing percentage values between third and fourth examination (Figure 1D).

Sprinters had significantly higher both absolute and percentage SMM than endurance athletes and controls in all training phases (Figure 1E,F; Table A1). There were no significant differences in SMM between endurance athletes and controls. In sprinters (but not endurance athletes and controls), absolute SMM significantly increased from the general to the specific and pre-competition phases (Figure 1E). During the annual training cycle, there was no significant change in percentage SMM in any of the three groups (Figure 1F).

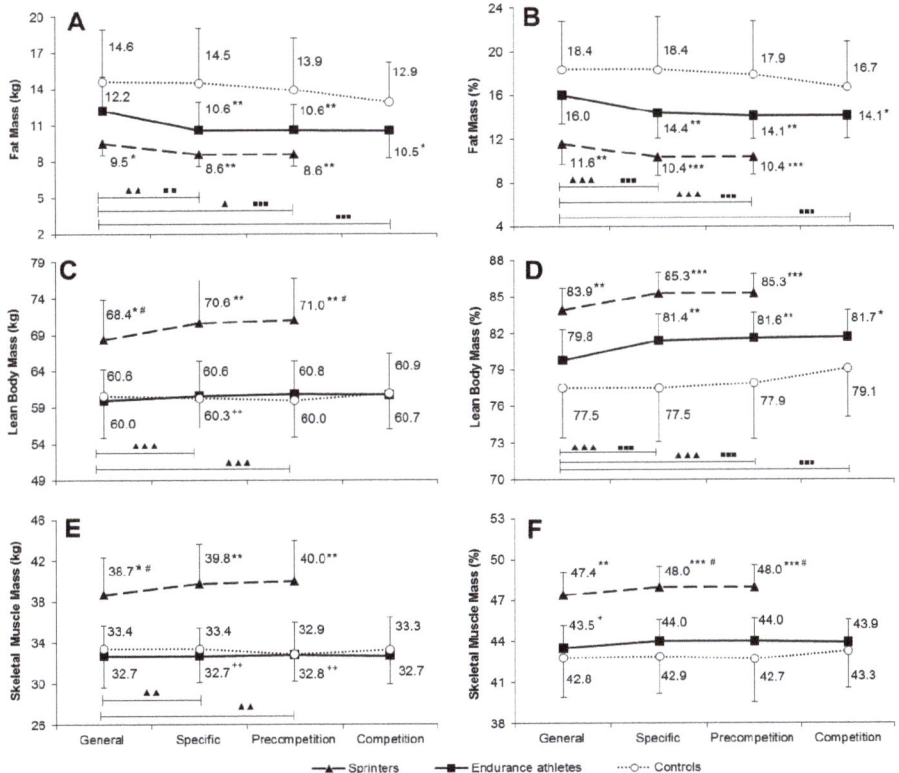

Figure 1. Changes in body composition expressed in absolute and percentage values between consecutive phases of the annual training cycle in athletic groups and controls. Panels (**A**,**B**)—fat mass; Panels (**C**,**D**)—lean body mass; Panels (**E**,**F**)—skeletal muscle mass. ▲ $p < 0.05$, ▲▲ $p < 0.01$, ▲▲▲ $p < 0.001$—significantly different from the general preparation phase in sprinters; ■■ $p < 0.01$, ■■■ $p < 0.001$—significantly different from the general preparation phase in endurance athletes; + $p < 0.05$, ++ $p < 0.01$—significantly different from sprinters at the same training phase; # $p < 0.01$—significantly different from endurance athletes at the same training phase; * $p < 0.05$, ** $p < 0.01$, *** $p < 0.001$—significantly different from controls at the same training phase.

3.2. Maximal Oxygen Uptake

Across the annual training cycle, a significant increase in all $\dot{V}O_2$max indicators (absolute, per total body mass, per LBM, or per SMM) was only observed in controls between the general and pre-competition or competition phase. In sprinters and endurance runners, none of the $\dot{V}O_2$max measures changed significantly (Figure 2A–D; Table A2).

Depending on the $\dot{V}O_2$max indicator used, the significance of the difference between speed-power, endurance, and amateur athletes varied. For absolute $\dot{V}O_2$max (mL·min^{-1}), the only significant difference was between endurance athletes and controls in the general preparation phase (Figure 2A, Table A2). For weight-adjusted $\dot{V}O_2$max, more pronounced differences were observed, i.e., endurance athletes significantly differed from speed-power and control groups in all training periods (Figure 2B; Table A2), however, sprinters and controls were not significantly different. Finally, when $\dot{V}O_2$max was adjusted for LBM and SMM, there emerged significant differences between sprinters and controls in addition to previous differences for weight-adjusted $\dot{V}O_2$max between endurance athletes and the other two groups. Consequently, the control group had higher LBM- and SMM-adjusted $\dot{V}O_2$max than sprinters in all training phases (Figure 2C,D; Table A2).

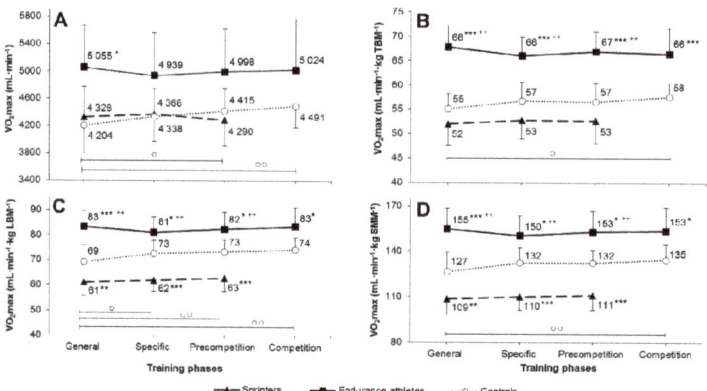

Figure 2. Changes in maximal oxygen uptake ($\dot{V}O_2$max) between consecutive phases of the annual training cycle in athletes and controls. (**A**)—absolute values; Panel (**B**)—calculated per weight or kilogram of total body mass (TBM); Panel (**C**)—calculated per kilogram of lean body mass (LBM); Panel (**D**)—calculated per kilogram of skeletal muscle mass (SMM.) $^\circ$ $p < 0.05$, $^{\circ\circ}$ $p < 0.01$—significantly different from the general preparation phase in the control group; $^{++}$ $p < 0.01$—significantly different from sprinters at the same training phase; $^{\#}$ $p < 0.01$—significantly different from endurance athletes at the same training phase; * $p < 0.05$, ** $p < 0.01$, *** $p < 0.001$—significantly different from controls at the same training phase.

4. Discussion

To our knowledge, this is the first study to analyze the changes in $\dot{V}O_2$max calculated per SMM across an annual training cycle in competitive athletes of different sports specializations. The major findings are that (i) the profile of change in SMM-adjusted $\dot{V}O_2$max in a 1-year training cycle is not different from the change in weight-adjusted $\dot{V}O_2$max and (ii) the between-group differences depend on the $\dot{V}O_2$max measure used, as shown by significant differences between sprinters and controls that emerged when SMM- or LBM-adjusted $\dot{V}O_2$max values were used.

4.1. Changes in $\dot{V}O_2$max between Training Phases

There is scarce research on $\dot{V}O_2$max expressed as relative values per kg of SMM [11,12]. Nevertheless, there were reasons to believe that the profile of the changes in SMM-adjusted $\dot{V}O_2$max across a 1-year training cycle would be different from that expressed as absolute and weight-adjusted values. However, this hypothesis has not been confirmed. In sprint- and endurance-trained athletes and controls, the profiles of change across training phases were very similar regardless of $\dot{V}O_2$max measure.

In endurance athletes, high $\dot{V}O_2$max is regarded as one of the necessary (although not sufficient) factors determining high endurance performance [16,17]. In response to years of intense training (apart from innate aptitudes), the level of $\dot{V}O_2$max is usually maximized and the observed seasonal changes can be negligible. Due to optimally high $\dot{V}O_2$max levels, endurance athletes are focused on other factors determining performance such as exercise response at lactate (anaerobic) threshold or exercise efficiency, e.g., "running economy" meaning the oxygen cost at a given running speed [16,18,19]. It seems that no indicator of maximal aerobic capacity, whether it be a weight- or SMM-adjusted one, is suitably sensitive to track training adaptations in highly trained athletes. On the other hand, the effect of body composition on endurance performance is still valid. For example, in male trained trial runners (age 36.1 ± 6.5 years), $\dot{V}O_2$max and fat mass percent were the two best predictors of race time among other physiological and body composition variables, explaining ~84% of the total variance in a multiple regression model [20]. Even if not considered in terms of cause and effect, the changes in body composition across training phases just accompany improvements in aerobic capacity and endurance performance as related physiological adaptations [21].

Available research indicates that body composition and its variations have a significant impact on $\dot{V}O_2$max. As mentioned in the introduction, absolute SMM in athletes is strongly directly proportional to absolute oxygen uptake (up to the suggested limit of ~45 kg of SMM). In highly trained male rowers (20 ± 2 years old), it was predicted based on a regression model that an increase in fat free mass by 1 kg should result in the gain in $\dot{V}O_2$max by 0.16 L·min^{-1} [22]. Also, it is known that body fat strongly negatively correlates with $\dot{V}O_2$max [13,23]. It can be assumed that body composition does matter in achieving high levels of aerobic capacity. However, our results showed that, despite reductions in absolute and percentage fat mass in endurance athletes across the training phases, there was no positive effect on $\dot{V}O_2$max. The likely explanation is that some determinants of $\dot{V}O_2$max, e.g., muscle adaptation to endurance training such as mitochondrial enzyme levels, capillary density or other central and peripheral factors [17,24,25], were maximized and could not be substantially improved in this highly trained group. Moreover, particular effects and relationships seem to depend on age, sex, training status, and athletic profile.

In controls, unlike in athletes, we observed significant changes in $\dot{V}O_2$max indicators between consecutive examinations, despite no significant change in body components. Zwaard et al. [4] suggested that in amateurs adaptive changes such as capillaries or the type of muscle fibers were not as one-sided directed as in endurance- or sprint-trained professional athletes. Central and peripheral adaptations supporting $\dot{V}O_2$max were not maximized in recreationally active individuals, thus our control group could have more strongly responded to training stimuli, even if their training loads were milder than in competitive athletes, because of their relatively low baseline level of $\dot{V}O_2$max (compared to the other two groups) at the start the annual cycle under consideration.

In sprinters, the expected lack of significant changes in $\dot{V}O_2$max between consecutive training phases (despite desired changes in body composition, i.e., fat mass reduction) results from their specific training and performance requirements. Sprint is an all-out high-intensity exercise and the distance covered during competition (including acceleration, achieving maximal velocity, and deceleration) lasts for up to several seconds [26]. It is recommended that elite sprinters should primarily focus on increasing their relative muscle power production using ballistic exercises to maximize speed performance [27]. It is clear that $\dot{V}O_2$max is not crucial for sprint performance. On the other hand, at the early stage of the annual training cycle (the general preparation phase), sprinters' workouts include a certain amount of aerobic exercise to reach an optimal level of aerobic capacity. This allows speed-power athletes to better tolerate training loads necessary for speed and speed endurance development [28]. Despite the significant decrease in body fat in sprinters, there was no positive effect on their $\dot{V}O_2$max. This may be associated with the simultaneous increase in SMM, the large amount of which is typical of sprinters. Our sprinters have approached the "upper limit" of SMM (~40 kg vs. the ~45 kg proposed by Beekley [13]), beyond which $\dot{V}O_2$max is plateauing or even decreasing. More importantly, skeletal muscles in speed-power athletes are characterized by a relatively low capillary density and mitochondrial density, resulting in lower O_2 extraction from the blood by contracting muscles and, consequently, in lower $\dot{V}O_2$max [4,29]. This athletic group focuses on training supporting anaerobic metabolic systems that are the main energy source for muscle activity during sprint running [30,31]. Such training results in a low content of aerobic enzymes in skeletal muscle [32,33].

4.2. Between-Group Differences in $\dot{V}O_2$max

In a few previous studies on the relationship between SMM and $\dot{V}O_2$max, it was suggested that $\dot{V}O_2$max normalized to skeletal muscle mass might be a more relevant index than simply weight-adjusted $\dot{V}O_2$max in the evaluation of aerobic power [11,12]. Moreover, Beekley et al. [13], developed the term "aerobic muscle quality", meaning the amount of oxygen consumed per 1 kg of SMM, to make better comparisons of $\dot{V}O_2$max between individuals of varying fat and total body mass or representing different sports.

In our study, significant differences in SMM- or LBM-adjusted $\dot{V}O_2$max were revealed between sprinters and controls, contrary to non-significant differences in absolute and weight-adjusted values. This can be affected by several factors. First, as other authors have suggested, adjustment of $\dot{V}O_2$max for fat-free mass or skeletal muscle mass is out the influence of adipose tissue [10]. In our sprinters, LBM and SMM significantly increased across the annual cycle, while these body components remained unchanged in controls. This caused significant differences between sprinters and controls in both SMM- and LBM-adjusted $\dot{V}O_2$max, while there was no significant change in absolute and weight-adjusted $\dot{V}O_2$max. Second, the control group consisted of recreationally active men whose physical activity was endurance-oriented. Endurance training modifies central (pulmonary diffusing capacity, maximal cardiac output, the oxygen-carrying capacity of the blood) and peripheral (skeletal muscle characteristics) factors affecting $\dot{V}O_2$max [16,18]. For example, skeletal muscles that undergo endurance training oxidize fat at a higher rate (thus sparing muscle glycogen and blood glucose) and contribute to the decrease in lactate production during exercise. Besides, more muscle mitochondria allow more oxygen to be extracted from the blood by contracting muscles [16,18]. Such typical muscle adaptations (occurring in endurance- but not sprint-trained individuals) may explain significant differences in SMM-adjusted $\dot{V}O_2$max that emerged between sprinters and controls, even though they were not detectable when standard $\dot{V}O_2$max measures were used.

In our participants, the percentage of LBM ranged between 78% and 85% of total body mass, whereas the percentage of SMM was between 43% and 48% (Figure 1). However, despite such a sizeable quantitative difference between these body components as regards their contribution to the total weight, adjusting $\dot{V}O_2$max for SMM only slightly (by mere ~2%) deepened the differences between sprinters and controls compared to LBM-adjusted values (Figure 2). In practical terms, it can be, therefore, assumed that LBM- and SMM-adjusted $\dot{V}O_2$max provide virtually the same information. Thus, calculating the SMM-adjusted $\dot{V}O_2$max to compare groups of different training status seems to be unnecessary. Using LBM, which itself contains about 55–57% SMM, to more precisely express the $\dot{V}O_2$max level, can be quite sufficient and easier.

5. Conclusions

In summary, our research has proven that in endurance- and sprint-trained competitive athletes and recreationally active individuals the profiles of 1-year changes in SMM-adjusted vs. weight-adjusted $\dot{V}O_2$max are not different. However, adjusting $\dot{V}O_2$max for LBM or SMM can uncover significant differences in maximal aerobic capacity between groups of different training specialization and status. In high-performance athletes, the use of the LBM- or SMM-adjusted $\dot{V}O_2$max as an index of "aerobic muscle quality" to track the changes in maximum aerobic capacity across consecutive training phases seems to be unjustified. In competitive athletes, the monitoring and control of maximum aerobic capacity across an annual training cycle can be successfully carried out using conventional (absolute and weight-adjusted) $\dot{V}O_2$max measures. Admittedly, the LBM- or SMM-adjusted $\dot{V}O_2$max can be useful as a tool to more precisely distinguish between groups or individuals differing in muscle adaptation to maximum oxygen uptake. It also seems that LBM- and SMM-adjusted $\dot{V}O_2$max measures provide equivalent information about maximum aerobic capacity. Finally, the limitation of our study is the participation of only male athletes, thus further research is needed to explore analogous patterns of change in different $\dot{V}O_2$max measures in female athletes.

Author Contributions: Conceptualization, J.T. and K.K.; methodology, J.T. and K.K.; software, not applicable; validation, J.T., J.Z. and K.K.; formal analysis, J.T.; investigation, J.T., J.Z. and K.K.; resources, J.T., K.K. and J.Z.; data curation, J.T.; writing—original draft preparation, J.T.; writing—review and editing, J.Z. and K.K.; visualization, J.T.; supervision, K.K.; project administration, K.K.; funding acquisition, K.K. All authors have read and agreed to the published version of the manuscript.

Funding: This research was funded by the National Science Centre, Poland, within the OPUS 14 program, application and grant number 2017/27/B/NZ7/02828.

Acknowledgments: The authors thank the coaches, athletes, and volunteers for their full participation in the study.

Conflicts of Interest: The authors declare that they have no conflicts of interest.

Appendix A

Table A1. Changes in body composition between consecutive phases of the annual training cycle in athletic groups and controls.

	General	Specific	Pre-Competition	Competition	ANOVA Btw. Phases	Effect Size η^2
Total Mass (kg)						
Sprint	81.6 ± 5.9	82.8 ± 6.3 ▲▲#	83.3 ± 6.3 ▲▲▲	-	<0.001	0.39
Endurance	75.4 ± 7.4 +	74.5 ± 6.5	74.6 ± 6.2 +	74.4 ± 6.7	0.138	0.12
Controls	78.4 ± 5.8	78.0 ± 6.2	77.1 ± 6.7	77.0 ± 5.6	0.165	0.17
ANOVA btw. Groups	0.033	0.006	0.019	0.179		
Effect Size η^2	0.32	0.43	0.36	0.19		
Fat Mass (kg)						
Sprinters	9.5 ± 1.5 *	8.6 ± 1.4 ▲▲▲**	8.6 ± 1.4 ▲**	-	0.002	0.32
Endurance	12.2 ± 2.8	10.6 ± 2.3 ■■■**	10.6 ± 2.1 ■■■**	10.54 ± 2.3 ■■■*	<0.001	0.46
Controls	14.6 ± 4.3	14.5 ± 4.5	13.9 ± 4.3	12.9 ± 3.3	0.109	0.20
ANOVA btw. Groups	0.011	<0.001	0.001	0.022		
Effect Size η^2	0.40	0.55	0.52	0.46		
Fat Mass (%)						
Sprinters	11.6 ± 1.9 **	10.38 ± 1.7 ▲▲▲***	10.36 ± 1.6 ▲▲▲***	-	<0.001	0.43
Endurance	16.00 ± 2.6	14.4 ± 2.3 ■■■**	14.1 ± 2.1 ■■■**	14.1 ± 2.1 ■■■*	<0.001	0.46
Controls	18.4 ± 4.4	18.4 ± 4.8	17.9 ± 4.9	16.7 ± 4.2	0.149	0.18
ANOVA btw. Groups	0.002	<0.001	<0.001	0.039		
Effect Size η^2	0.51	0.64	0.65	0.39		
Lean Body Mass (kg)						
Sprinters	68.4 ± 5.5 #*	70.6 ± 5.9 ▲▲▲***	71.0 ± 5.8 ▲▲▲#**	-	<0.001	0.72
Endurance	60.0 ± 5.2	60.6 ± 4.8 ++	60.8 ± 4.6	60.7 ± 4.7	0.140	0.12
Controls	60.6 ± 3.6	60.3 ± 4.1	60.0 ± 5.1	60.9 ± 5.5	0.511	0.08
ANOVA btw. Groups	0.002	<0.001	<0.001	0.61		
Effect Size η^2	0.49	0.60	0.55	0.03		

Table A1. Cont.

	General	Training Phases Specific	Pre-Competition	Competition	ANOVA Btw. Phases	Effect Size η^2
		Lean Body Mass (%)				
Sprinters	83.9 ± 1.8 **	85.3 ± 1.7 ▲▲▲***	85.3 ± 1.6 ▲▲▲***	-	<0.001	0.48
Endurance	79.8 ± 2.5	81.4 ± 2.2 ■■**	81.6 ± 2.1 ■■**	81.7 ± 2.2 ■■■*	<0.001	0.47
Controls	77.5 ± 4.1	77.5 ± 4.4	77.9 ± 4.6	79.1 ± 4.0	0.165	0.17
ANOVA btw. groups	0.001	<0.001	<0.001	0.036		
Effect size η^2	0.52	0.66	0.67	0.40		
		Skeletal Muscle Mass (kg)				
Sprinters	38.7 ± 3.6 #*	39.8 ± 3.8 ▲▲**	40.0 ± 4.0 ▲▲**	-	<0.001	0.37
Endurance	32.7 ± 3.1	32.7 ± 2.6 ++	32.8 ± 2.6 ++	32.7 ± 2.8	0.961	0.01
Controls	33.4 ± 2.3	33.4 ± 2.1	32.9 ± 3.1	33.3 ± 3.2	0.561	0.07
ANOVA btw. Groups	0.002	<0.001	<0.001	0.503		
Effect Size η^2	0.51	0.64	0.60	0.05		
		Skeletal Muscle Mass (%)				
Sprinters	47.4 ± 1.7 **	48.0 ± 1.5 #***	48.0 ± 1.6 #***	-	0.198	0.10
Endurance	43.5 ± 1.7 +	44.0 ± 1.6	44.0 ± 1.7	43.9 ± 1.7	0.108	0.13
Controls	42.8 ± 2.9	42.9 ± 2.7	42.7 ± 3.2	43.3 ± 2.7	0.631	0.06
ANOVA btw. Groups	0.001	<0.001	<0.001	0.036		
Effect Size η^2	0.52	0.62	0.70	0.24		

▲ $p < 0.05$, ▲▲ $p < 0.01$, ▲▲▲ $p < 0.001$—significantly different from the general preparation phase in a sprinters group; ■ $p < 0.01$, ■■■ $p < 0.001$—significantly different from the general preparation phase in endurance group; + $p < 0.05$, ++ $p < 0.01$—significantly different from sprinters at the same training phase, # $p < 0.01$—significantly different from endurance athletes at the same training phase, * $p < 0.05$, ** $p < 0.01$, *** $p < 0.001$—significantly different from controls at the same training phase.

Table A2. Changes in maximal oxygen uptake (absolute and relative values) between consecutive phases of the annual training cycle in athletic groups and controls.

	Training Phases			ANOVA Btw. Phases	Effect Size η^2
	General	Specific	Pre-Competition	Competition		
$\dot{V}O_2max$ (mL·min^{-1})						
Sprint	4328 ± 438	4368 ± 370	4290 ± 381	–	0.268	0.08
Endurance	5055 ± 615 *	4939 ± 628.15	4998 ± 628	5024 ± 753	0.628	0.04
Controls	4204 ± 419	4338 ± 365	4415 ± 335 ○	4491 ± 315 ○○	0.001	0.45
ANOVA btw. Groups	0.022	0.232	0.077	0.487		
Effect Size η^2	0.34	0.15	0.25	0.06		
$\dot{V}O_2max$ (mL·min^{-1}·kg TBM^{-1})						
Sprinters	52.1 ± 4.5	52.8 ± 3.7	52.7 ± 4.6	–	0.406	0.05
Endurance	67.9 ± 4.3 +++++	66.1 ± 3.9 +++++	66.9 ± 4.1 +++++	66.5 ± 5.3 ***	0.467	0.06
Controls	54.6 ± 3.4	56.4 ± 3.9	56.7 ± 3.7	57.4 ± 2.8 ○	0.033	0.27
ANOVA btw. Groups	>0.001	>0.001	>0.001	>0.001		
Effect Size η^2	0.86	0.78	0.76	0.78		
$\dot{V}O_2max$ (mL·min^{-1}·kg LBM^{-1})						
Sprinters	61.1 ± 5.4 **	62.0 ± 4.5 ***	62.7 ± 5.4 ***	–	0.077	0.15
Endurance	83.2 ± 6.4 +++++	81.0 ± 6.1 +++	82.4 ± 6.9 +++	83.4 ± 7.8 *	0.321	0.08
Controls	69.2 ± 6.7	72.5 ± 5.2 ○	73.3 ± 4.7 ○○	74.2 ± 4.0 ○○	0.001	0.47
ANOVA btw. Groups	>0.001	>0.001	>0.001	0.011		
Effect Size η^2	0.83	0.81	0.79	0.53		
$\dot{V}O_2max$ (mL·min^{-1}·kg SMM^{-1})						
Sprinters	108.6 ± 10.6 **	110.2 ± 9.2 ***	111.2 ± 10.1 ***	–	0.306	0.07
Endurance	154.8 ± 13.4 +++++	150.5 ± 13.1 +++	152.7 ± 14.0 +++	153.4 ± 15.7 *	0.404	0.07
Controls	126.7 ± 12.9	132.4 ± 9.9	132.4 ± 8.4	134.7 ± 10.0 ○	0.005	0.37
ANOVA btw. Groups	>0.001	>0.001	>0.001	0.023		
Effect Size η^2	0.82	0.83	0.80	0.45		

Abbreviations: LBM = lean body mass; SMM = skeletal muscle mass; $\dot{V}O_2max$ = maximal oxygen uptake; ○ $p < 0.05$, ○○ $p < 0.01$—significantly different from the general preparation phase in a controls group; ++ $p < 0.001$—significantly different from sprinters at the same training phase; * $p < 0.05$, ** $p < 0.01$, *** $p < 0.001$—significantly different from controls at the same training phase.

References

1. Costill, D.; Thomason, H.; Roberts, E. Fractional utilization of the aerobic capacity during distance running. *Med. Sci. Sports* **1973**, *5*, 248–252. [CrossRef]
2. Hill, A.; Long, C.; Lupton, H. Muscular exercise, lactic acid and the supply and utilisation of oxygen: Parts VII-VIII. *Proc. R. Soc. B* **1924**, *97*, 155–176.
3. Ranković, G.; Mutavdžić, V.; Toskić, D.; Preljević, A.; Kocić, M.; Nedin-Ranković, G.; Damjanović, N. Aerobic capacity as an indicator in different kinds of sports. *Bosn. J. Basic Med. Sci.* **2010**, *10*, 44–48. [CrossRef]
4. Zwaard, S.; Laarse, W.; Weide, G.; Bloemers, F.; Hofmijster, M.; Levels, K.; Noordhof, D.; Koning, J.; Ruiter, C.; Jaspers, R. Critical determinants of combined sprint and endurance performance: An integrative analysis from muscle fiber to the human body. *FASEB J.* **2018**, *32*, 2110–2123. [CrossRef] [PubMed]
5. Kim, J.; Wang, Z.; Heymsfield, S.; Baumgartner, R.; Gallagher, D. Total-body skeletal muscle mass: Estimation by a new dual-energy X-ray absorptiometry method. *Am. J. Clin. Nutr.* **2002**, *76*, 378–383. [CrossRef] [PubMed]
6. Andreato, L.; Esteves, J.; Gomes, T.; Andreato, T.; Alcantara, B.; Almeida, D.; Franzói De Moraes, S. Morphological profile of Brazilian jiu-jitsu athletes from different competitive level. *Rev. Bras. Med. Esporte* **2010**, *18*, 46–50. [CrossRef]
7. Delaney, J.; Thornton, H.; Scott, T.; Ballard, D.; Duthie, G.; Wood, L.; Dascombe, B. Validity of skinfold-based measures for tracking changes in body composition in professional rugby league players. *Int. J. Sports Physiol. Perform.* **2016**, *11*, 261–266. [CrossRef] [PubMed]
8. González-Mendoza, R.; Gaytán-González, A.; Jiménez-Alvarado, J.; Villegas-Balcázar, M.; Jáuregui-Ulloa, E.; Torres-Naranjo, F.; López-Taylor, J. Accuracy of anthropometric equations to estimate DXA-derived skeletal muscle mass in professional male soccer players. *J. Sports Med.* **2019**, *1*, 4387636. [CrossRef]
9. Martín-Matillas, M.; Valadés, D.; Hernández-Hernández, E.; Olea-Serrano, F.; Sjöström, M.; Delgado-Fernández, M.; Ortega, F. Anthropometric, body composition and somatotype characteristics of elite female volleyball players from the highest Spanish league. *J. Sports Sci.* **2014**, *32*, 137–148. [CrossRef]
10. Milanese, C.; Cavedon, V.; Corradini, G.; De Vita, F.; Zancanaro, C. Seasonal DXA-measured body composition changes in professional male soccer players. *J. Sports Sci.* **2015**, *33*, 1219–1228. [CrossRef]
11. Proctor, D.; Joyner, M. Skeletal muscle mass and the reduction of VO2max in trained older subjects. *J. Appl. Physiol.* **1997**, *82*, 1411–1415. [CrossRef] [PubMed]
12. Sanada, K.; Kearns, C.; Kojima, K.; Abe, T. Peak oxygen uptake during running and arm cranking normalized to total and regional skeletal muscle mass measured by magnetic resonance imaging. *Eur. J. Appl. Physiol.* **2005**, *93*, 687–693. [CrossRef] [PubMed]
13. Beekley, M.; Abe, T.; Kondo, M.; Midorikawa, T.; Yamauchi, T. Comparison of normalized maximum aerobic capacity and body composition of sumo wrestlers to athletes in combat and other sports. *J. Sports Sci. Med.* **2006**, *5*, 13–20. [PubMed]
14. Nana, A.; Slater, G.J.; Hopkins, W.G.; Burke, L.M. Effects of daily activities on DXA measurements of body composition in active people. *Med. Sci. Sports Exerc.* **2012**, *44*, 180–189. [CrossRef]
15. Edvardsen, E.; Hem, E.; Anderssen, S. End criteria for reaching maximal oxygen uptake must be strict and adjusted to sex and age: A cross-sectional study. *PLoS ONE* **2014**, *9*, e85276. [CrossRef]
16. Bassett, D.R., Jr.; Howley, E. Limiting factors for maximum oxygen uptake and determinants of endurance performance. *Med. Sci. Sports Exerc.* **2000**, *32*, 70–84. [CrossRef]
17. Joyner, M. Physiological limits to endurance exercise performance: Influence of sex. *J. Physiol.* **2017**, *595*, 2949–2954. [CrossRef]
18. Jacobs, R.; Rasmussen, P.; Siebenmann, C.; Díaz, V.; Gassmann, M.; Pesta, D.; Gnaiger, E.; Nordsborg, N.; Robach, P.; Lundby, C. Determinants of time trial performance and maximal incremental exercise in highly trained endurance athletes. *J. Appl. Physiol.* **2011**, *111*, 1422–1430. [CrossRef]
19. Joyner, M.; Coyle, E. Endurance exercise performance: The physiology of champions. *J. Physiol.* **2008**, *586*, 35–44. [CrossRef]
20. Alvero-Cruz, J.; Parent, V.; Garcia, J.; Albornoz-Gil, M.; Benítez-Porres, J.; Ordóñez, F.; Rosemann, T.; Nikolaidis, P.; Knechtle, B. Prediction of performance in a short trail running race: The role of body composition. *Front. Physiol.* **2019**, *10*, 1306. [CrossRef]
21. Venkata, Y.; Surya, M.V.L.; Sudhakar, S.; Balakrishna, N. Effect of changes in body composition profile on VO2max and maximal work performance in athletes. *J. Exerc. Physiol. Online* **2004**, *7*, 34–39.

22. Durkalec-Michalski, K.; Nowaczyk, P.M.; Podgórski, T.; Kusy, K.; Osiński, W.; Jeszka, J. Relationship between body composition and the level of aerobic and anaerobic capacity in highly trained male rowers. *J. Sports Med. Phys. Fit.* **2019**, *59*, 1526–1535. [CrossRef] [PubMed]
23. Shete, A.; Bute, S.; Deshmukh, P. A study of VO2max and body fat percentage in female athletes. *J. Clin. Diagn. Res.* **2014**, *8*, BC01–BC03. [CrossRef] [PubMed]
24. Andersen, P.; Henriksson, J. Capillary supply of the quadriceps femoris muscle of man: Adaptive response to exercise. *J. Physiol.* **1977**, *270*, 677–690. [CrossRef] [PubMed]
25. Holloszy, J.; Coyle, E. Adaptations of skeletal muscle to endurance exercise and their metabolic consequences. *J. Appl. Physiol.* **1984**, *56*, 831–838. [CrossRef]
26. Haugen, T.; Seiler, S.; Sandbakk, Ø.; Tønnessen, E. The training and development of elite sprint performance: An integration of scientific and best practice literature. *Sports Med. Open* **2019**, *5*, 44. [CrossRef]
27. Loturco, I.; Kobal, R.; Kitamura, K.; Fernandes, V.; Moura, N.; Siqueira, F.; Cal Abad, C.; Pereira, L. Predictive factors of elite sprint performance: Influences of muscle mechanical properties and functional parameters. *J. Strength Cond. Res.* **2019**, *33*, 974–986. [CrossRef]
28. Bompa, T.; Buzzichelli, C. *Periodization Training for Sports*; Human Kinetics: Champaign, IL, USA, 2015.
29. Torok, D.; Duey, W.; Bassett, D.R., Jr.; Howley, E.; Mancuso, P. Cardiovascular responses to exercise in sprinters and distance runners. *Med. Sci. Sports Exerc.* **1995**, *27*, 1050–1056. [CrossRef]
30. Duffield, R.; Dawson, B.; Goodman, C. Energy system contribution to 100-m and 200-m track running events. *J. Sci. Med. Sport* **2004**, *7*, 302–313. [CrossRef]
31. Kusy, K.; Zarębska, E.; Ciekot-Sołtysiak, M.; Janowski, M.; Zieliński, J. Cardiorespiratory response and energy system contribution during speed endurance workout in a highly trained sprinter: A preliminary report. Antropomotoryka. *J. Kinesiol. Exerc. Sci.* **2015**, *70*, 27–36.
32. Bompa, T.; Haff, G. *Periodization: Theory and Methodology of Training*; Human Kinetics: Champaign, IL, USA, 2009.
33. Ross, A.; Leveritt, M. Long-term metabolic and skeletal muscle adaptations to short-sprint training implications for sprint training and tapering. *Sports Med.* **2001**, *31*, 1063–1082. [CrossRef] [PubMed]

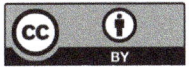

© 2020 by the authors. Licensee MDPI, Basel, Switzerland. This article is an open access article distributed under the terms and conditions of the Creative Commons Attribution (CC BY) license (http://creativecommons.org/licenses/by/4.0/).

Article

Dietary Acid-Base Balance in High-Performance Athletes

Marius Baranauskas [1,*], Valerija Jablonskienė [1], Jonas Algis Abaravičius [1], Laimutė Samsonienė [2] and Rimantas Stukas [3]

1. Department of Physiology, Biochemistry, Microbiology and Laboratory Medicine of the Faculty of Medicine, Institute of Biomedical Sciences, Vilnius University, 01513 Vilnius, Lithuania; valerija.jablonskiene@mf.vu.lt (V.J.); algis.abaravicius@mf.vu.lt (J.A.A.)
2. Department of Rehabilitation, Physical and Sports Medicine, Institute of Health Sciences of the Faculty of Medicine, Vilnius University, 01513 Vilnius, Lithuania; laimute.samsoniene@mf.vu.lt
3. Department of Public Health, Institute of Health Sciences of the Faculty of Medicine, Vilnius University, 01513 Vilnius, Lithuania; rimantas.stukas@mf.vu.lt
* Correspondence: marius.baranauskas9@gmail.com

Received: 8 July 2020; Accepted: 22 July 2020; Published: 24 July 2020

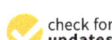

Abstract: Physical exercise leads to metabolic changes that affect the acid-base balance in skeletal muscles and other tissues. Nutrition is one of the factors that may influence the acid-base balance in the body. Keeping alkaline circumstances in the body is important not only for health and athletic performance in training but also during competition in many sport events. This is especially significant for athletes who practice in sport at the highest level of competition. The aim of the study was to determine the dietary acid-base balance in competitive Lithuanian high-performance athletes, and to evaluate the effect of actual diets of athletes on NEAP (net endogenous acid production), muscle mass and body mineral content during a four-year Olympic cycle. The research participants were 18.1 ± 3.3-year-old Lithuanian high performance athletes (n = 323). The actual diet was investigated using the 24 h recall dietary survey method. The measurements of body composition were performed using BIA (bioelectrical impedance analysis). The potential renal acid load of the diets of athletes (dietary PRAL) and NEAP were calculated. In 10.2% of athletes, NEAP exceeds 100 mEq·day^{-1} and is on average 126.1 ± 32.7 mEq·day^{-1}. Higher NEAP in athletes is associated with lower muscle mass (β -1.2% of body weight, p < 0.001) but has no effect on the amount of minerals in the body (β 0.01% of body weight, p = 0.073). Overall, 25–30% of Lithuanian high-performance athletes use high-protein diets (2.0–4.8 g·kg^{-1}·day^{-1}) leading to a dietary acid-base imbalance as well as an excessive production of endogenous acids in the body. Athletes are recommended to consume higher amounts of potassium and magnesium. An increase in calcium intake up to 1500 mg per day is recommended. In exceptional cases, periodised nutrition for athletes may involve diets complemented with bicarbonate and/or beta-alanine supplements.

Keywords: high-performance athletes; actual nutrition; eating habits; diet; body composition; acid-base balance

1. Introduction

Acid-base balance homeostasis is essential for ensuring health and physical performance indicators. Organic acids are produced in the body during basal metabolism, while physical exercise can lead to additional acid production in the body [1]. When engaged in sports, even submaximal exercise induces metabolic changes that affect the acid-base balance in the skeletal muscles and other tissues [2]. Exercise intensity can lower blood pH from 7.4 to 6.9. It is noteworthy that the lowest blood pH reading

(6.80–6.90) due to endogenous acids production was found in runners after a simulated 400 m race [3,4]. The increased H^+ levels in myocytes during high-intensity exercise lead to acidosis and fatigue [1,5]. Muscle fatigue occurs due to H^+ accumulation because the mitochondrial function and enzymatic activity are impaired. As a consequence, the production of glycolytic energy is disrupted [6,7]. It has also been proven that the concentration of H^+ ions leads to the accumulation of interstitial K^+, where proteins bind H^+ ions instead of K^+ ions. This causes the hyperpolarisation of cells, inhibits the rate of the nerve impulse propagation, triggers the changes in the membrane potential and, as a result, disrupts the muscle function [8]. HCO_3^- in extracellular fluids is the major H^+ buffer [9]. Therefore, the maintenance of a higher concentration of HCO_3^- results in a faster removal of H^+ from muscle cells [5]. Thus, an increase in the capacity of the acid buffer system improves the anaerobic [10,11] and aerobic [12] fitness of athletes. The maintenance of alkalinity in intracellular fluids enables a faster removal of H^+ from muscle cells resulting in a delayed muscle fatigue which occurs due to increased acidosis [1].

Nutrition is one of the factors that can affect the acid-base balance in the body. This was confirmed by research that showed a strong relationship between the chemical composition of dietary intake and the urine pH range [13]. In this context, the possible influence of the intake of different foods on the potential renal acid load (PRAL) was assessed. The PRAL index that shows the potential renal acid load indicates the presence of milliequivalents (mEq) of H^+ ions per 100 g of food. Most fruits and vegetables have a negative PRAL index because the biologically active substances found in them act as H^+ buffers in the body. Meanwhile, foods high in protein and phosphorus have a positive PRAL index, which means that their consumption stimulates H^+ production in the body.

According to the research, the dietary habits of the population in the developed countries with the typical Western diet are dominated by protein foods of animal origin (fish, meat, eggs), leading to high levels of metabolic acidosis in the body [14]. The similarity in problems such as high protein and fat intakes was found among athletes from many countries. Based on the research data reported in the scientific literature, it has been stated that a diet high in protein and fat, but low in carbohydrates was adopted by professional athletes from countries such as Poland [15,16], Iran [17], Kuwait [18], England [19,20], Brazil [21], Greece [22], Australia [23–25], France [26,27] Finland [28], China [29,30], Ireland [31], Netherlands [32], Spain [33,34], the United States of America (USA) [35], South Africa [36], Canada [37]. It has also been found that if athletes consume large amounts of protein and their diets are low in carbohydrates, they can suffer from metabolic acidosis which can adversely affect their physical performance [13,38–40]. In addition, insufficient consumption of potassium and magnesium with vegetables and fruits increases the risk of acidosis which may result in the reduced physical working capacity of athletes [41].

It should be noted that the presence of persistent acidosis in the body may trigger the impairment of the muscle function leading to the inhibition of muscle protein synthesis. Part of the amino acids from the degraded muscle proteins can be used for glutamine synthesis in the liver and, in later stages, for acid neutralisation. As a consequence, the increased acid production can lead to a decrease in muscle mass [42–45]. In addition, regular acidic diet may trigger a reduction in bone mineralisation, an increase in urinary calcium excretion and pose a risk of bone fractures [46].

There are no scientifically grounded data on how the diets of high-performance athletes impact their body's acid-base balance, muscle mass and body mineral content. The aim of the study was to determine the dietary acid-base balance in competitive Lithuanian high-performance athletes, and to evaluate the effect of the actual diets of athletes on NEAP (net endogenous acid production), muscle mass and body mineral content during a four-year Olympic cycle.

2. Materials and Methods

2.1. Study Population

High-performance sport or elite sport is sport at the highest level of competition. The target population for the survey was high-performance athletes ($n = 341$) included in the lists, approved under the orders the National Olympic Committee of Lithuania. The main inclusion criteria for study participants was qualification standards that have been previously met by athletes.

Only those athletes that had already obtained an Olympic qualification quota place or the athletes who had participated in the European Athletics Championships and/or the World Athletics Championships for the purposes of Olympic qualification were investigated. Those athletes who had not participation in sports competitions on a professional level were excluded from the survey. The size of the sample group ($n = 338$) was selected using the OpenEpi Sample Size Calculator with a margin of error of 5% and probability of 99.9%. Over the period from 2017 through 2018, during a preparatory phase of training (macrocycle), 96% of the candidates ($n = 323$) to the Lithuanian Olympic team were included in study and investigated. The athletes ranged in age from 16 to 33 (the average mean age of the athletes was 18.1 ± 3.3 years) and were tested during the research and the training status of the athletes corresponded to 7.9 ± 3.8 years, while workouts were done 5.8 ± 0.8 days a week, with an average workout time of 175.6 ± 60.6 min a day. The dimensions of the training workload of athletes fully complied with the training plans approved by the Lithuanian Sports Centre and the National Olympic Committee of Lithuania. The training plans were specified in the Tokyo 2020 and PyeongChang 2018 programmes. The research sample included 72.4% ($n = 234$) men and 27.6% ($n = 89$) women. According to the dominant energy expenditure methods, the subjects were divided into anaerobic 40.2% ($n = 130$) and aerobic 59.8% ($n = 193$) fitness athletes [47]. The group of anaerobic athletes comprised weightlifters ($n = 6$), gymnasts ($n = 3$), discus, javelin throwers, shot put athletes ($n = 6$), jumpers ($n = 4$), basketball players ($n = 52$), boxers ($n = 14$), Greco-Roman wrestlers ($n = 29$), judo wrestlers ($n = 12$), and taekwondo wrestlers ($n = 4$). The group of athletes of aerobic fitness involved representatives of academic rowing ($n = 36$), road cyclists ($n = 50$), swimmers ($n = 66$), skiers ($n = 17$), biathletes ($n = 20$), long-distance runners ($n = 13$), representatives of modern pentathlon ($n = 12$) and representatives of figure skating ($n = 2$). A more detailed analysis of the study recruitment process and study procedures is provided in Figure 1.

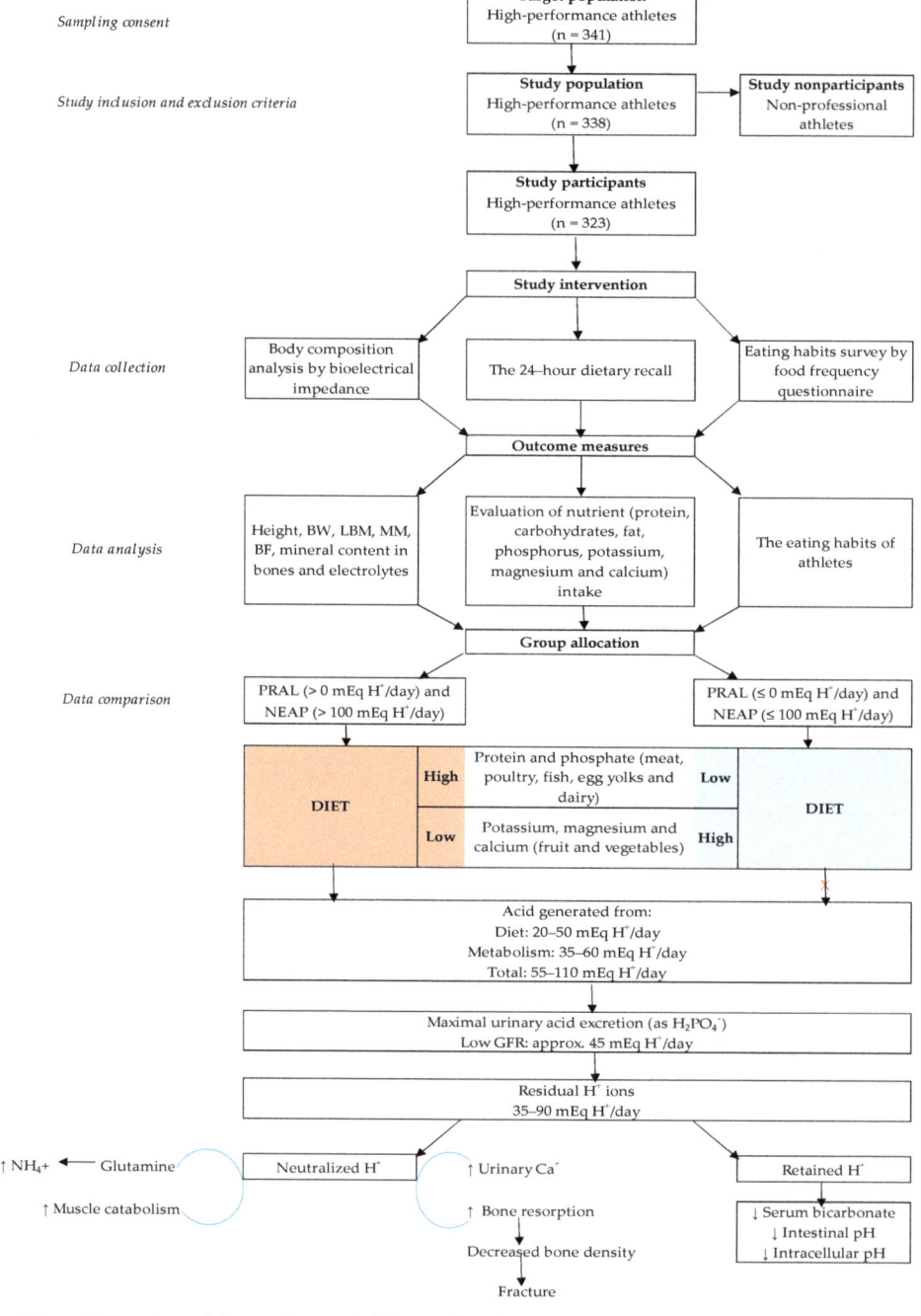

Figure 1. Flowchart of the enrollment of athletes and study procedures. BW—body weight; LBM—lean body mass; MM—muscle mass; BF—body fat; PRAL—potential renal acid load; NEAP—net endogenous acid production; GFR—glomerular filtration rate.

2.2. Anthropometric Measures

The height measurements in athletes were taken at the Lithuanian Sports Medicine Centre using a stadiometer (± 0.01 m). The measurements of the body weight and the individual weight components (body weight (BW), lean body mass (LBM) (in kg and %), muscle mass (MM) (in kg and %), body fat (BF) (in kg and %) and mineral content in bones and electrolytes) (in kg and %) were performed at the Lithuanian Sports Centre using the bioelectrical impedance analysis (BIA) tetra-polar electrodes (13 lot 21 block with certification EN ISO (an international standard is adopted by the European Union) 13488; Jinryang Industrial Complex, Kyungsan City, South Korea) and resistivity was measured with 8–12 tangent electrodes at different frequencies of the signal: 5, 50, 250, 550 and 1000 kHz [47,48]. LBM, MM and mineral content were assessed according to the norms set for men and women. LBM norm for men is 75–85%, for women 70–80%; MM norm for men is 74–80%, for women 64–80%; mineral norm for men ranges between 5.8–6.0%, for women 5.5–6.0%. The muscle and fat mass index (MFMI) of each athlete was determined by dividing the weight of the muscle (in kg) by weight (in kg). The BF and the ratio of muscle and fat mass were evaluated according to the standards presented in Table 1 (MFMI) [47].

Table 1. Body fat (BF) percentage and muscle and fat mass index (MFMI) scale for athletes (by gender).

BF			MFMI		
Value	Males	Females	Value	Male Athletes	Female Athletes
Too low	<5%	<15%	Insufficient	<2	<1.8
Lean	5–9%	15–19%	Too small	2.1–3.39	1.9–2.89
Optimal	10–14%	20–24%	Moderate	3.4–4.69	3–3.99
Acceptable	15–19%	25–29%	Extensive	4.7–6.0	4–5
Excessive	20–24%	30–34%	Maximum	>6	>5

BF—body fat; MFMI—muscle and fat mass index.

2.3. Energy Requirements

The basal metabolic rate (BMR), daily energy expenditure (DEE), training energy expenditure (TEE) were estimated in all the subjects. BMR was calculated using the Harris and Benedict formulas [49]. We collected 24-h records of physical activity on the same day when the participants recorded their dietary energy intake (EI). The physical activity levels and lifestyle variables (regular and non-regular activities, sedentary activities and sleeping habits) conform to the standards specified by the American Dietetic Association, Dietitians of Canada, and the American College of Sports Medicine [50]. These measures (the activity codes and metabolic equivalents (METs) (in kcal/kg/h) for physical activities) were supported by the studies of Ainsworth et al. [51] and the data were processed according to the specific activity.

2.4. Dietary Intake and Eating Habits

The 24-h actual nutrition survey method was employed to assess the actual nutrition in athletes [52–54]. The respondents were surveyed through the direct interview carried out by a specially trained interviewer at the Lithuanian Sports Centre. The actual nutrition survey method facilitated the compilation of the data on the amounts of food, meals, food supplements consumed by each athlete. To capture all foods and meals eaten, and their amounts, a special atlas of photos with different portions of foods and meals weighted in grams was used [55]. We evaluated the average daily food sets consumed by athletes on the basis of which the chemical composition and energy value of food rations were determined in line with the chemical composition tables [56]. The consumption of carbohydrates, proteins and fats was assessed taking into account the recommendations provided in the scientific literature [57,58]. The amount of carbohydrates recommended for athletes is 5–8 $g\cdot kg^{-1}\cdot day^{-1}$, protein content is 1.4–2.0 $g\cdot kg^{-1}\cdot day^{-1}$. The percentage of energy provided by fat should be between 20% and 35%. The daily intake of minerals and their compliance with the reference daily intake (RDI) was assessed according to the RDI of vitamins and minerals approved in Lithuania [59]. To study the eating habits, we designed and used a validated questionnaire originally constructed by M. Baranauskas [60]. The respondents participated in direct interviews. The questionnaire comprised questions about the socio-demographics (gender, age, place of residence, sport, sporting experience, etc.) and eating habits of athletes.

2.5. Potential Renal Acid Load (PRAL), Net Endogenous Acid Production (NEAP) and the Diets

The following formula was used to estimate the NEAP [61]: NEAP was estimated according to the equation (mEq·day^{-1}) = PRAL^1 (mEq·day^{-1}) + OA^2 (mEq·day^{-1}) where PRAL shows the potential renal acid load of the estimated diet and OA (organic anions) shows the urinary organic anions under analysis, with the 2 components calculated as follows:

PRAL^1 (mEq·day^{-1}) = (0.49 × protein (g·day^{-1})) + (0.037 × phosphorus (mg·day^{-1})) − (0.021· potassium (mg·day^{-1})) − (0.026 × magnesium (mg·day^{-1})) − (0.013 × calcium (mg·day^{-1})).

OA^2 (mEq·day^{-1}) = individual body surface area ^{3}·41/1.73.

The body surface area was calculated according to the formula proposed by Du Bois and Du Bois [62]: ^{3} Individual body surface area (m^2) = 0.007184 · height (cm)$^{0.725}$ · weight (kg)$^{0.425}$.

2.6. Statistical Analysis

All the normally distributed continuous variables are presented as means ± standard deviations (SD), whereas the qualitative variables are presented as relative frequencies (in %). The normality of variable distribution was tested by the Shapiro–Wilk W test. When normality was confirmed, the *t*-tests of the independent samples were used to assess the differences observed between the groups. Pearson (*r*) correlation coefficient were used to determine the strength of the relationship between the variables under analysis. The correlation coefficient r can range in value from −1 to +1. A higher degree of the absolute value of the coefficient shows a stronger the relationship between the variables. The correlations above 0.4 are considered to be relatively strong; the correlations between 0.2 and 0.4 are moderate, and those below 0.2 are weak.

The multiple linear regression analysis was used to determine the association between the dietary intake and NEAP. The model was adjusted for gender and type of sport. Logarithmic or inverse square transformations were used to improve normality. By using a stepwise multivariate logistic regression method, we determined which eating habits of athletes depended on their sport. The stepwise multivariate logistic regression method was used to establish which eating habits determined PRAL ≤ 0 and PRAL > 0. The method of parameter estimation used in this study was maximum likelihood, and several techniques were employed to assess the appropriateness, adequacy and usefulness of the model using the likelihood-ratio test, Hosmer and Lemeshow (H-L) test statistic, Wald (W) statistic, and Nagelkerke R^2 statistic. During the next stages, we calculated the logistic regression coefficients (β), odds ratios (OR) and their 95% confidence intervals (CIs) for each variable under analysis. All the reported *p*-values are based on two-sided tests and compared to a significance level of 5%. The statistical analysis was performed using Stata version 12.1 (StataCorp, College Station, TX, USA), SPSS V.25 for Windows (International Business Machines Corporation, Armonk, NY, USA) and Microsoft Excel (Microsoft Corporation, Redmond, WA, USA).

2.7. Ethics Statement

Prior to the research, all the organisational issues regarding the survey were discussed with the Lithuanian Sports Centre and the Bioethics Committee. The study was conducted in accordance with a permit to carry out biomedical research, issued by the Lithuanian Bioethics Committee (No. 158200-11-113-25, of 3 November 2009). Prior to testing, all the athletes provided a written consent and the study protocols were approved by the Institutional Review Board of the Lithuanian Sports Medicine Centre. The biomedical research was conducted according to the principles expressed in the Declaration of Helsinki.

3. Results

3.1. Characteristics of Respondents

The body composition (BW, LBM, BF MM, and MFMI) of athletes was examined as shown in Table 2. The height, BW, LBM, MM, and the mineral content (in bones and electrolytes) fluctuated within the norms. BF in male athletes (16.7 ± 4.7%) was acceptable (15–19%) while MFMI (5.2 ± 2.5) was high (4.7–6.0). Meanwhile, the BF and MFMI in female athletes differed in the groups of different sports. BF of female athletes involved in sports of anaerobic fitness was 24.9 ± 4.8%, which was acceptable (25–29%) and higher than BF of athletes of aerobic fitness which was 22.2 ± 3.6% and corresponded to the optimal FM (20–24%) ($p = 0.005$). In addition, MFMI (2.9 ± 0.8) in anaerobic female athletes corresponded to the low one (1.9–2.9). Meanwhile, a higher MFMI observed in aerobic women involved (3.4 ± 0.8, corresponding to the average of 3.0–3.9) confirms a more optimal body composition ($p = 0.012$).

Table 2. Body composition of athletes (by sport and gender).

Body Composition	Anaerobic Sports		Aerobic Sports	
	Male	Female	Male	Female
Height (m)	1.83 ± 0.15	1.73 ± 0.11	1.83 ± 0.08	1.67 ± 0.06
BW (kg)	77.5 ± 17.4	67.4 ± 14.3	75.0 ± 11.6	59.7 ± 7.5
LBM (kg)	63.8 ± 11.4	50.1 ± 7.9	62.2 ± 7.7	46.3 ± 4.7
LBM (% of BW)	83.3 ± 5.3	75.2 ± 4.9	83.3 ± 4.2	77.6 ± 3.7
MM (kg)	59.3 ± 10.5	46.2 ± 7.2	57.9 ± 7.0	42.8 ± 4.3
MM (% of BW)	77.4 ± 5.2	69.4 ± 4.8	77.6 ± 4.1	72.1 ± 3.6
MFMI	5.3 ± 2.4	2.9 ± 0.8	5.2 ± 2.6	3.4 ± 0.8
BF (kg)	13.7 ± 7.1	17.6 ± 7.1	12.9 ± 4.7	13.4 ± 3.5
BF (% of BW)	16.7 ± 5.3	24.9 ± 4.8	16.7 ± 4.2	22.2 ± 3.6
Minerals (kg) [1]	4.5 ± 1.0	3.9 ± 0.8	4.4 ± 0.7	3.4 ± 0.4
Minerals (% of BW) [1]	5.8 ± 0.1	5.8 ± 0.1	5.8 ± 0.1	5.8 ± 0.1

BW—body weight; LBM—lean body mass; MM—muscle mass; MFMI—muscle and fat mass index; BF—body fat; [1]—mineral composed of bone and electrolyte. The data is normally distributed and presented as means ± standard deviation (SD).

3.2. Dietary Intake and Energy Expenditure

The examination of the actual diet of athletes revealed that the EI amounts to 3343 ± 1133 kcal and corresponds to DEE by 91.4 ± 27.8% (Table 2).

The evaluation of the nutrient intake showed that regardless of the type of sport, when training 175.6 ± 60.6 min per day, the amount of carbohydrates consumed (5.5 $g \cdot kg^{-1} \cdot day^{-1}$) conforms to the minimum requirements (5–8 $g \cdot kg^{-1} \cdot day^{-1}$). Nutrient imbalances in the diets of athletes are caused by an excessive fat intake. Irrespective of the type of sport, the share of energy value of fat in the diet of athletes (39.0 ± 7.8%) exceeds what is recommended (by 20–35%).

The average amount of protein of 1.7 ± 0.6 $g \cdot kg^{-1} \cdot day^{-1}$ found in the diets of all types of athletes (anaerobic and aerobic) corresponds to what is recommended (1.4–2.0 $g \cdot kg^{-1} \cdot day^{-1}$). The protein content recommended for athletes is no more than 2.0 $g \cdot kg^{-1} \cdot day^{-1}$. However, according to our study, 29.2% of the athletes who develop anaerobic fitness consume 2.0–4.8 $g \cdot kg^{-1} \cdot day^{-1}$ protein, and 24.4% of the athletes training for aerobic fitness consume 2.0–3.9 $g \cdot kg^{-1} \cdot day^{-1}$ protein.

The consumption of phosphorus, potassium, magnesium and calcium by athletes exceed the recommended amounts. In contrast to aerobic athletes, anaerobic athletes consumed more phosphorus ($p = 0.014$), calcium ($p = 0.022$), and magnesium ($p = 0.012$). In terms of RDI, the anaerobic athletes consumed more phosphorus, calcium and magnesium by 2.9, 1.2 and 1.5 times respectively. Meanwhile, the amounts of phosphorus, calcium and magnesium in the diets of aerobic athletes exceeded RDI by 2.6, 1.4 and 1.4 times, respectively. Regardless of the sport, the amount of potassium consumed by the athletes was 1.5 times higher than RDI. In addition, the dietary amounts of calcium and phosphorus were unbalanced. This was confirmed by the calcium to phosphorus ratio (Ca/P) (0.6 ± 0.2) which was below the recommended 0.75 and resulted from the excessive dietary intake of phosphorus (Table 3).

Table 3. Dietary intake of athletes.

Nutrition Profile	Anaerobic Sports [1]	Aerobic Sports [2]	t-Test[1/2]	
	Mean ± SD		t	p
DEE (kcal·day^{-1})	3894 ± 876	3595 ± 864	3.032	0.003
EI (kcal·day^{-1})	3457 ± 1280	3266 ± 1020	1.486	0.138
EI (kcal·kg^{-1}·day^{-1})	47 ± 16	47 ± 15	−0.230	0.818
CHO (g·kg^{-1}·day^{-1})	5.4 ± 2.0	5.5 ± 2.2	−0.268	0.789
CHO (%)	46.5 ± 7.3	46.3 ± 8.9	0.206	0.837
PRO (g·kg^{-1}·day^{-1})	1.7 ± 0.6	1.7 ± 0.6	0.084	0.933
FAT (%)	38.9 ± 7.1	39.1 ± 8.2	−0.270	0.788
K (mg·day^{-1})	5189.7 ± 2341.8	4790.6 ± 1984.5	1.647	0.100
Ca (mg·day^{-1})	1254.0 ± 580.2	1113.9 ± 501.9	2.310	0.022
Mg (mg·day^{-1})	522.7 ± 240.7	461.6 ± 191.0	2.534	0.012
P (mg·day^{-1})	1999.0 ± 788.1	1806.9 ± 600.1	2.483	0.014
Ca/P ratio	0.6 ± 0.2	0.6 ± 0.2	0.680	0.497
PRAL (mEq·day^{-1})	10.7 ± 42.1	9.3 ± 35.9	0.305	0.761
NEAP (mEq·day^{-1})	56.9 ± 43.3	53.7 ± 37.1	0.725	0.469

The values are expressed as mean ± SD; EI—energy intake; DEE—daily energy expenditure; BW—body weight; PRO—protein; CHO—carbohydrate; FAT—fat; Ca—calcium; P—phosphorus; Mg—magnesium; K—potassium; PRAL—potential renal acid load; NEAP—net endogenous acid production. Significant differences set by independent samples Student's t-test between groups: [1]—group 1, [2]—group 2.

3.3. Eating Habits and the PRAL

Lithuanian high-performance athletes rarely consume foods that should be found in their diets every day. The study revealed that 49.8% of athletes consumed bakery products, 29.6%—cereals, 43.7%—fresh vegetables, 43.7%—fresh fruits, and 36.8%—dairy products four to seven days a week. Dried fruits and boiled potatoes are consumed less frequently—25.9% and 40.1% of the athletes consumed dried fruit and boiled potatoes 2 days a week, 12.1% and 37.6% from 2 to 7 days a week, respectively.

In terms of the frequency of consumption of protein found in meat and fish products, 41.3% of the athletes chose poultry 2–4 days a week, while eggs (53.6%), beef (46.2%), pork (49%), fish (44.9%) and meat preparations (42.1%) were consumed less frequently, from 1 to 2 days a week.

The eating habits of athletes are likely to determine the potential renal acid load (PRAL) of their diets. After evaluating PRAL of athletes' diets, it was found that more than half (65.9%) of the examined diets had a positive PRAL. PRAL (10.7 ± 42.1 mEq·day^{-1}) of the diets of anaerobic athletes did not differ from PRAL (9.3 ± 35.9 mEq·day^{-1}) of aerobic athletes and was also positive (PRAL > 0 mEq·day^{-1}) ($p = 0.761$) (Table 3).

A stepwise multivariate logistic regression method was used to determine which eating habits of athletes determine the PRAL of their diets. Table 4 presents the OR estimating the association between the different food intakes by athletes and the dietary acid load among the participants who were identified with dietary PRAL ≤ 0 mEq·day^{-1}. The final built logit model was tested with the Hosmer and Lemeshow goodness-of-fit test statistic (Nagelkerke $R^2 = 0.28$; H-L stat $\chi^2 = 14.5$, $p < 0.006$). As indicated in Table 4, the probability of PRAL in the diets of athletes increased 1.4 times (OR 1.4) to become ≤ 0 mEq·day^{-1}, when dairy products ($p = 0.05$), fresh vegetables ($p = 0.048$) and dried fruits ($p = 0.046$) were consumed more frequently. Specifically, milk and fresh vegetables were consumed more frequently by athletes in PRAL ≤ 0 group (47.7% and 52.3%, respectively) 4–7 days per week compared to athletes in PRAL > 0 group (31.1% and 39.1%, respectively). Similarly, more athletes (47.8%) with PRAL ≤ 0 consumed dried fruit more frequently (2–7 days a week) compared to the group of PRAL > 0 athletes (32.9%). In contrast, PRAL of the athletes who consumed more grain products was higher than 0 mEq·day^{-1} (OR 0.7, $p = 0.050$). Specifically, the athletes in PRAL > 0 group (71.4%) consumed grain products more frequently (2–7 days a week) compared to athletes in PRAL ≤ 0 group (62.6%).

Table 4. Effects of athletes' eating habits on their dietary PRAL.

PRAL ≤ 0 (mEq · day^{-1})[a]	β	SE	W	p	Exp (β) (95% CI)
Grain products	−0.3	0.2	3.5	0.050	0.7 (0.5; 1,1)
Dairy products	0.3	0.2	3.7	0.050	1.4 (1.0; 2.0)
Fresh vegetables	0.3	0.2	3.3	0.048	1.4 (1.0; 2.0)
Dried fruits	0.3	0.2	3.6	0.046	1.4 (1.0; 2.0)
Constant	−2.2	0.8	7.6	0.006	0

[a]—reference category is PRAL > 0 mEq·day^{-1}; β—is the estimated coefficient, with standard error SE (<5); W is the Wald test statistic; Nagelkerke $R^2 = 0.28$; Exp (β) is the predicted change in odds for a unit increase in the predictor (odds ratio (OR)); CI—confidence interval. The final model was tested with the Hosmer and Lemeshow goodness-of-fit test statistic (H-L stat $\chi^2 = 14.5$, $p < 0.006$).

3.4. Acid-Base Balance and Diets

Aiming to determine whether the chemical composition of the athlete diets was suitable for maintaining the body's acid-base balance, the study assessed the effect of nutrition on the body's net endogenous acid production (NEAP). It is important for athletes that NEAP did not exceed 100 mEq·day^{-1} for a longer period of time.

Although, according to our study, the average NEAP in anaerobic athletes (56.9 ± 43.3 mEq·day^{-1}) did not differ from NEAP observed in aerobic athletes (53.7 ± 37.1 mEq·day^{-1}) ($p = 0.469$), in 10.2% of Lithuanian high-performance athletes NEAP is higher than 100 mEq·day^{-1} and on average amounts to 126.1 ± 32.7 mEq·day^{-1}.

After using a multivariate linear regression method, we found that with a 95% confidence level of the consumption of larger amounts of protein, phosphorus, and carbohydrates, NEAP increases from 34.1 to 167.2 mEq·day^{-1} ($p < 0.001$). Meanwhile, with the increased consumption of potassium, calcium, and magnesium with food, NEAP decreases from −9.1 to −100.4 mEq·day^{-1} ($p < 0.05$) (Table 5).

Table 5. Effects of carbohydrates, proteins, phosphorous, potassium, calcium, magnesium consumed by athletes on their net endogenous acid production (NEAP).

NEAP (mEq · day^{-1})	β	95% CI	p
PRO (g·kg^{-1}·day^{-1}) (ln)	34.1	(23.0; 45,1)	<0.001
CHO (g·kg^{-1}·day^{-1}) (ln)	21,5	(11.0; 31.8)	<0.001
P (mg·day^{-1}) (ln)	167.2	(152.4; 181.9)	<0.001
K (mg·day^{-1}) (ln)	−100.4	(−108.3; −92.6)	<0.001
Ca (mg·day^{-1}) (ln)	−39.2	(−45.6; −32.8)	<0.001
Mg (mg·day^{-1}) (ln)	−9.1	(−17.9; −0.2)	0.044
EI (kcal·kg^{-1}·day^{-1}) (ln)	−69.2	(−85.6; −52.8)	<0.001

The influence of dietary intake on NEAP (mEq·day^{-1}) is estimated controlling for athlete sport and gender (adjusted for sports type and gender). $F (9, 313) = 201.2$, $p < 0.0001$, $R^2 = 0.85$. PRO—protein; CHO—carbohydrate; Ca—calcium; P—phosphorus; Mg—magnesium; K—potassium; EI—energy intake; CI—confidence interval.

A more detailed analysis of the results showed that the daily protein intake (2.6 ± 0.8 and 2.4 ± 0.7 g·kg^{-1}·day^{-1}) of anaerobic and aerobic athletes with NEAP > 100 mEq·day^{-1} exceeds the maximum recommended amounts by 1.3 times, and phosphorus content (2907.3 ± 892.2 and 2402.7 ± 516.3 mg·day-1)—by 4.1–3.4 times.

The correlation analysis also confirmed a moderate relationship between the protein intake and NEAP in the group of anaerobic athletes ($r = 0.482$, $p < 0.001$) and a weak relationship in the group of aerobic athletes ($r = 0.274$, $p < 0.001$) (Figures 2 and 3).

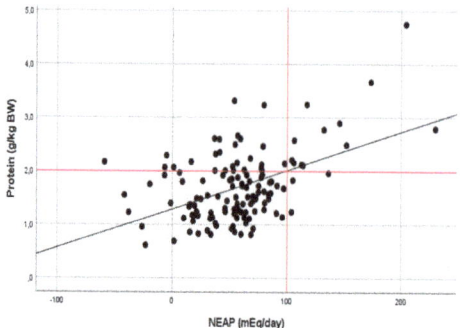

Figure 2. Relationship between the dietary protein intake (g·kg^{-1}·day^{-1}) and NEAP (mEq·day^{-1}) in athletes of anaerobic sports (r = 0.482, $p < 0.001$).

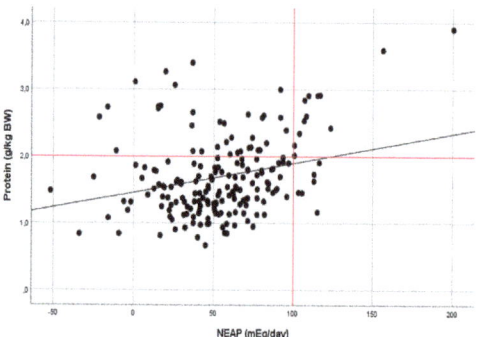

Figure 3. Relationship between the dietary protein intake (g·kg^{-1}·day^{-1}) and NEAP (mEq·day^{-1}) in athletes of aerobic sports (r = 0.274, $p < 0.001$).

The consumption of more protein foods, lower dietary PRAL and lower NEAP can be achieved by consuming sufficient amounts of the minerals—potassium, calcium and magnesium. According to the study, the consumption of potassium (4834.8 ± 1642.3 mg·day^{-1}), calcium (1375.1 ± 562.3 mg·day^{-1}) and magnesium (525.8 ± 150.8 mg·day^{-1}) in athletes with NEAP > 100 mEq·day^{-1} did not significantly differ ($p > 0.05$) from those found in athletes with NEAP < 100 mEq·day^{-1}, and exceeded RDI by 1.4, 1.5, and 1.5 times, respectively.

3.5. The Effect of Acid-Base Balance on the Muscle Mass and Body Mineral Content of Athletes

As indicated in Table 6, after applying the method of linear multivariate regression, it was found that the amount of muscle mass in athletes depended on the protein and phosphorus consumption, and the resulting NEAP in the body. At higher NEAP, the muscle mass (% of BW) was significantly lower by 1.2% ($p < 0.001$). However, only the excess phosphorus intake was associated with lower muscle mass (β −10.2% of BW, $p < 0.001$). Meanwhile, the athletes taking an increased amount of protein are characterized by an increase of 12.6% in the muscle mass of BW ($p < 0.001$).

Table 6. Effects of athletes' NEAP, protein and phosphorus consumption on their muscle mass (% of BW).

Muscle Mass (% of BW)	β	95% CI	p
NEAP (mEq·day^{-1}) (ln)	−1.2	(−1.8; −0.7)	<0.001
PRO (g·kg^{-1}·day^{-1}) (ln)	12.6	(10.8; 14.5)	<0.001
P (mg·day^{-1}) (ln)	−10.2	(−12.1; −8.2)	<0.001

Muscle mass (% of body weight) is estimated controlling for athlete sport and gender (adjusted for sports type and gender). $F_{(5, 295)} = 78.1$, $p < 0.0001$, $R^2 = 0.56$. BW—body weight; NEAP—net endogenous acid production; PRO—protein; P—phosphorus; CI—confidence interval.

The analysis of NEAP and the impact made on NEAP by nutrient components as well as their influence on the body mineral content (in bones and electrolytes) revealed no effects of NEAP (β −0.01%, $p = 0.073$). The results of our study showed that the body mineral content (% of BW) of athletes was increasing with higher protein (β 0.15%, $p < 0.001$) and calcium (β 0.06%, $p = 0.04$) consumption. Meanwhile, with higher amounts of phosphorus intake, lower amounts of body mineral content were observed (β −0.16%, $p < 0.001$) (Table 7).

Table 7. Effects of athletes' NEAP, protein, phosphorus, and calcium consumption on their body mineral content (% of BW).

Body Mineral (% of BW) [1]	β	95% CI	p
NEAP (mEq·day^{-1}) (ln)	−0.01	(−0.03; −0.001)	0.073
PRO (g·kg^{-1}·day^{-1}) (ln)	0.15	(0.10; 0.19)	<0.001
P (mg·day^{-1}) (ln)	−0.16	(−0.23; −0.09)	<0.001
Ca (mg·day^{-1}) (ln)	0.06	(0.02; 0.09)	0.004

Body mineral content (% of body weight) is estimated controlling for athlete sport and gender (adjusted for sports type and gender). $F_{(6, 294)} = 12.6$, $p < 0.0001$, $R^2 = 0.20$. NEAP—net endogenous acid production; PRO—protein; P—phosphorus; Ca—calcium; CI—confidence interval. [1]—minerals in bones and electrolytes.

4. Discussion

Daily high-intensity exercise causes stress to the body's buffer systems. Even moderate-intensity exercise causes metabolic changes that affect the acid-base balance in skeletal muscles and other tissues. Intense exercise can lower blood pH from 7.4 to 6.9 in 1 min leading to very rapid muscle fatigue [1,3,4]. Another factor influencing the acid-base balance in the body is diet [13] which can lead to low-grade metabolic acidosis (MA) (arterial blood pH is close to 7.35) [63]. Low-grade MA is typical when NEAP reaches about 50 mEq·day^{-1}. In other countries, Remer et al. [64] and Lemann [65] found that NEAP for young people was 40.1–50 mEq·day^{-1}. Similar data were obtained in our study. The average NEAP for anaerobic athletes was 56.9 mEq·day^{-1}, and that for aerobic athletes—53.7 mEq·day^{-1}. However, as many as 10.2% of Lithuanian high-performance athletes had NEAP higher than 100 mEq·day^{-1} which averaged to 126.1 ± 32.7 mEq·day^{-1}. Long-term NEAPs of 100–120 mEq·day^{-1} or more results in kidney overload with acid and thus a decreased availability of bicarbonates in the blood [66].

The research suggests that a high-protein, low-carbohydrate diet can lead to low-grade MA, high NEAP and have an adverse effect on physical performance [38–40]. We have obtained conflicting results confirming that athletes' NEAP was driven by higher protein (β 34.1 mEq·day^{-1}) and carbohydrate (β 21.5 mEq·day^{-1}) intake. According to our study, the more frequent consumption of grain products by athletes acidified their dietary PRAL (OR 0.7). PRAL of concentrated carbohydrate grain products are positive due to their amino acids (PRAL 4.5–8.0) which determined the acid load [61]. Meanwhile, the impact of carbohydrate-containing products on higher NEAP, as identified by scientists, was based only on the consumption of fruit and vegetables [67]. Nonetheless, carbohydrate intake (5.5 g·kg^{-1}·day^{-1}) among the athletes that we studied was relatively low for meeting the daily energy needs of 3600–3900 kcal having a 175-min workout [57]. The consumption of grain products, vegetables, fresh and dried fruits by the Lithuanian athletes is too low and infrequent. This can lead to insufficient levels of glycogen stores in the liver and muscles between sports practice sessions, an increased risk of overtraining, and a weakened immune system [68].

It should be emphasized that 25–30% of Lithuanian high-performance athletes consume 2.0–4.8 g·kg^{-1}·day^{-1} proteins per day, which exceeds the recommendations. There is still a debate as to whether an increased long-term protein intake among physically inactive, incapacitated people can impair their kidney function [69,70]. According to some studies, a long-term acidogenic diet combined with physical exertion results in the initial impairment of the renal function. The glomerular filtration rate has been shown to decrease with the diet of moderate PRAL for 12 weeks in physically active men and women [71]. Other data suggest that a long-term use of 2.5 to 3.5 g·kg^{-1}·day^{-1} protein did not impair the renal and hepatic functions in weightlifters [72–75].

Scientific studies have shown that low-grade MA caused by an excessive protein and phosphorus intake increases cortisol secretion (hypercortisolism), proteolysis and inhibits protein synthesis [76–78]. The rate of anabolism of muscle proteins is inversely proportional to the amount of acids present [79]. The results of our study confirmed that at higher NEAP, athletes had a significantly lower muscle mass, by 1.2% of BW. It is noteworthy that at low-grade MA, more muscle protein is broken down in order to neutralize dietary acids [80]. After the breakdown of muscle proteins, part of the amino acids released into the plasma is used for glutamine synthesis in the liver. Glutamine is further metabolised and degraded in the proximal renal tubules to alpha-ketoglutarate (AKG^{2-}) and ammonium. AKG^{2-} metabolism to glucose (or O$_2$ and CO$_2$) consumes two H$^+$ ions, which reduces the acid load. As a consequence, the use of amino acids for glutamine synthesis may result in a lack of amino acids for the synthesis of new proteins in the muscles and a decrease in muscle mass [80]. According to the data in our study, a higher protein intake leads to a higher muscle mass (β 12.6% of BW), has no association with muscle loss and is sufficient to ensure a positive nitrogen balance in athletes' bodies. Higher protein intakes for athletes are essential to promote muscle hypertrophy during the workout process [81].

Theoretically, protein and phosphorus in diets may lead to an increased acid load and increased calcium excretion, which may increase the risk of osteoporosis [42]. We have not determined the effect of NEAP on the body mineral content of our subjects (β −0.01% of BW). In contrast, higher amounts of body minerals (in bones and electrolyte) depend on higher protein and calcium intakes (β 0.15 and 0.06 % of BW, respectively) and lower phosphorus consumption (β −0.16% of BW). Our results are consistent with the data obtained from other researchers suggesting that a high protein intake increases the intestinal calcium absorption, insulin-like growth factor-1 (IGF-1) concentration in the blood, and lowers parathyroid hormone levels. In this way, protein compensates for the negative protein-induced acid load on urinary calcium excretion [82]. To prevent osteoporosis, with an increased protein intake (2.0 g·kg^{-1}·day^{-1}), higher amounts (>600 mg·day^{-1}) of calcium are recommended [83]. Also, similar data from epidemiological studies suggest that high levels of phosphorus do not have adverse effects on bone metabolism when an adequate calcium quantity is consumed [84]. An adequate (1170.2 ± 538.3 mg·day^{-1}) calcium intake is confirmed by the actual nutrition results of the athletes that we have studied. However, calcium and phosphorus in the diets of athletes are unbalanced (Ca/P 0.6; should be 0.75) due to an excessive phosphorus intake. Therefore, Lithuanian athletes are recommended to increase the calcium intake to 1500 mg·day^{-1} as recommended by the International Olympic Committee (IOC) [85], and to consume milk and dairy products more frequently.

The research has shown that the dietary intake to reduce NEAP requires adequate potassium and magnesium intakes with fruits and vegetables. Switching from a moderate-protein (1.3 g·kg^{-1}·day^{-1}) diet to a high-protein (2.1 g·kg^{-1}·day^{-1}) diet with a low intake of vegetables and fruits has been shown to significantly reduce blood pH and HCO^{3-} concentration. Therefore, high-performance athletes who are advised to consume increased protein (1.4–2.0 g·kg^{-1}·day^{-1}) amounts are also advised to consume sufficient amounts of fresh vegetables and fruits (at least 400 g) [81]. In our study, lower potassium and magnesium intakes resulted in higher NEAP (β −100.4 and −39.2 mEq·day^{-1}, respectively). On the other hand, our study showed that the athletes with high NEAP consumed the amount of potassium higher than RDI by 1.4 times. This suggests that potassium RDI in athletes is too low to ensure the neutral dietary PRAL. In addition, no tolerable upper intake level (UL) has been established [86,87]. In this regard, potassium levels recommended for athletes may be 2–3 times higher than RDI.

Thus, the eating habits of the athletes we have studied and those of the population of other countries are characterized by a high consumption of protein foods of animal origin, which is associated with low-grade MA [14]. In this case, MA can be normalized by changing the eating habits (ensuring low PRAL) [88] or by taking dietary supplements [89]. However, there are no scientific studies demonstrating the benefits of a short-term (4–9 days) vegetarian low-protein diet for aerobic physical working capacity. No change was observed in recording the increased respiratory exchange ratio (RER) in athletes due to an increase in "non-metabolic" CO_2 during submaximal exercise [90]. Studies justifying the effects of low PRAL diets on RER relate only to long-term eating habits with a high intake of vegetables and fruits [1,91]. Additionally, studies have shown that high doses of sodium bicarbonate (150 mEq·day^{-1}) neutralize food acids and minimize the total excretion of acids caused by ammonium. [14]. Thus, in exceptional cases, to increase the capacity of the buffer system while performing repeated bouts of exercise for 0.5–7 min, Lithuanian high-performance athletes are recommended to use sodium bicarbonate in doses of 0.30 g·kg^{-1}·day^{-1} 120–150 min before workouts [92]. To reduce intracellular acidification during 1–4 min repeated bout physical exercise, athletes are recommended to enrich their diets with beta-alanine supplements (65 mg·kg^{-1}·day^{-1}) for 10–12 weeks [92,93]. On the other hand, food supplements with buffering characteristics cannot replace conventional foods that lower PRAL.

In summary, while athletes may require a higher protein intake, high-protein diets can promote metabolic changes due to the production of additional acids in the body and lead to very rapid muscle fatigue during exercise. Dietary acid-base balance is also important for variables such as skeletal muscle protein metabolism and bone mineralisation. According to our study results, an excessive production of endogenous acids in the body in athletes is associated with lower muscle mass and has no effect on the amount of minerals in the body. It is clear then that the interaction between the dietary acid-base balance and exercise in athletes needs to be further studied in order to better and more accurately assess the contribution of alkaline diet in athletic performance and the variables like the rate of protein synthesis and the breakdown and bone density. Therefore, further research is needed to assess the impact of higher fruit and vegetable consumption by athletes on the indicators of their physical performance between workouts.

Actual nutrition data combined with objective readings of body composition of athletes allow us to predict and implement targeted measures and recommendations for optimising the athlete nutrition for the next Olympic cycle. The data and recommendations of our study can be applied in practice by including them in the current sports training programmes like Tokyo 2020 and Beijing 2022. In the future, continuous investigation and monitoring of body composition and actual nutrition should be carried out during each 4-year Olympic cycle.

However, in the course of our study, we did not include selection criteria such as comorbidities, because professional athletes in Lithuania do not have long-term health-related clinical symptoms or their combinations and they are completely healthy. The athletes' health monitoring is carried out every three months at the Lithuanian Sports Medicine Center. The health professionals ensure good health indicators of athletes in Lithuania. If serious health problems are identified during the monitoring process, the athlete is officially prohibited from exercising and participating in any level of competition. Therefore, the limitations of our study are related to the fact that while conducting our study we did not add the inclusion and exclusion criteria of this study such as the economic status, health indicators of the athletes (e.g., exercise-related injuries, iron deficiency anaemia, short-term renal impairments due to rapid bodyweight reduction among wrestlers and/or boxers). These variables may have associations with the actual diet or eating habits of athletes and these are the directions for further research. Another limitation of our study is that it was only a 24-h dietary recall survey of actual nutrition during the pre-competition period. Thus, in the future, in cooperation with the Lithuanian Sports Medicine Center

(LSMC), it is necessary to monitor the actual nutrition and other health indicators of high-performance athletes for a period of three to seven days during the preparatory and competition periods.

5. Conclusions

Regardless of the type of sport, the diets of Lithuanian high-performance athletes do not meet requirements. The diets of athletes are too high in fat. Even 25–30% of athletes practice high protein (2.0–4.8 g·kg^{-1}·day^{-1}) diets which result in dietary acid-base imbalance as well as excessive production of endogenous acids in the body. Higher NEAP in athletes is associated with lower muscle mass and has no effect on the body mineral content.

The training of athletes in different sports needs to be very individualised in terms of mesocycling of sports goals, including changes in the body composition, giving priority to the formation of eating habits. The eating habits of athletes need to be changed and carefully planned in practice to ensure acid-alkaline balance in the body by consuming alkaline-producing foods. In order to ensure the optimal dietary acid-base balance and to maximize muscle adaptation to exercise, athletes are recommended to consume higher amounts of potassium and magnesium found in fresh vegetables and dried fruits—twice as much as RDI. A more frequent consumption of milk and dairy products is recommended in order to increase calcium intake to 1500 mg per day. In exceptional cases, the diets of athletes should be enriched with bicarbonate and/or beta-alanine supplements.

Author Contributions: Conceptualization, M.B. and V.J.; methodology, M.B. and L.S.; data curation, M.B., L.S., V.J. and J.A.A.; software, M.B. and R.S.; investigation, M.B. and V.J.; writing—original draft preparation, M.B., R.S., J.A.A. and V.J.; writing—review and editing, all authors. All authors have read and agreed to the published version of the manuscript.

Funding: This research received no external funding.

Acknowledgments: We hereby express our acknowledgement to the Lithuanian Sports Centre and the Lithuanian Sports Medicine Centre for their assistance in performing the athlete body composition and nutritional survey.

Conflicts of Interest: The authors declare no conflict of interest. The funders played no role in the design of the study, or the collection, analyses, interpretation of the data; in the writing of the manuscript; or in the decision to publish the results.

References

1. Robergs, R.A.; Ghiasvand, F.F.; Parker, D. Biochemistry of exercise-induced metabolic acidosis. *Am. J. Physiol. Regul. Integr. Comp. Physiol.* **2004**, *287*, R502–R516. [CrossRef]
2. Lindinger, M.I. Origins of [H$^+$] changes in exercising skeletal muscle. *Can. J. Appl. Physiol.* **1995**, *20*, 357–368. [CrossRef]
3. Vilmi, N.; Äyrämö, S.; Nummela, A.; Pullinen, T.; Linnamo, V.; Häkkinen, K.; Mero, A. Oxygen uptake, acid-base balance and anaerobic energy system contribution in maximal 300–400 m running in child, adolescent and adult athletes. *J. Athl. Enhanc.* **2016**, *5*, 3. [CrossRef]
4. Hanon, C.; Lepretre, P.M.; Bishop, D.; Thomas, C. Oxygen uptake and blood metabolic responses to a 400 m run. *Eur. J. Appl. Physiol.* **2010**, *109*, 233–240. [CrossRef]
5. Lancha Junior, A.H.; de Salles Painelli, V.; Saunders, B.; Artioli, G.G. Nutritional strategies to modulate intracellular and extracellular buffering capacity during high-intensity exercise. *Sports Med.* **2015**, *45*, 71–81. [CrossRef]
6. Hollidge-Horvat, M.G.; Parolin, M.L.; Wong, D.; Jones, N.L.; Heigenhauser, G.J.F. Effect of induced metabolic alkalosis on human skeletal muscle metabolism during exercise. *Am. J. Physiol. Endocrinol. Metab.* **2000**, *278*, E316–E329. [CrossRef]
7. Jubrias, S.A.; Crowther, G.J.; Shankland, E.G.; Gronka, R.K.; Conley, K.E. Acidosis inhibits oxidative phosphorylation in contracting human skeletal muscle in vivo. *J. Physiol.* **2003**, *553*, 589–599. [CrossRef]
8. Street, D.; Nielsen, J.; Bangsbo, J.; Juel, C. Metabolic alkalosis reduces exercise-induced acidosis and potassium accumulation in human skeletal muscle interstitium. *J. Physiol.* **2005**, *566*, 481–489. [CrossRef]
9. McNaughton, L.R.; Siegler, J.; Midgley, A. Ergogenic effects of sodium bicarbonate. *Curr. Sports Med. Rep.* **2008**, *7*, 230–236. [CrossRef]

10. Mero, A.A.; Keskinen, K.L.; Malvela, M.T.; Sallinen, J.M. Combined creatine and sodium bicarbonate supplementation enhances interval swimming. *J. Strength Cond. Res.* **2004**, *18*, 306–310.
11. Wilkes, D.; Gledhill, N.; Smyth, R. Effect of acute induced metabolic alkalosis on 800-m racing time. *Med. Sci. Sport. Exerc.* **1983**, *15*, 277–280. [CrossRef]
12. Ööpik, V.; Saaremets, I.; Medijainen, L.; Karelson, K.; Janson, T.; Timpmann, S. Effects of sodium citrate ingestion before exercise on endurance performance in well trained college runners. *Br. J. Sport Med.* **2003**, *37*, 485–489. [CrossRef]
13. Remer, T. Influence of nutrition on acid–base balance—Metabolic aspects. *Eur. J. Nutr.* **2001**, *40*, 214–220. [CrossRef]
14. Sebastian, A.; Frassetto, L.A.; Sellmeyer, D.E.; Merriam, R.L.; Morris, R.C., Jr. Estimation of the net acid load of the diet of ancestral preagricultural *Homo sapiens* and their hominid ancestors. *Am. J. Clin. Nutr.* **2002**, *76*, 1308–1316. [CrossRef]
15. Zapolska, J.; Witczak, K.; Manczuk, A.; Ostrowska, L. Assessment of nutrition, supplementation and body composition parameters on the example of professional volleyball players. *Rocz. Panstw. Zakl. Hig.* **2014**, *65*, 235–242.
16. Pilis, K.; Michalski, C.; Zych, M.; Pilis, A.; Jelonek, J.; Kaczmarzyk, A.; Pilis, W. A Nutritional Evaluation of Dietary Behaviour in Various Professional Sports. *Rocz. Panstw. Zakl. Hig.* **2014**, *65*, 227–234.
17. Daneshvar, P.; Hariri, M.; Ghiasvand, R.; Askari, G.; Darvishi, L.; Iraj, B.; Mashhadi, N.S. Dietary behaviours and nutritional assessment of young male isfahani wrestlers. *Int. J. Prev. Med.* **2013**, *4*, S48–S52.
18. Ghloum, K.; Hajji, S. Comparison of diet consumption, body composition and lipoprotein lipid values of Kuwaiti fencing players with international norms. *J. Int. Soc. Sports Nutr.* **2011**, *8*, 13. [CrossRef]
19. Tooley, E.; Bitcon, M.; Briggs, M.A.; West, D.J.; Russell, M. Estimates of energy intake and expenditure in professional rugby league players. *Int. J. Sports Sci. Coach.* **2015**, *10*, 551–560. [CrossRef]
20. Martin, L.; Lambeth, A.; Scott, D. Nutritional practices of National female soccer players: Analysis and recommendations. *J. Sports Sci. Med.* **2006**, *5*, 130–137.
21. Cabral Costa, C.A.; Paixao Rosado, G.; Osorio Silva, C.H.; Bouzas Marins, J.C. Diagnosis of the nutritional status of the weight lifting permanent Olympic team of the Brazilian Olympic Committee. *Rev. Braz. Sports Med.* **2006**, *12*, 308e–312e.
22. Farajian, P.; Kavouras, S.A.; Yannakoulia, M.; Sidossis, L.S. Dietary intake and nutritional practices of elite Greek aquatic athletes. *Int. J. Sport Nutr. Exerc. Metab.* **2004**, *14*, 574–585. [CrossRef] [PubMed]
23. Burke, L.M.; Slater, G.; Broad, E.M.; Haukka, J.; Modulon, S.; Hopkins, W.G. Eating patterns and meal frequency of elite Australian athletes. *Int. J. Sport Nutr. Exerc. Metab.* **2003**, *13*, 521–538. [CrossRef] [PubMed]
24. Andrews, M.C.; Itsiopoulos, C. Room for improvement in nutrition knowledge and dietary intake of male football (Soccer) players in Australia. *Int. J. Sport Nutr. Exerc. Metab.* **2016**, *26*, 55–64. [CrossRef] [PubMed]
25. Devlin, B.L.; Leveritt, M.D.; Kingsley, M.; Belski, R. Dietary intake, body composition, and nutrition knowledge of Australian football and soccer players: Implications for sports nutrition professionals in practice. *Int. J. Sport Nutr. Exerc. Metab.* **2017**, *27*, 130–138. [CrossRef]
26. Leblanc, J.C.H.; Gall, F.L.E.; Grandjean, V.; Verger, P.H. Nutritional intake of French soccer players at the clairefontaine training center. *Int. J. Sport. Nutr. Exerc. Metab.* **2002**, *12*, 268–280. [CrossRef]
27. Filaire, E.; Maso, F.; Degoutte, F.; Jouanel, P.; Lac, G. Food Restriction, performance, psychological state and lipid values in judo athletes. *Int. J. Spots Med.* **2001**, *22*, 454–459. [CrossRef]
28. Fogelholm, G.M.; Himberg, J.J.; Alopaeus, K.; Gref, C.G.; Laakso, J.T.; Lehto, J.J.; Mussalo-Rauhamaa, H. Dietary and biochemical indices of nutritional status in male athletes and controls. *J. Am. Coll. Nutr.* **1992**, *11*, 181–191.
29. Nutrition, Physical Activity and Bone Mineral Density of Hong Kong Elite Athletes. Available online: https://www.hksi.org.hk/f/publication/589/rh201203_1e.pdf (accessed on 16 July 2020).
30. Chen, J.D.; Wang, J.F.; Li, K.J.; Zhao, Y.W.; Wang, S.W.; Jiao, Y.; Hou, X.Y. Nutritional problems and measures in elite and amateur athletes. *Am. J. Clin. Nutr.* **1989**, *49*, 1084–1089. [CrossRef]
31. Barry, A.; Cantwell, T.; Doherty, F.; Folan, J.C.; Ingoldsby, M.; Kevany, J.P.; O'Broin, J.D.; O'Connor, H.; O'Shea, B.; Ryan, B.A.; et al. A Nutritional study of Irish Athletes. *Br. J. Sports Med.* **1981**, *15*, 99–109. [CrossRef]

32. Bettonviel, A.E.O.; Brinkmans, N.Y.J.; Russcher, K.; Wardenaar, F.C.; Witard, O.C. Nutritional status and daytime pattern of protein intake on match, post-match, rest and training days in senior professional and youth elite soccer players. *Int. J. Sport Nutr. Exerc. Metab.* **2016**, *26*, 285–293. [CrossRef] [PubMed]
33. Conejos, C.; Giner, A.; Mañes, J.; Soriano, J.M. Energy and nutritional intakes in training days of soccer players according to their playing positions. *Arch. Med. Deporte* **2011**, *28*, 29–35.
34. Gravina, L.; Ruiz, F.; Diaz, E.; Lekue, J.A.; Badiola, A.; Irazusta, J.; Gil, S.M. Influence of nutrient intake on antioxidant capacity, muscle damage and white blood cell count in female soccer players. *J. Int. Soc. Sports Nutr.* **2012**, *9*, 32. [CrossRef] [PubMed]
35. Kirwan, R.D.; Kordick, L.K.; McFarland, S.; Lancaster, D.; Clark, K.; Miles, M.P. Dietary, anthropometric, blood-lipid, and performance patterns of American college football players during 8 weeks of training. *Int. J. Sport Nutr. Exerc. Metab.* **2012**, *22*, 444–451. [CrossRef] [PubMed]
36. Potgieter, S.; Visser, J.; Croukamp, I.; Markides, M.; Nascimento, J.; Scott, K. Body composition and habitual and match-day dietary intake of the FNB Maties Varsity Cup rugby players. *S. Afr. J. Sports Med.* **2014**, *26*, 35–43. [CrossRef]
37. Vermeulen, T. Seven Day Dietary Intakes of Female Varsity Ice Hockey Players. Master's Thesis, The University of Guelph, Guelph, ON, Canada, 2017.
38. Maughan, R.J.; Greenhaff, P.L.; Leiper, J.B.; Ball, D.; Lambert, C.P.; Gleeson, M. Diet composition and the performance of high-intensity exercise. *J. Sport Sci.* **1997**, *15*, 265–275. [CrossRef]
39. Greenhaff, P.L.; Gleeson, M.; Maughan, R.J. The effects of dietary manipulation on blood acid–base status and the performance of high intensity exercise. *Eur. J. Appl. Physiol. Occup. Physiol.* **1987**, *56*, 331–337. [CrossRef]
40. Berardi, J.M.; Logan, A.C.; Rao, A.V. Plant based dietary supplement increases urinary pH. *J. Int. Soc. Sports Nutr.* **2008**, *5*, 20. Available online: http://www.jissn.com/content/5/1/20 (accessed on 15 April 2020). [CrossRef]
41. Remer, T. Influence of diet on acid-base balance. *Semin. Dial.* **2000**, *13*, 221–226. [CrossRef]
42. Passey, C. Reducing the Dietary Acid Load: How a More Alkaline Diet Benefits Patients with Chronic Kidney Disease. *J. Ren. Nutr.* **2017**, *27*, 151–160. [CrossRef]
43. Welch, A.A.; MacGregor, A.J.; Skinner, J.; Spector, T.D.; Moayyeri, A.; Cassidy, A. A higher alkaline dietary load is associated with greater indexes of skeletal muscle mass in women. *Osteoporos. Int.* **2013**, *24*, 1899–1908. [CrossRef] [PubMed]
44. Chan, R.; Leung, J.; Woo, J. Association between estimated net endogenous acid production and subsequent decline in muscle mass over four years in ambulatory older Chinese People in Hong Kong: A prospective cohort study. *J. Gerontol. Biol. Sci. Med. Sci.* **2015**, *70*, 905–911. [CrossRef] [PubMed]
45. Faure, A.M.; Fischer, K.; Dawson-Hughes, B.; Egli, A.; Bischoff-Ferrari, H.A. Gender-specific association between dietary acid load and total lean body mass and its dependency on protein intake in seniors. *Osteoporos Int.* **2017**, *28*, 3451–3462. [CrossRef] [PubMed]
46. De Jonge, E.A.L.; Koromani, F.; Hofman, A.; Uitterlinden, A.G.; Franco, O.H.; Rivadeneira, F.; Kiefte-de Jong, J.C. Dietary acid load, trabecular bone integrity, and mineral density in an ageing population: The Rotterdam study. *Osteoporos. Int.* **2017**, *28*, 2357–2365. [CrossRef] [PubMed]
47. Skernevičius, J.; Milašius, K.; Raslanas, A.; Dadelienė, R. Sporto treniruotė (*Fitness Training*). In *Sportininkų Gebėjimai ir jų Ugdymas (Athlete Skills and Training Them)*, 1st ed.; Čepulėnas, A., Saplinskas, J., Paulauskas, R., Eds.; Lithuanian University of Educational Sciences Press: Vilnius, Lithuania, 2011; pp. 165–217.
48. Lukaski, H.C.; Bolonchuk, W.W. (Eds.) *Theory and Validation of the Tetrapolar Bioelectrical Impedance Method to Assess Human Body Composition*; Institute of Physical Science and Medicine: London, UK, 1987.
49. Harris, J.; Benedict, F. *A Biometric Study of Basal Metabolism in Man*; Lippincott: Philadelphia, PA, USA, 1919.
50. American Dietetic Association; Dietitians of Canada; American College of Sports Medicine; Rodriguez, N.R.; Di Marco, N.M.; Langley, S. American College of Sports Medicine position stand, Nutrition and Athletic Performance. *Med. Sci. Sports Exerc.* **2009**, *41*, 709–731.
51. Ainsworth, B.E.; Haskell, W.L.; Herrmann, S.D.; Meckes, N.; Bassett, D.R.; Tudor-Locke, C., Jr.; Greer, J.L.; Vezina, J.; Whitt-Glover, M.C.; Leon, A.S. Compendium of physical activities: A second update of codes and MET values. *Med. Sci. Sports Exerc.* **2011**, *43*, 1575–1581. [CrossRef]

52. Deakin, V.; Kerr, D.; Boushey, C. Measuring nutritional status of athletes: Clinical and research perspectives. In *Clinical Sports Nutrition*, 5th ed.; Burke, L.M., Deakin, V., Eds.; McGraw-Hill: North Ryde, NSW, Australia, 2015; pp. 27–53.
53. Elmadfa, I.; Meyer, A.; Nowak, V.; Hasenegger, V.; Putz, P.; Verstraeten, R.; Remaut-DeWinter, A.M.; Kolsteren, P.; Dostalova, J.; Dlouhy, P.; et al. European Nutrition and Health Report 2009. *Forum Nutr.* **2009**, *62*, 1–405. [CrossRef]
54. Pomerleau, J.; McKee, M.; Robertson, A.; Vaasc, S.; Kadziauskiene, K.; Abaravicius, A.; Bartkeviciute, R.; Pudule, I.; Grinberga, D. Physical inactivity in the Baltic countries. *Prev. Med.* **2000**, *31*, 665–672. [CrossRef]
55. Barzda, A.; Bartkevičiūtė, R.; Viseckienė, V.; Abaravičius, A.J.; Stukas, R. *Maisto Produktų ir Patiekalų Porcijų Nuotraukų Atlasas (Atlas of Foodstuffs and Dishes)*; Republican Nutrition Center: Vilnius, Lithuania; Vilnius University Faculty of Medicine: Vilnius, Lithuania, 2007; pp. 7–42. Available online: http://www.smlpc.lt/media/file/Skyriu_info/Metodine_medziaga/Maisto%20prod%20atlasas%202007.pdf (accessed on 14 April 2020).
56. Sučilienė, S.; Abaravičius, A. *Maisto Produktų Sudėtis (Food Product Composition)*; Ministry of Health of the Republic of Lithuania: Vilnius, Lithuania, 2002; pp. 10–315.
57. Kerksick, C.M.; Wilborn, C.D.; Roberts, M.D.; Smith-Ryan, A.; Kleiner, S.M.; Jäger, R.; Collins, R.; Cooke, M.; Davis, J.N.; Galvan, E.; et al. ISSN exercise & sports nutrition review update: Research & recommendations. *J. Int. Soc. Sports Nutr.* **2018**, *15*, 8. [CrossRef]
58. Thomas, D.T.; Erdman, K.A.; Burke, L.M. American College of Sports Medicine Joint Position Statement. Nutrition and Athletic Performance. *Med. Sci. Sports Exerc.* **2016**, *48*, 543–568.
59. Ministry of Health of the Republic of Lithuania. *2016 June 23 order No. V-836 of Minister of Health of the Republic of Lithuania. Recommended Daily Intake for Energy and Nutrients*; Ministry of Health of the Republic of Lithuania: Vilnius, Lithuania, 2016. Available online: https://www.e-tar.lt/portal/lt/legalAct/4bd890f0428011e6a8ae9e1795984391 (accessed on 14 April 2020).
60. Baranauskas, M. Assessment of Actual Nutrition and Dietary Habits of Athletes during the 2008–2012 Olympic Period. Ph.D. Thesis, Faculty of Medicine of Vilnius University, Vilnus, Lithuania, 2012; pp. 229–233.
61. Remer, T.; Manz, F. Potential Renal Acid Load of Foods and its influence on Urine pH. *J. Am. Diet. Assoc.* **1995**, *95*, 791–797. [CrossRef]
62. Du Bois, D.; Du Bois, E.F. A formula to estimate the approximate surface area if height and weight be known. *Arch. Int. Med.* **1916**, *17*, 863–871. [CrossRef]
63. Carnauba, R.A.; Baptistella, A.B.; Paschoal, V.; Hübscher, G.H. Diet-induced low-grade metabolic acidosis and clinical outcomes: A review. *Nutrients* **2017**, *25*, 538. [CrossRef] [PubMed]
64. Remer, T.; Manz, F. Estimation of the renal net acid excretion by adults consuming diets containing variable amounts of protein. *Am. J. Clin. Nutr.* **1994**, *59*, 1356–1361. [CrossRef]
65. Lemann, J., Jr. Relationship between urinary calcium and net acid excretion as determined by dietary protein and potassium: A review. *Nephron* **1999**, *81*, 18–25. [CrossRef]
66. Remer, T.; Dimitriou, T.; Manz, F. Dietary potential renal acid load and renal net acid excretion in healthy, free-living children and adolescents. *Am. J. Clin. Nutr.* **2003**, *77*, 1255–1260. [CrossRef]
67. Osuna-Padilla, I.A.; Leal-Escobar, G.; Garza-García, C.A.; Rodríguez-Castellanos, F.E. Dietary Acid Load: Mechanisms and evidence of its health repercussions. *Nefrologia* **2019**, *39*, 343–354. [CrossRef]
68. Burke, L.M. Fuelling strategies to optimize performance: Training high or training low? *Scand. J. Med. Sci. Sports.* **2010**, *20*, 48–58. [CrossRef]
69. Knight, E.L.; Stampfer, M.J.; Hankinson, S.E.; Spiegelman, D.; Curhan, G.C. The impact of protein intake on renal function decline in women with normal renal function or mild renal insufficiency. *Ann. Int. Med.* **2003**, *138*, 460–467. [CrossRef]
70. Rhee, C.M.; You, A.S.; Parsons, T.K.; Tortorici, A.R.; Bross, R.; St-Jules, D.E.; Jing, J.; Lee, M.L.; Benner, D.; Kovesdy, C.P.; et al. Effect of high-protein meals during hemodialysis combined with lanthanum carbonate in hypoalbuminemic dialysis patients: Findings from the FrEDI randomized controlled trial. *Nephrol. Dial. Transplant.* **2017**, *1*, 1233–1243. [CrossRef]
71. Hietavala, E.M.; Stout, J.R.; Frassetto, L.A.; Puurtinen, R.; Pitkänen, H.; Selänne, H.; Suominen, H.; Mero, A.A. Dietary acid load and renal function have varying effects on blood acid-base status and exercise performance across age and sex. *Appl. Physiol. Nutr. Metab.* **2017**, *42*, 1330–1340. [CrossRef] [PubMed]

72. Antonio, J.; Ellerbroek, A.; Silver, T.; Orris, S.; Scheiner, M.; Gonzalez, A.; Peacock, C.A. A high protein diet (3.4 g/kg/d) combined with a heavy resistance training program improves body composition in healthy trained men and women–a follow-up investigation. *J. Int. Soc. Sports Nutr.* **2015**, *12*, 39. [CrossRef] [PubMed]
73. Antonio, J.; Ellerbroek, A.; Silver, T.; Vargas, L.; Peacock, C. The effects of a high protein diet on indices of health and body composition—A crossover trial inresistance-trained men. *J. Int. Soc. Sports Nutr.* **2016**, *13*, 3. [CrossRef] [PubMed]
74. Antonio, J.; Ellerbroek, A.; Silver, T.; Vargas, L.; Tamayo, A.; Buehn, R.; Peacock, C.A. A high protein diet has no harmful effects: A one-year crossover study in resistance-trained males. *J. Nutr. Metab.* **2016**, *2016*, 9104792. [CrossRef] [PubMed]
75. Antonio, J.; Peacock, C.A.; Ellerbroek, A.; Fromhoff, B.; Silver, T. The effects of consuming a high protein diet (4.4 g/kg/d) on body composition inresistance-trained individuals. *J. Int. Soc. Sports Nutr.* **2014**, *11*, 19. [CrossRef]
76. Williams, R.S.; Kozan, P.; Samocha-Bonet, D. The role of dietary acid load and mild metabolic acidosis in insulin resistance in humans. *Biochimie* **2016**, *124*, 171–177. [CrossRef] [PubMed]
77. Simmons, P.S.; Miles, J.M.; Gerich, J.E.; Haymond, M.W. Increased proteolysis: An effect of increases in plasma cortisol within the physiologic range. *J. Clin. Investig.* **1984**, *73*, 412–420. [CrossRef]
78. Caso, G.; Garlick, P.J. Control of muscle protein kinetics by acid–base balance. *Curr. Opin. Clin. Nutr. Metab. Care* **2005**, *8*, 73–76. [CrossRef]
79. Garibotto, G.; Russo, R.; Sofia, A.; Sala, M.R.; Robaudo, C.; Moscatelli, P.; Deferrari, G.; Tizianello, A. Skeletal muscle protein synthesis and degradation in patients with chronic renal failure. *Kidney Int.* **1994**, *45*, 1432–1439. [CrossRef]
80. Ballmer, P.E.; McNurlan, M.A.; Hulter, H.N.; Anderson, S.E.; Garlick, P.J.; Krapf, R. Chronic metabolic acidosis decreases albumin synthesis and induces negative nitrogen balance in humans. *J. Clin. Investig.* **1995**, *95*, 39–45. [CrossRef]
81. Jäger, R.; Kerksick, C.M.; Campbell, B.I.; Cribb, P.J.; Wells, S.D.; Skwiat, T.M.; Purpura, M.; Ziegenfuss, T.N.; Ferrando, A.A.; Arent, S.M.; et al. International Society of Sports Nutrition position stand: Protein and exercise. *J. Int. Soc. Sports Nutr.* **2017**, *14*, 20. [CrossRef] [PubMed]
82. Cao, J.J. High Dietary Protein Intake and Protein-Related Acid Load on Bone Health. *Curr. Osteoporos. Rep.* **2017**, *15*, 571–576. [CrossRef] [PubMed]
83. Bonjour, J.P. Protein intake and bone health. *Int. J. Vitam. Nutr. Res.* **2011**, *81*, 134–142. [CrossRef] [PubMed]
84. Lee, A.W.; Cho, S.S. Association between phosphorus intake and bone health in the NHANES population. *Nutr. J.* **2015**, *14*, 28. [CrossRef] [PubMed]
85. Mountjoy, M.; Sundgot-Borgen, J.; Burke, L.; Carter, S.; Constantini, N.; Lebrun, C.; Meyer, N.; Sherman, R.; Steffen, K.; Budgett, R.; et al. The IOC consensus statement: Beyond the Female Athlete Triad–Relative Energy Deficiency in Sport (RED-S). *Br. J. Sports Med.* **2014**, *48*, 491–497. [CrossRef]
86. Sebastian, A.; Frassetto, L.A.; Sellmeyer, D.E.; Morris, R.C. The evolution-informed optimal dietary potassium intake of human beings greatly exceeds current and recommended intakes. *Semin. Nephrol.* **2006**, *26*, 447–453. [CrossRef]
87. Institute of Medicine, Food and Nutrition Board. *Dietary Reference Intakes for Water, Potassium, Sodium, Chloride, and Sulfate*; The National Academies Press: Washington, DC, USA, 2005.
88. Pizzorno, J.; Frassetto, L.A.; Katzinger, J. Diet-induced acidosis: Is it real and clinically relevant? *Br. J. Nutr.* **2010**, *103*, 1185–1194. [CrossRef]
89. Derave, W.; Everaert, I.; Beeckman, S.; Baguet, A. Muscle carnosine metabolism and beta-alanine supplementation in relation to exercise and training. *Sports. Med.* **2010**, *40*, 247–263. [CrossRef]
90. Hietavala, E.M.; Puurtinen, R.; Kainulainen, H.; Mero, A.A. Low-protein vegetarian diet does not have a short-term effect on blood acid-base status but raises oxygen consumption during submaximal cycling. *J. Int. Soc. Sports Nutr.* **2012**, *26*, 50. [CrossRef]
91. Niekamp, K.; Zavorsky, G.S.; Fontana, L.; McDaniel, J.L.; Villareal, D.T.; Weiss, E.P. Systemic acid load from the diet affects maximal-exercise RER. *Med. Sci. Sports Exerc.* **2012**, *44*, 709–715. [CrossRef]

92. Maughan, R.J.; Burke, L.M.; Dvorak, J.; Larson-Meyer, D.E.; Peeling, P.; Phillips, S.M.; Rawson, E.S.; Walsh, N.P.; Garthe, I.; Geyer, H.; et al. IOC consensus statement: Dietary supplements and the high-performance athlete. *Br. J. Sports Med.* **2018**, *52*, 439–455. [CrossRef] [PubMed]
93. Trexler, E.T.; Smith-Ryan, A.E.; Stout, J.R.; Hoffman, J.R.; Wilborn, C.D.; Sale, C.; Kreider, R.B.; Jäger, R.; Earnest, C.P.; Bannock, L.; et al. International society of sports nutrition position stand: Beta-Alanine. *J. Int. Soc. Sports Nutr.* **2015**, *12*, 30. [CrossRef] [PubMed]

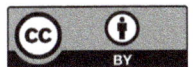

© 2020 by the authors. Licensee MDPI, Basel, Switzerland. This article is an open access article distributed under the terms and conditions of the Creative Commons Attribution (CC BY) license (http://creativecommons.org/licenses/by/4.0/).

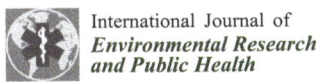

Article

Bone Mineral Reference Values for Athletes 11 to 20 Years of Age

Irina Kalabiska [1], Annamária Zsakai [2,*], Robert M. Malina [3] and Tamas Szabo [1]

[1] Research Center for Sport Physiology, University of Physical Education, Alkotas u. 44, 1123 Budapest, Hungary; kalabiskai@gmail.com (I.K.); szabo.tamas@tf.hu (T.S.)
[2] Department of Biological Anthropology, Eotvos Lorand University, Pazmany P. s. 1/c, 1117 Budapest, Hungary
[3] Department of Kinesiology and Health Education, University of Texas, Austin, TX 78712, USA; rmalina@1skyconnect.net
* Correspondence: zsakaia@elte.hu; Tel.: +36-20-355-7036

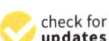

Received: 8 June 2020; Accepted: 6 July 2020; Published: 8 July 2020

Abstract: Objectives. Training for sport is associated with the development of bone minerals, and the need for reference data based on athletes is often indicated. The purpose of this study was to develop a reference for bone mineral density (BMD) and content (BMC) specific for youth athletes of both sexes participating in several sports. Methods DEXA (dual energy X-ray absorptiometry) was used for total body measurements of bone minerals in 1385 athletes 11 to 20 years, 1019 males and 366 females. The athletes were training in several sports at Hungarian academies. Reference values for total bone mineral density and bone mineral content, and also BMD excluding the head (total body less head, TBLH) were developed using the LMS chartmaker pro version 2.3. Results. The centile distributions for BMD and BMC of the athletes differed significantly from those of the age- and sex-specific references for the general population. The youth athletes had higher BMD and BMC than those of the reference for the general population. Conclusion. The potential utility of the DEXA reference for male and female youth athletes may assist in monitoring changes in the BMC and BMD associated with normal growth and maturation, and perhaps more importantly, may be useful in monitoring changes specific to different phases of sport-specific training protocols.

Keywords: DEXA; bone mineral; bone development; youth athletes

1. Introduction

Concern for bone health, specifically bone mineral density (BMD) and bone mineral content (BMC), is a major concern given age and gender variation [1,2]. In this context, reference data for a population are routinely used for screening purposes; as such, they are a reference for comparison [1,3,4]. Given changes in BMD and BMC during the course of growth and maturation, there is increased interest in the bone health of children and youth, especially in the context of beneficial effects of regular physical activity on BMC [5–7]. Evidence is also consistent in showing beneficial effects of systematic training for sport on BMC [8,9]. Mechanical loading associated with regular training has a significant influence on skeletal development and bone maintenance. Regular intensive exercise with considerable mechanical loading in athletes is associated with an increase in absolute and relative bone dimensions and structural parameters. In contrast, inadequate bone development per se and some practices associated with specific sports, e.g., extreme weight control measures and disordered eating, can negatively influence performance and can increase the risk for bone stress injuries. Understanding bone development in young athletes may inform training practices, leading to success in sport, facilitate the diagnosis of structural abnormalities in bone, and contribute to the prevention of skeletal injuries [10–12].

The bone health of athletes, specifically BMD and BMC status, is generally evaluated relative to reference data for the general population [13–15]. Such a reference may have limitations with athletes given the selectivity of sport in general, sport-specific training demands, and dietary pressures associated with specific sports [16,17]. Moreover, measures of BMD and BMC among athletes often fall outside normal ranges for the general population [18–20].

DEXA (dual energy X-ray absorptiometry) technology provides measures of total body bone area (cm^2), BMC (g), and BMD (g/cm^2) [21]. However, evaluation of BMC and BMD requires appropriate reference data that allow for chronological age, body size, pubertal status, ethnicity, and sex, and perhaps demands of specific sports [22–24]. The preferred indicator of BMD is the total body, excluding the head [25]. Evidence suggests that age, height, and weight were better predictors of total body BMD excluding the head (total body less head (TBLH) BMD) in contrast to total body BMD [26]. Use of the subtotal BMD result, excluding the head region, is preferred as the skull does not develop in a proportionally similar manner to body mass and to the weight of other organs in children and adolescents. In addition, the head constitutes a large portion of the total body bone mass but changes little with growth, activity, or disease. Thus, including the skull may mask gains or losses at other skeletal sites [21].

The purpose of this study was to develop reference values for BMC, BMD, and TBLH BMD based on DEXA in a sample of Hungarian youth athletes of both sexes.

2. Material and Methods

The project was approved by the Ethics Committee of the University of Physical Education in Budapest, Hungary. Parents of athletes <18 years and also the athletes were informed of the details of the project; both provided written informed consent. Details of the project were also given to older athletes who also provided informed written consent.

Participants were 1385 athletes, 1019 males and 366 females, 11–20 years of age, who volunteered to participate in this cross-sectional study. The athletes represented several Hungarian sport academies, primarily basketball, football, and handball with smaller numbers for ice hockey and several individual sports including pentathlon, rhythmic gymnastics, swimming, athletics, fencing, kayak, canoe, rowing, wrestling, karate, and weight-lifting. All of the participants in the study were considered elite and most began training at 6–7 years of age. The athletes trained daily for approximately two hours per day through most of the year and had at least one competition per week. The respective academies delegated the athletes for the body structural and DEXA examinations. Exclusion criteria for DEXA scans included the lack of written consent, body weight >130 kg, height >200 cm, pregnancy, non-removable objects (e.g., prostheses or implants) in the past one-half year, and inability of an athlete to attain correct position and/or to remain motionless during the scan.

The research was conducted between September 2015 and March 2019. Whole body bone mineral density (BMD), bone mineral content (BMC), and total body less head (TBLH BMD) were measured with a GE Lunar Prodigy dual-energy X-ray scanner. The scanner was located in the Research Center for Sport Physiology, University of Physical Education, Budapest, Hungary, and the first Author (IK) made the DEXA measurements. The data were processed with enCORE Version 16 software. The Lunar Prodigy reference data were based on an international sample of healthy children and adults from the general population in several regions of the world in the 1990s and early 2000s. The sample was free of people with chronic diseases affecting bone structure and development and those taking bone-altering medications. The enCORE software of the scanner permits comparison of a subject's results to a selected reference population considering ethnicity (Black, White, Asian, or Hispanic; White was chosen in the case of the Hungarian young athletes). The athletes were grouped into single year chronological age groups with the whole year as the midpoint, i.e., 11 years = 10.50 to 11.49,

12 years = 11.50 to 12.49, etc. Sample sizes and descriptive statistics for age, height, and weight of male and female athletes are summarized by age groups in Tables 1 and 2, respectively.

Table 1. Sample sizes and descriptive statistics (means (M) and standard deviations (SD)) for age, height, and weight of male athletes by age group.

Age Group (years)	Sample n	Age M	Age SD	Height M	Height SD	Weight M	Weight SD
11	25	11.56	0.28	157.62	6.28	43.19	6.23
12	28	12.63	0.26	166.89	9.05	50.75	12.72
13	63	13.55	0.28	173.04	10.57	57.65	11.55
14	98	14.57	0.30	177.09	8.86	63.98	10.67
15	200	15.50	0.27	180.08	8.79	69.12	11.94
16	237	16.48	0.29	181.87	9.19	71.27	9.48
17	174	17.49	0.28	184.74	9.65	76.65	11.09
18	123	18.43	0.29	182.27	8.21	76.52	12.19
19	42	19.53	0.32	180.76	7.39	76.13	6.50
20	29	20.34	0.27	177.40	6.00	78.91	11.95

Table 2. Sample sizes and descriptive statistics (means (M) and standard deviations (SD)) for age, height, and weight of female athletes by age group.

Age Group (years)	Sample n	Age M	Age SD	Height M	Height SD	Weight M	Weight SD
13	25	13.60	0.23	168.24	8.86	57.27	10.32
14	79	14.51	0.24	171.47	7.06	63.76	9.36
15	86	15.55	0.30	173.46	7.26	67.11	11.36
16	49	16.54	0.30	172.70	7.08	65.35	8.96
17	63	17.37	0.32	173.00	7.01	66.98	12.78
18	27	18.52	0.32	174.46	8.14	66.10	7.31
19	27	19.43	0.24	174.16	6.69	70.14	9.64
20	10	20.65	0.24	167.38	8.14	63.53	7.16

Age- and sex-specific means and standard deviations, and selected percentiles (10th, 25th, 50th, 75th, 90th) were calculated for BMD, BMC, and TBLH BMD using the LMS chart maker pro version 2.3. The bone mineral parameters of each athlete were converted to z-scores relative to age- and sex-specific reference values specified by the Lunar Prodigy type dual-energy X-ray scanner manual. The distributions of BMD and BMC parameters in the athletes were compared to standard reference centile distributions by using individual z-scores of bone mineral parameters in young athletes on the basis of the reference centile distribution (reference L, M, S parameters). Single sample t-tests were used to evaluate the distribution of z-scores in each age-group of males and females, i.e., to compare age and sex-specific z-scores for BMD and BMC of the athletes to the Lunar Prodigy reference for youth. The normality of z-scores for BMD and BMC was tested by the Kruskal–Wallis test. Hypotheses were tested at a 5% level of random error.

Ethical Approval Information

The Research Ethics Committee of the University of Physical Education (Budapest, Hungary) approved the study (ID of approval: TE-KEB/No42/2019). The investigations were carried out following the rules of the Declaration of Helsinki of 1975 (https://www.wma.net/what-we-do/medical-ethics/declaration-of-helsinki/), revised in 2013.

3. Results

Sex differences in the selected bone mineral parameters are apparent at 14 years and older; total BMD, TBLH BMD, and BMC of male athletes are greater than corresponding values in their female age-peers except for total BMD (tBMD) at 13, 14, 19, and 20 years, and TBLH BMD at 20 years. At each indicated age, the BMD parameters do not differ between boys and girls (Table 3).

Table 3. Significance levels for sex differences in BMD and bone mineral content (BMC) parameters among athletes (significant values in italics).

Age (years)	Total BMD (g/cm^2)	TBLH BMD (g/cm^2)	BMC (g)
12	0.378	0.669	0.505
13	0.421	0.468	0.806
14	*<0.001*	*<0.001*	*0.009*
15	0.157	*0.009*	*<0.001*
16	0.127	*0.012*	*<0.001*
17	*0.012*	*<0.001*	*<0.001*
18	*0.015*	*<0.001*	*<0.001*
19	0.384	*0.024*	*0.002*
20	0.557	0.773	*0.004*

The total BMD of male athletes is considerably higher than that of the age-specific reference for males (Figure 1, $p < 0.001$ in each age-group). The median BMD curve exceeds the 90th percentiles of the reference. Although the data are cross-sectional, the adolescent increase in BMD occurs at a somewhat later age among the athletes.

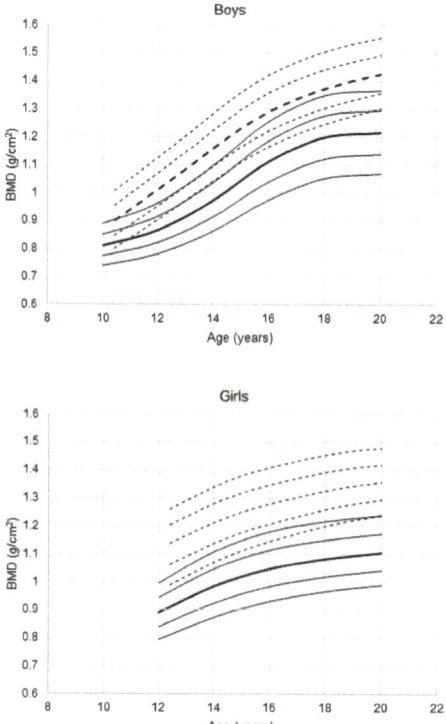

Figure 1. Total bone mineral density (BMD) in youth male and female athletes 11 to 20 years of age; percentiles (- - -) for athletes estimated with the LMS method, are plotted relative to the DEXA (dual energy X-ray absorptiometry) reference (—) percentiles (10th, 25th, 50th, 75th, 90th; the 50th percentiles are in bold).

The corresponding trend for total BMD among female athletes also indicates higher BMD (Figure 1, $p < 0.001$ in all age groups except 20 years, $p = 0.02$). Of interest, the 25th percentile for female athletes is higher than the 90th percentile of the reference. Nevertheless, the percentiles for female athletes parallel those of the reference.

Percentiles for BMD excluding the head (TBLH BMD in male athletes are higher than those of the reference beginning at 11 years (Figure 2, $p < 0.001$ in all age groups), while the 25th percentiles of the athletes approximate the 90th percentiles of the reference. In contrast to total body BMD, the adolescent spurt in TBLH BMD appears to be somewhat earlier in athletes compared to that of the reference.

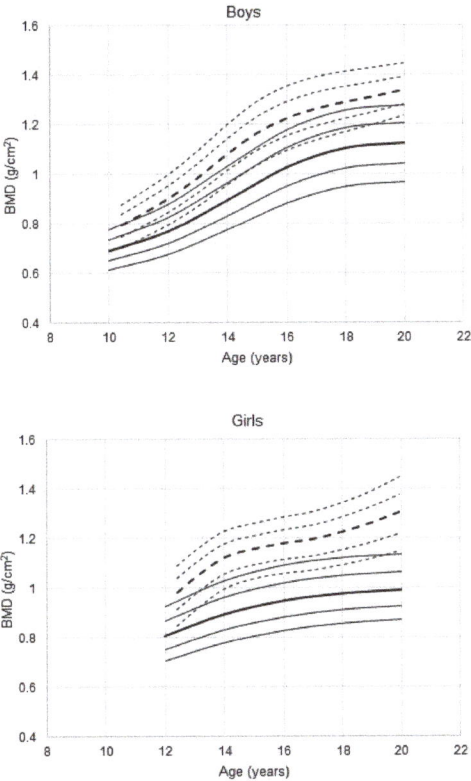

Figure 2. Total body less head (TBLH) BMD in youth male and female athletes 11 to 20 years of age; percentiles (- - -) for athletes, estimated with the LMS method, are plotted relative to the DEXA reference (—) percentiles (10th, 25th, 50th, 75th, 90th; the 50th percentiles are in bold).

The trend in TBLH BMD percentiles of female athletes is similar to that in males (Figure 2, $p < 0.001$ in all age groups except 13 years, $p = 0.04$). The cross-sectional data also suggest a more intense adolescent spurt in female athletes.

Percentiles for BMC among male athletes are also consistently higher than those of the reference (Figure 3, $p < 0.001$ in all age groups). The medians for athletes approximate the 90th percentiles of the reference across the age range except at 12 years when the 25th percentile of the athletes approximated the 90th percentile of reference.

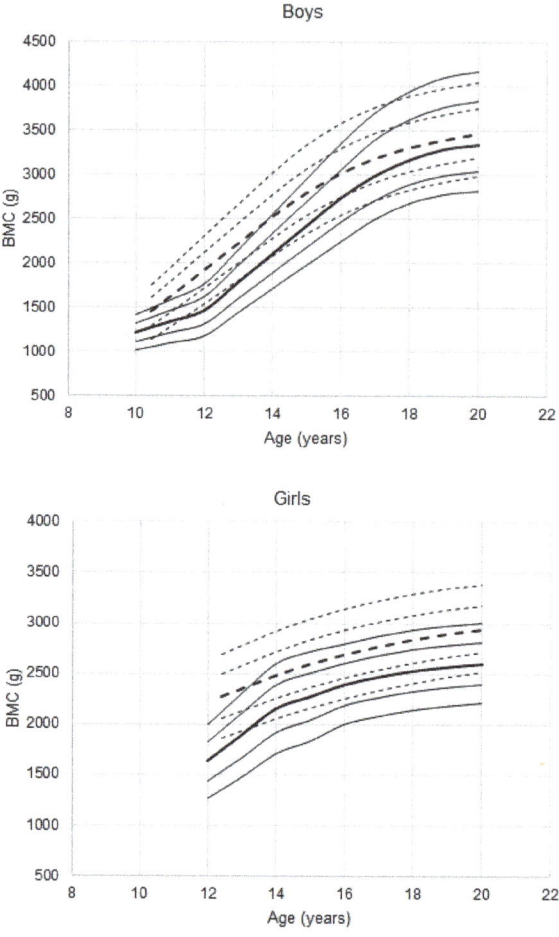

Figure 3. Total BMC in youth male and female athletes 11 to 20 years of age; percentiles (- - -) for athletes, estimated with the LMS method, are plotted relative to the DEXA reference (—) percentiles (10th, 25th, 50th, 75th, 90th; the 50th percentiles are in bold).

The corresponding trends for BMC of female athletes generally parallel those of the reference percentiles from 14 years on, but are significantly higher than those of the reference (Figure 3, $p < 0.001$ in all age groups except 13 years, $p = 0.04$).

Examples of the application of the reference percentiles for athletes in the evaluation of individual BMDs are shown in Figure 4. The athletes were selected from a longitudinal study of bone structure in youth athletes. In the male athlete (Figure 4, left), the BMD of the athlete is higher than the 90th percentile of the general population at each observation, but relative to the reference for athletes, the BMD shifts from the median at observation 1 to the 75th percentile at observation 2, suggesting that BMD continued to increase between 17 and 19 years. In the example of the female athlete (Figure 4, right), BMD values are higher than the 90th percentile of the general population reference across the age interval considered, but are below the reference median for athletes and gradually decline over time to <25th percentile of the athlete reference by 20 years of age. Such a decline in BMD relative to the athlete reference suggests the need for attention from the trainers as to potential factors associated with the decline.

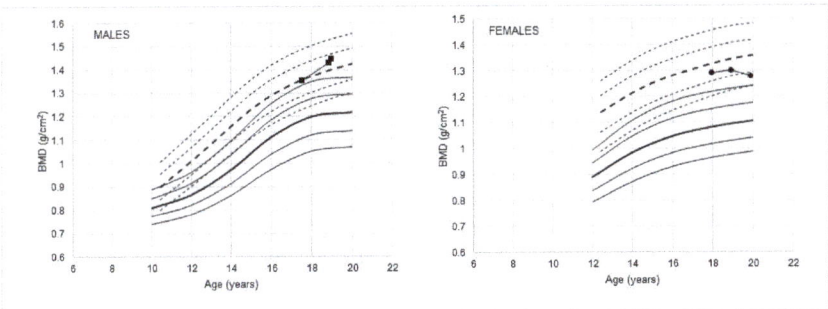

Figure 4. BMD of two athletes, a female handball player and a male football player, is shown relative to the percentiles (- - -) for athletes and the DEXA reference (—) percentiles (10th, 25th, 50th, 75th, 90th; the 50th percentiles are in bold).

4. Overview

Comparison of the percentiles of DEXA measurements of total BMD, BMD TBLH, and BMC of athletes 11–20 years in several sports (Appendix A, Tables A1–A3) with the corresponding Lunar Prodigy reference percentiles highlighted the contrast in bone development between athletes and the reference, and by inference suggested a need for reference values specific for youth athletes. References data for DEXA bone parameters for athletes are limited [27]. As such, the reference values for athletes in the present study may aid in the understanding of bone development in actively training youth athletes.

Relative to age- and sex-peers in the general population [28], BMD and BMC are better developed among the youth athletes. The results were consistent with earlier studies of youth athletes, and highlighted the importance of regular physical activity associated with specific sports on bone structure, density, and morphology [12,29–31]. Intensive physical activity associated with systematic training was associated with increased BMC and BMD. The data, however, were based on a combined sample of athletes in a variety of sports, and in the context of the literature, highlight the need to evaluate BMD and BMC in specific sports and also in sports characterized by variation in impact forces, e.g., high-impact (gymnastics, judo, karate, volleyball, etc.), odd-impact (soccer, basketball, step-aerobics, etc.), and non-impact or negative-impact (cycling, swimming, water polo, etc.) stresses. In addition to BMD and BMC, it is also important to consider variation in bone geometry in anatomic regions specific to variation in loading patterns by sport.

5. Limitations of the Study

Given the limited number of female athletes, the analysis of sex differences in BMD and BMC should be evaluated with caution. The lack of an indicator of maturity status in the younger athletes is also a limitation.

6. Summary

- Reference values for DEXA measures of BMD, TBLH BMD, and BMC were developed for a relatively large sample of youth athletes 11–20 years of age.
- Compared to reference values for the general population (White ethnicity), BMD and BMC of the youth athletes were better developed.
- By inference, comparison of DEXA observations of athletes with reference values for the general population must be done with care to avoid potential misinterpretations.

Author Contributions: I.K. participated in the data collection, bone development estimation, statistical analyses and the interpretation of the results, manuscript construction. A.Z. participated in statistical analyses and the interpretation of the results, manuscript construction. R.M.M. participated in the interpretation of the results, preparation of the manuscript. T.S. participated in statistical analyses and the interpretation of the results, manuscript construction. All authors have read and agreed to the published version of the manuscript.

Funding: The project was supported by the Scientific Excellence Program 2019 at the University of Physical Education, Innovation and Technology Ministry, Hungary (project number: TUDFO/51757/2019-ITM).

Acknowledgments: We would like to thank the sports clubs for their cooperation and engagement. Also, we thank the participants for their valuable time during the tests.

Conflicts of Interest: The authors declare that they have no conflict of interest.

Appendix A

Table A1. Basic statistical parameters (mean, SD, and 10th, 25th, 50th, 75th, and 90th percentiles) for total BMD (g/cm^2) in youth male and female athletes.

Age (year)	Mean	SD	P10	P25	P50	P75	P90
			Males				
11	0.962	0.062	0.837	0.885	0.942	0.996	1.048
12	0.997	0.063	0.902	0.952	1.012	1.069	1.124
13	1.063	0.095	0.971	1.023	1.085	1.145	1.202
14	1.158	0.098	1.041	1.096	1.160	1.223	1.283
15	1.248	0.105	1.109	1.165	1.232	1.297	1.359
16	1.296	0.101	1.166	1.223	1.292	1.358	1.423
17	1.335	0.109	1.212	1.269	1.338	1.405	1.471
18	1.372	0.093	1.248	1.305	1.374	1.441	1.506
19	1.378	0.085	1.278	1.334	1.402	1.469	1.534
20	1.412	0.112	1.303	1.359	1.426	1.492	1.557
			Females				
13	1.085	0.130	1.020	1.092	1.168	1.233	1.290
14	1.239	0.106	1.071	1.139	1.214	1.280	1.340
15	1.240	0.087	1.113	1.178	1.251	1.318	1.380
16	1.278	0.119	1.146	1.209	1.280	1.348	1.410
17	1.296	0.096	1.175	1.235	1.305	1.371	1.435
18	1.326	0.087	1.202	1.259	1.328	1.393	1.456
19	1.357	0.105	1.224	1.280	1.346	1.410	1.472
20	1.377	0.177	1.240	1.294	1.358	1.420	1.480

Table A2. Basic statistical parameters (mean, SD, and 10th, 25th, 50th, 75th, and 90th percentiles) of TBLH BMD (g/cm^2) in youth male and female athletes.

Age (year)	Mean	SD	P10	P25	P50	P75	P90
			Males				
11	0.846	0.062	0.734	0.780	0.831	0.876	0.917
12	0.899	0.090	0.796	0.845	0.900	0.951	0.997
13	0.973	0.107	0.870	0.923	0.984	1.040	1.092
14	1.084	0.105	0.957	1.014	1.079	1.141	1.199
15	1.177	0.106	1.038	1.096	1.165	1.230	1.293
16	1.220	0.098	1.096	1.154	1.224	1.291	1.356
17	1.261	0.117	1.137	1.194	1.262	1.328	1.394
18	1.290	0.095	1.171	1.224	1.289	1.353	1.417
19	1.298	0.087	1.203	1.252	1.312	1.373	1.433
20	1.318	0.103	1.235	1.280	1.336	1.392	1.448
			Females				
13	0.994	0.133	0.906	0.972	1.040	1.097	1.147
14	1.143	0.116	0.995	1.057	1.122	1.178	1.227
15	1.143	0.083	1.036	1.094	1.156	1.211	1.259
16	1.180	0.113	1.057	1.116	1.179	1.235	1.284
17	1.192	0.094	1.070	1.130	1.195	1.253	1.305
18	1.220	0.094	1.092	1.155	1.224	1.286	1.342
19	1.241	0.115	1.118	1.186	1.261	1.329	1.391
20	1.339	0.211	1.146	1.219	1.302	1.377	1.445

Table A3. Basic statistical parameters (mean, SD, and 10th, 25th, 50th, 75th, and 90th percentiles) for BMC (g) in youth male and female athletes.

Age (year)	Mean	SD	P10	P25	P50	P75	P90
				Males			
11	1691.0	216.3	1281.4	1446.2	1625.3	1800.8	1956.1
12	1886.5	343.6	1539.6	1720.9	1923.5	2127.3	2311.7
13	2136.9	459.0	1807.7	2003.2	2227.2	2458.0	2671.3
14	2537.4	433.1	2079.2	2285.8	2527.6	2782.4	3022.8
15	2883.5	447.9	2331.8	2545.3	2799.4	3072.3	3334.6
16	3030.0	401.7	2543.0	2759.1	3019.6	3303.1	3579.7
17	3219.2	461.4	2708.0	2924.1	3186.5	3474.8	3758.7
18	3300.5	451.4	2830.5	3045.9	3308.2	3597.4	3883.4
19	3328.7	403.1	2918.7	3134.1	3396.1	3684.7	3969.8
20	3321.2	422.3	2986.0	3203.2	3466.3	3754.8	4038.4
				Females			
13	2073.0	386.1	1937.0	2135.8	2356.4	2576.8	2775.0
14	2580.8	375.0	2055.7	2258.9	2485.4	2712.6	2917.7
15	2551.6	321.3	2162.6	2368.5	2598.9	2830.9	3041.1
16	2722.9	370.8	2254.9	2461.6	2693.7	2928.5	3141.9
17	2729.8	340.7	2334.6	2540.5	2772.7	3008.4	3223.2
18	2818.1	345.4	2406.0	2610.2	2841.3	3076.6	3291.8
19	2899.2	461.5	2468.0	2669.5	2898.2	3131.9	3346.2
20	2687.9	865.3	2518.5	2716.2	2941.4	3172.0	3384.2

References

1. Ward, K.A.; Ashby, R.L.; Roberts, S.A.; Adams, J.E.; Mughal, M.Z. UK reference data for the Hologic QDR Discovery dual-energy x ray absorptiometry scanner in healthy children and young adults aged 6–17 years. *Arch. Dis. Child.* **2007**, *92*, 53–59. [CrossRef] [PubMed]
2. Elhakeem, A.; Frysz, M.; Tilling, K.; Tobias, J.H.; Lawlor, D.A. Association between age at puberty and bone accrual from 10 to 25 years of age. *JAMA Netw. Open* **2019**, *2*, e198918. [CrossRef]
3. Baroncelli, G.I. Quantitative ultrasound methods to assess bone mineral status in children: Technical characteristics, performance, and clinical application. *Pediatric Res.* **2008**, *63*, 220–228. [CrossRef] [PubMed]
4. Golden, N.H.; Abrams, S.A. Optimizing bone health in children and adolescents. *Pediatrics* **2014**, *134*, e1229–e1243. [CrossRef] [PubMed]
5. Soininen, S.; Sidoroff, V.; Lindi, V.; Mahonen, A.; Kröger, L.; Kröger, H.; Jaaskelainenf, J.; Atalaya, M.; Laaksonenai, E.D.; Laitinen, T.; et al. Body fat mass, lean body mass and associated biomarkers as determinants of bone mineral density in children 6–8 years of age—The Physical Activity and Nutrition in Children (PANIC) study. *Bone* **2018**, *108*, 106–114. [CrossRef]
6. Larsen, M.N.; Nielsen, C.M.; Helge, E.W.; Madsen, M.; Manniche, V.; Hansen, L.; Hansen, P.R.; Bangsbo, J.; Krustrup, P. Positive effects on bone mineralisation and muscular fitness after 10 months of intense school-based physical training for children aged 8–10 years: The FIT FIRST randomised controlled trial. *Br. J. Sports Med.* **2018**, *52*, 254–260. [CrossRef]
7. Strong, W.B.; Malina, R.M.; Blimkie, C.J.; Daniels, S.R.; Dishman, R.K.; Gutin, B.; Hergenroeder, A.C.; Must, A.; Nixon, P.A.; Pivarnik, J.M.; et al. Evidence based physical activity for school-age youth. *J. Pediatrics* **2005**, *146*, 732–737. [CrossRef]
8. Malina, M.R.; Coelho-e-Silva, J.M. Physical activity, growth and maturation of youth. In *Body Composition: Health and Performance in Exercise and Sport*; Lukaski, H., Ed.; CRC Press (Taylor and Francis Group): Boca Raton, FL, USA; Abingdon, UK, 2017; pp. 69–88.
9. Herbert, A.J.; Williams, A.G.; Hennis, P.J.; Erskine, R.M.; Sale, C.; Day, S.H.; Stebbings, G.K. The interactions of physical activity, exercise and genetics and their associations with bone mineral density: Implications for Injury Risk in Elite Athletes. *Eur. J. Appl. Physiol.* **2019**, *119*, 29–47. [CrossRef]
10. Carbuhn, A.F.; Fernandez, T.E.; Bragg, A.F.; Green, J.S.; Crouse, S.F. Sport and training influence bone and body composition in women collegiate athletes. *J. Strength Cond. Res.* **2010**, *24*, 1710–1717. [CrossRef]

11. Tenforde, A.S.; Carlson, J.L.; Chang, A.; Sainani, K.L.; Shultz, R.; Kim, J.H.; Fredericson, M.; Kim, J.H.; Cutti, P.; Golden, N.H.; et al. Association of the female athlete triad risk assessment stratification to the development of bone stress injuries in collegiate athletes. *Am. J. Sport. Med.* **2017**, *45*, 302–310. [CrossRef]
12. Vlachopoulos, D.; Barker, R.A.; Ubago-Guisado, E.; Ortega, B.F.; Krustrup, P.; Metcalf, B.; Pinero, C.J.; Ruiz, R.J.; Knapp, M.K.; Williams, A.C.; et al. The effect of 12-month participation in osteogenic and non-osteogenic sports on bone development in adolescent male athletes. The PRO-BONE study. *J. Sci. Med. Sport* **2018**, *21*, 404–409. [CrossRef]
13. Csakvary, V.; Puskas, T.; Oroszlan, G.; Lakatos, P.; Kalman, B.; Kovacs, G.L.; Toldy, E. Hormonal and biochemical parameters correlated with bone densitometric markers in prepubertal Hungarian children. *Bone* **2013**, *54*, 106–112. [CrossRef] [PubMed]
14. Sioen, I.; Lust, E.; Henauw, S.; Moreno, A.L.; Jiménez-Pavon, D. Associations between body composition and bone health in children and adolescents: A systematic review. *Calcif. Tissue Int.* **2016**, *99*, 557–577. [CrossRef] [PubMed]
15. Gordon, C.M.; Zemel, B.S.; Wren, T.A.; Leonard, M.B.; Bachrach, L.K.; Rauch, F.; Gilsanz, V.; Rosen, C.J.; Winer, K.K. The determinants of peak bone mass. *J. Pediatric* **2017**, *180*, 261–269. [CrossRef] [PubMed]
16. Mountjoy, M.; Sundgot-Borgen, J.; Burke, L.; Carter, S.; Constantini, N.; Lebrun, C.; Meyer, N.; Sherman, R.; Steffen, K.; Budgett, R.; et al. The IOC consensus statement: Beyond the female athlete triad–Relative Energy Deficiency in Sport (RED-S). *Br. J. Sports. Med.* **2014**, *48*, 491–497. [CrossRef] [PubMed]
17. Mountjoy, M.; Sundgot-Borgen, J.K.; Burke, L.M.; Ackerman, K.E.; Blauwet, C.; Constantini, N.; Lebrun, C.; Lundy, B.; Melin, A.K.; Meyer, N.L.; et al. IOC consensus statement on relative energy deficiency in sport (RED-S): 2018 update. *Br. J. Sports. Med.* **2018**, *52*, 687–697. [CrossRef]
18. Malina, C.; Bouchard, C.; Bar-Or, O. *Growth, Maturation, and Physical Activity*, 2nd ed.; Human Kinetics: Champaign, IL, USA, 2004.
19. Tenforde, S.A.; Sainani, L.K.; Sayres, C.L.; Milgrom, C.; Fredericson, M. Participation in ball sports may represent a prehabilitation strategy to prevent future stress fractures and promote bone health in young athletes. *PM&R* **2015**, *7*, 222–225. [CrossRef]
20. Faigenbaum, D.A.; Lloyd, S.R.; MacDonald, J.; Myer Citius, G.; Altius, D. Fortius: Beneficial effects of resistance training for young athletes: Narrative review. *Br. J. Sports. Med.* **2016**, *50*, 3–7. [CrossRef]
21. Liu, J.; Wang, L.; Sun, J.; Liu, G.; Yan, W.; Xi, B.; Xiong, F.; Ding, W.; Huang, G.; Heymsfield, S.; et al. Bone mineral density reference standards for Chinese children aged 3–18: Cross-sectional results of the 2013–2015 China Child and Adolescent Cardiovascular Health (CCACH) Study. *BMJ Open* **2017**, *7*, e014542. [CrossRef]
22. Neu, C.M.; Manz, F.; Rauch, F.; Merkel, A.; Schoenau, E. Bone densities and bone size at the distal radius in healthy children and adolescents: A study using peripheral quantitative computed tomography. *Bone* **2001**, *28*, 227–232. [CrossRef]
23. Schoenau, E.; Neu, C.M.; Rauch, F.; Manz, F. Gender-specific pubertal changes in volumetric cortical bone mineral density at the proximal radius. *Bone* **2002**, *31*, 110–113. [CrossRef]
24. Bachrach, L.K.; Gordon, C.M. Section on endocrinology. Bone densitometry in children and adolescents. *Pediatrics* **2016**, *138*, e20162398. [CrossRef] [PubMed]
25. Crabtree, N.J.; Arabi, A.; Bachrach, L.K.; Fewtrell, M.; Fuleihan, G.E.H.; Kecskemethy, H.H.; Jaworski, M.; Gordon, C.M. Dual-energy X-ray absorptiometry interpretation and reporting in children and adolescents: The revised 2013 ISCD Pediatric Official Positions. *J. Clin. Densitom.* **2014**, *17*, 225–242. [CrossRef] [PubMed]
26. Taylor, A.; Konrad, P.T.; Norman, M.E.; Harcke, H.T. Total body bone mineral density in young children: Influence of head bone mineral density. *J. Bone Miner. Res.* **1997**, *12*, 652–655. [CrossRef]
27. Andreoli, A.; Monteleone, M.; Loan, M.; Promenzio, L.; Tarantino, U.; Lorenzo, A. Effects of different sports on bone density and muscle mass in highly trained athletes. *Med. Sci. Sports Exerc.* **2001**, *33*, 507–511. [CrossRef]
28. General Electric Healthcare. *Lunar X-ray Bone Densitometer with Encore v18 Software-User Manual*; LU46000EN-2EN Revision; General Electric: Boston, MA, USA, 2019.
29. Peer, K.S. Bone Health in Athletes: Factors and Future Considerations. *Orthop. Nurs.* **2004**, *23*, 174–181. [CrossRef]

30. Quiterio, A.L.D.; Carnero, E.A.; Baptista, F.M.; Sardinha, L.B. Skeletal mass in adolescent male athletes and nonathletes: Relationships with high-impact sports. *J. Strength. Condition. Res.* **2011**, *25*, 3439–3447. [CrossRef]
31. Tenforde, A.S.; Fredericson, M. Influence of sports participation on bone health in the young athlete: A review of the literature. *PMR* **2011**, *3*, 861–867. [CrossRef]

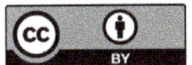

© 2020 by the authors. Licensee MDPI, Basel, Switzerland. This article is an open access article distributed under the terms and conditions of the Creative Commons Attribution (CC BY) license (http://creativecommons.org/licenses/by/4.0/).

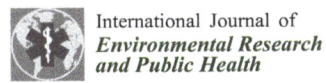

Article

Sex Differences in Body Composition Changes after Preseason Training in Elite Handball Players

Ireneusz Cichy [1], Andrzej Dudkowski [1], Marek Kociuba [2], Zofia Ignasiak [3], Anna Sebastjan [3,*], Katarzyna Kochan [3], Slawomir Koziel [4], Andrzej Rokita [1] and Robert M. Malina [5]

1. Department of Team Sport Games, University School of Physical Education in Wrocław, Al. I. J. Paderewskiego 35, 51-612 Wroclaw, Poland; ireneusz.cichy@awf.wroc.pl (I.C.); andrzej.dudkowski@awf.wroc.pl (A.D.); andrzej.rokita@awf.wroc.pl (A.R.)
2. Department of Physical Education, Military University of Technology, ul. gen. Sylwestra Kaliskiego 2, 00–908 Warsawa, Poland; marekkociuba@wp.pl
3. Department of Biostructure, University School of Physical Education in Wroclaw, Al. I. J. Paderewskiego 35, 51-612 Wrocław, Poland; zofia.ignasiak@awf.wroc.pl (Z.I.); kkochan2@wp.pl (K.K.)
4. Department of Anthropology, Hirszfeld Institute of Immunology and Experimental Therapy, Polish Academy of Sciences, ul. Rudolfa Weigla 12, 53-114 Wrocław, Poland; slawomir.koziel@hirszfeld.pl
5. Department of Kinesiology and Health Education, University of Texas, Main Building (MAI), 110 Inner Campus Drive, Austin, TX 78505, USA; rmalina@1skyconnect.net
* Correspondence: Anna.sebastjan@awf.wroc.pl

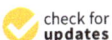

Received: 17 April 2020; Accepted: 28 May 2020; Published: 30 May 2020

Abstract: The purpose of this study was to evaluate changes in the estimated body composition of elite female and male Polish handball players during a five-week preseason training camp. Height and weight were measured, while body composition was estimated with bioelectrical impedance in 18 male and 17 female handball players before and after the five-week training protocol. Components of body composition included total body water (TBW), fat-free mass (FFM), muscle mass (MM), and absolute and relative fat mass (FM). Weight and body mass index (BMI) did not change in males, but declined in females after five weeks of training. FM and %FM declined, while estimated TBW, FFM, and MM increased significantly after training in both males and females. In contrast, comparisons of log transformed ratios for changes in weight, the BMI and body composition in males and females, respectively, suggested that estimated TBW, FFM, and MM increased relatively more in females than in males, while FM and %FM decline relatively more in males than females. Overall, the five-week preseason training program modified the body composition of male and female handball players. FM and %FM decreased, while estimated TBW, FFM, and MM increased, in both males and females after the preseason training program. Comparisons of log transformed ratios for changes in body composition in males and females suggested sexual dimorphism in response to intensive preseason training.

Keywords: handball; athletes; bioelectrical impedance; preseason training

1. Introduction

Body composition is often viewed as central to success in sport at many levels [1]. Although the two-compartment model of body composition—body weight = fat-free mass (FFM) + fat mass (FM)—was used in many early studies of body composition among athletes, often with a specific focus on estimates of relative FM (FM%), body composition can be approached at several levels [1], and advances in technology *per se* and methods have facilitated assessment so that FFM *per se* and lean tissue mass (LTM) and bone mineral content (BMC) or bone mineral density (BMD) components can be readily estimated, in addition to FM [2,3]. Among methodological developments, dual energy X-ray absorptiometry (DXA) and bioelectrical impedance analysis (BIA) are increasingly used in studies of body composition among athletes [4–6]. Nevertheless, no single method is the "gold standard".

The demands of specific sports vary considerably, and must accommodate variation associated with the extremes of size and mass in some sports and/or positions within a sport. As such, attention is commonly focused on endurance sports [7]; strength; speed and power sports [8]; and weight-sensitive sports, i.e., sports associated with low adiposity, fluctuation in weight, weight categories, dieting, and/or disordered eating [9]. Team sports are often included among strength, speed, and power sports, but must accommodate the demands of specific positions within a sport and the overall demands of the sport, e.g., size and mass variation in American football by position, height *per se* in basketball, etc. In addition, attention is often focused on the changes in body composition associated with training for sport in children and adolescents [10,11] and in young adults [12].

Estimates of the body composition of handball players have been largely based on several anthropometric protocols [13–20] that are associated with a considerable degree of variability, e.g., inter- and intra-technician measurement variability *per se* [21] and errors associated with specific prediction equations [12]. In contrast, estimates for handball players based on current technology, specifically BIA and DXA, are limited at present [22–24]. Nevertheless, many of the studies are largely descriptive and comparative, while few address training effects.

Although training methods have changed over time, often with a focus on specialization, expectations of athletes and coaches may differ relative to body mass and composition, especially in the context of absolute and relative fatness. Moreover, changes in estimated body composition prior to a season are of interest as both players and coaches prepare for the new season. In the context of the preceding, the purpose of this study is to evaluate changes in the estimated body composition of elite female and male Polish handball players during a five-week preseason training camp.

2. Materials and Methods

The study was conducted according to the Declaration of Helsinki, and the project was approved by the Research Bioethics Committee of the Faculty Senate of the University School of Physical Education in Wrocław, Poland (No. 4/2020; adopted in 05/03/2020; Chairperson prof. Marek Mędraś). The participants were elite Polish handball players (MKS Zagłębie Lubin Handball Team, Super Liga), 17 women (27.5 ± 4.5 years) with 16±4 years of experience in the sport, and 18 men (24.2 ± 3.3 years) with 12 ± 5 years of experience in the sport. All athletes provided written informed consent to have body composition estimated on the first and then on the final day of a five-week preseason training program, i.e., prior to the competitive season.

2.1. Anthropometry and Body Composition

All athletes were measured under similar conditions in the morning (10 a.m. to 1 p.m.) and afternoon (2 and 5 p.m.) before and after the preseason training program (see below). Measurements consisted of body height (anthropometer, GPM, Zurich, Switzerland) and body weight (InBody 230 system, Tanita, Tokyo, Japan). The body mass index (BMI, kg/m^2) was calculated. Based on BIA, InBody 230 system provides estimates of body composition, specifically total body water (TBW), fat-free mass (FFM), lean body mass (LBM), muscle mass (MM), and absolute and relative fat mass (kg, FM; %FM).

2.2. Training Protocol

The training program for both males and females began six weeks before the start of the Polish Superliga season. The training cycle spanned 36 days and included similar daily routines for men and women, with 5 and 4 free days for women and men, respectively. The program included 56 training sessions and 12 control games for women, and 50 training sessions and 9 control games for men. Training sessions were conducted outdoors, in the gymnasium or indoor arena, and/or swimming pool, and were held twice per day. Sessions were specifically focused on the development of endurance, static and dynamic strength, speed, individual techniques, and tactics, and included internal controlled games and time for recovery. About 38% and 48% of training time was devoted to techniques and tactics in women and men, respectively. Estimated intensities of the training sessions are summarized in Table 1. The camp concluded seven days before the start of the league season.

Table 1. Number of training sessions by intensity as noted by the coaches of the respective teams.

	Low	Moderate	High	Submaximal	Maximal
Women	1	13	27	6	9
Men	1	15	20	6	7

2.3. Analysis

Descriptive statistics (means, standard deviations, and medians) were calculated for body size and components of body composition before and after the preseason training program. Sex-specific Student t-tests for dependent groups were initially calculated to evaluate the significance of changes associated with training. Changes in each component of body composition were also calculated as ratios using the following formula: $\log^2$ (post-training/pre-training value). Transformation of the raw values at each observation has two advantages: (1) pre- and post-training changes in body composition are independent of pre-training levels in each individual, and (2) changes in different components are in turn comparable between sexes and among individuals since they are expressed as ratios and not as absolute or relative units. The transformed ratio was compared to a "0" value for changes in each component separately for each sex.

In addition, sex-specific zero order, rank order (Spearman rho), and partial correlations, controlling for age and for both age and age squared, between preseason indicators of body mass and composition, and change scores after the training program were also calculated. Given the age range of the samples (females 19–38 years, males 19–36 years), age *per se* is an important covariate, and age-squared controls for the nonlinear distribution of age in the samples.

3. Results

Body mass and the BMI did not change among males, while body mass increased slightly but significantly and the BMI did not change among females after the five-week training program. In contrast, the specific components of body composition changed significantly after the training program (Table 2). FM and %FM declined significantly, while estimated TBW, FFM, and MM increased significantly after training in both males and females. Consistent with other studies, FM and %FM were higher in females than males, while TBW, FFM, and MM were higher in males than females.

The transformed values for changes in body mass, the BMI, and specific components of body composition from pre- to post-training for males and females are presented in Table 3. Body weight and the BMI did not change, while all estimates of body composition changed significantly with intensive training among males. In contrast, all variables changed significantly with intensive training in females. In both sexes, MM and FFM increased, and FM and %FM decreased with training.

Comparisons of the transformed ratios for change in weight, BMI, and body composition in males and females, respectively (Table 3, far right column), suggested that estimated TBW, FFM, and MM increased relatively and significantly more in females than in males, while FM and %FM declined relatively more, though not significantly so, in males than females. By inference, training-associated changes in weight and the BMI of males were associated with a decline in fatness and a moderate increase in FFM and MM, while corresponding training-associated changes in weight and the BMI among females were associated primarily with an increase in FFM and MM and a moderate decline in fatness.

Table 2. Descriptive statistics (means [M], standard deviations [SD], and medians [Md]) for body mass and estimates of body composition among male and female handball players before and after training, and results of t-tests comparing pre- and post-training measures.

	Pre-Training			Post-Training			
	Mean	SD [#]	Median	Mean	SD	Median	t
	Males ($n = 18$)						
Height, cm	188.8	4.9	187				
Weight, kg	92	9.8	92.1	91.9	10.2	91.7	0.5
BMI, kg/m^2	25.8	2.1	25.1	25.7	2.2	25.1	0.54
TBW, kg	60	5.4	59.9	61.1	6	61	3.49 *
FFM, kg	81.9	7.4	81.7	83.4	8.3	83.3	3.57 *
FM, kg	10.1	4.6	9.4	8.5	4	7.3	4.13 *
FM, %	10.8	4.1	10.5	9.1	3.6	8.4	4.34 *
MM, kg	47.2	4.4	47.1	48.1	4.9	48.3	3.63 *
	Females ($n = 17$)						
Height, cm	176.3	7	176.2				
Weight, kg	70.6	8.9	69	71.4	8.6	70	3.70 *
BMI, kg/m^2	22.6	1.7	22.2	22.9	1.6	22.4	3.73
TBW, kg	41.7	4	40.8	43.4	4	42.8	11.02 *
FFM, kg	56.9	5.4	55.6	59.3	5.5	58.5	11.18 *
FM, kg	13.7	4.1	12.6	12.1	3.9	11.9	8.25 *
FM, %	19.1	3.6	18.9	16.7	3.6	16.6	10.24 *
MM, kg	31.9	3.1	31.5	33.3	3.1	33	11.17 *

* $p < 0.01$; [#] standard deviation.

Table 3. Transformed values (M, SD) changes in body mass, body mass index (BMI), and estimates of body composition after the five week training program among male and female handball players and results of the t-tests. The transformed values are compared relative to "0". Results for the comparison of transformed values of males and females are also indicated along with results of t tests for independent samples).

$\log_2(t_2/t_1)$ of	Males ($n = 18$)			Females ($n = 17$)			t Sex Comparison
	M	SD	t	M	SD	t	
Weight	−0.31	2.26	−0.58	1.62	1.74	3.84 **	−2.28 **
BMI	−0.31	2.26	−0.58	1.62	1.74	3.84 **	−2.82 **
TBW	2.43	2.90	3.55 **	5.77	2.23	10.67 ***	−3.80 **
FFM	2.43	2.85	3.62 **	5.89	2.27	10.71 ***	−3.95 **
FM	−25.69	23.11	−4.72 ***	−18.77	9.20	−8.42 ***	−1.15
%FM	−25.06	21.81	−4.87 ***	−20.44	8.93	−9.44 ***	−0.81
Muscle	2.65	3.08	3.64 **	6.52	2.58	10.44 ***	−4.02 **

** $p < 0.01$; *** $p < 0.001$.

Correlations between pre-training body weight and composition and subsequent changes after five weeks of intensive training are summarized in Table 4. Among males, changes in FM and %FM were significantly but negatively correlated with pre-training levels of fatness, i.e., players with higher levels of fatness at baseline experienced greater declines in FM and %FM after the training program. Among females, only the partial correlation for body weight is significant, while the other correlations for weight and those for FM are similar in magnitude but not significant. The direction of the correlations for females suggests that players with higher levels of body weight and absolute fatness tended to show larger declines in weight and FM after the training program.

Table 4. Correlations between pre-training values and respective changes (deltas) in weight and components of body composition after five weeks of training.

	Males (n = 18)			Females (n = 17)		
	Zero Order	Partial †	Spearman	Zero Order	Partial †	Spearman
Weight, kg	0.22	0.31	0.1	−0.37	−0.44 **	−0.30
Muscle, kg	0.37	0.27	0.34	−0.10	−0.28	−0.21
FFM, kg	0.41 **	0.31	0.28	−0.00	−0.17	−0.07
FM, kg	−0.52 *	−0.57 *	−0.50 *	−0.36	−0.35	−0.27
FM, %	−0.47 *	−0.54 *	−0.44	−0.09	−0.12	−0.11

† Partial correlations controlling for age and age2, * $p \leq 0.05$, ** $p \leq 0.10$.

4. Discussion

The results highlight changes in body composition associated with an intensive preseason training program among elite female and male handball players. On average, absolute and relative fat mass declined significantly and the lean components of body mass increased significantly. The direction of changes was generally consistent with expectations of coaches and athletes. In contrast, changes in body mass associated with the five-week training program were negligible and not significant in males, and relatively small but significant in females. The BMI was not affected by the preseason training protocol, which was consistent with the literature and highlighted the limitations of the BMI with among athletes. In males, mean BMIs before and after the training program (Table 2) were in the lower range of overweight ($25.0 \leq BMI < 30.0$ kg/m^2), which likely reflected the significant development of and gains in lean tissue mass associated with training. In females, on the other hand, mean BMIs were within the normal range and changed negligibly with training. Consistent with the literature [1,6,21,25], the findings highlight the limited utility of the BMI in female and male handball players.

Studies of changes in body composition associated with systematic training have a relatively long history [1,11,12], and results of the present study of female and male handball players were generally consistent with the literature, although corresponding studies of handball players using current technology are limited. A decline in FM, estimated with BIA, was noted among adolescent female handball players following eight weeks of high-intensity interval training, whereas players following a standard training protocol showed no significant change in FM [22]. Compared to a sample of 85 female players from six teams participating in the Italian national championship, the sample of Polish players (Table 2, based on BIA) was, on average, older, taller, and heavier, and had a lower FM of 13.7 kg, compared to 16.7 kg in the Italians sample, which was based on DXA [23].

As noted earlier, many studies of handball players have focused on characteristics of players by level of competition and by position, and on comparisons of handball players with athletes in other sports. The current sample of male players was, on average, younger, shorter, and slightly lighter than the Polish team participating in the 2013 Handball World Championship [26]. Elite male handball players in several studies were taller and heavier, had a higher lean tissue mass, and had a lower fat mass, than players at lower competitive levels [13–15]. The estimates of body composition in the comparative studies were based on anthropometry. Among females, elite players were, on average, taller and heavier, and had a considerably lower %FM and a higher lean tissue mass, especially of the upper limbs (based on DXA), compared to sub-elite players [24]. A similar trend was also apparent among junior (16 years) top elite, elite and non-elite handball players, although body composition was estimated anthropometrically [16].

The heights, weights, and anthropometric estimates of body composition of female and male handball players from several teams participating in the 12th Asian games (1994, Hiroshima, Japan) were compared [17,18]. Among 60 female players, differences among players from China, Japan, Kazakhstan, and South Korea were relatively small, but players from China were tallest with a larger estimated muscle mass, while those from Japan were shortest, lightest, and lowest in estimated FM [17]. In the comparison with male players, those from China, Japan, and South Korea (labeled East Asia) were, on average, slightly taller and heavier than players from Kuwait and Saudi Arabia (labeled West Asia), while predicted %FM was slightly less and predicted muscle mass was higher in the East than the West Asian players [18]. Among the East Asian male players, those from China were significantly taller, while those from South Korea were lighter.

Several studies of male handball players suggested variation in body size by position [17–30]. Wings were, on average, shortest with one exception, while backs tended to be tallest, though not in all samples; pivots, though not much shorter than backs, were intermediate. For body weight, pivots tended to be heaviest with backs slightly lighter; wings, in contrast, were lightest. Overall, there was considerable overlap between backs and pivots. Although data are less extensive, body size showed similar variation by position among female handball players [24]. It is likely that the size and the demands of specific playing positions in handball contribute to variation in body composition and regional variation in body composition (especially in the upper limbs) among players by position [28]. This is particularly noticeable in female and male pivot players, where greater muscle mass facilitates direct competition with the defender, allowing, perhaps, for a better position prior to throwing at the goal.

Compared to elite male basketball players, elite male handball players were, on average, shorter and lighter, while differences in anthropometric estimates of relative muscle, bone, and fat between players in the two sports were relatively small [31]. Among male junior players (16–17 years) in four sports, volleyball and basketball players were, average, tallest heaviest, followed by handball and then soccer players [32]. In contrast, anthropometric estimates of muscle and bone content overlapped considerably among players in the four sports, while handball players had, on average, a higher estimated fatness than players in the three other sports. Among national level Greek female athletes, volleyball players were, average, tallest, followed by basketball and then handball players. In contrast, the handball players had a higher anthropometric estimate of FM than players in the other two sports [20].

Allowing for variation in body size *per se* and variation among methods for estimating body composition, it is likely that sport-specific demands, especially by position, and training protocols contribute to variation in body composition among athletes in the respective sports. Handball is a sport that involves frequent contact with opponents and many high-intensity actions. Knowledge of the physical characteristics of players, including body composition, may assist in the identification individual aptitudes of athletes, which in turn may affect behaviour and effectiveness during play, and perhaps facilitate a profile for sports training [18].

5. Summary

Weight and BMI did not change during the preseason training program in males, but declined in females. Estimated MM and FFM increased, while FM and %FM decreased after training in both males and females. The absolute increases in TBW and MM and the declines in FM and %FM with five-weeks of intensive training were slightly greater in males than in females. However, comparisons of log-transformed ratios for changes in weight, BMI, and body composition in males and females, respectively, suggested that estimated TBW, FFM, and MM increased relatively more in females than in males. By inference, there appeared to be a sexual dimorphism in response to intensive preseason training.

The study is not without limitations. The duration of the preseason training program was limited to five weeks. This was a decision of the coaches. In addition, the number of players was relatively small, which limited the utility of comparisons of players by position.

Author Contributions: Conceptualization, Z.I., S.K., A.R., R.M.M.; Data curation, I.C., A.D., M.K., A.S., K.K.; Formal analysis: S.K.; Investigation, I.C., A.D., M.K., Z.I., A.S., K.K., S.K., A.R., R.M.M.; Methodology, I.C., A.D., M.K., Z.I., A, K.K., S.K., A.R., R.M.M.; Project Administration, I.C.; Software, S.K.; Supervision, Z.I., S.K., A.R.; Writing – original draft, I.C., Z.I.; Writing – review & editing, I.C., A.D., M.K., Z.I., A.S., K.K., S.K., A.R., R.M.M. All authors have read and agreed to the published version of the manuscript.

Funding: This research received no external founding.

Conflicts of Interest: The authors declare no conflict of interest.

References

1. Malina, R.M. Body composition in athletes: assessment and estimated fatness. *Clin. Sports Med.* **2007**, *26*, 37–68. [CrossRef] [PubMed]
2. Heymsfield, S.B.; Lohman, T.G.; Wang, Z.; Going, S.B. *Human Body Composition*, 2nd ed.; Human Kinetics: Champaign, IL, USA, 2005.
3. Lukaski, H.C. *Body Composition: Health and Performance in Exercise and Sport*; Taylor and Francis Group: Boca Raton, FL, USA, 2017.
4. Chumlea, W.C.; Sun, S.S. Bioelectrical impedance analysis. In *Human Body Composition*, 2nd ed.; Heymsfield, S.B., Lohman, T.G., Wang, Z., Going, S.B., Eds.; Human Kinetics: Champaign, IL, USA, 2005.
5. Moon, J.R. Body composition in athletes and sports nutrition. *Eur. J. Clin. Nutr.* **2013**, *67*, 54–59. [CrossRef] [PubMed]
6. Gatterer, H.; Schenk, K.; Burtscher, M. Assessment of human body composition: Methods and limitations. In *Body Composition: Health and Performance in Exercise and Sport*; Taylor and Francis Group: Boca Raton, FL, USA, 2017.
7. Moon, J.R.; Kendall, K.L. Endurance athletes. In *Body Composition: Health and Performance in Exercise and Sport*; Taylor and Francis Group: Boca Raton, FL, USA, 2017.
8. Fukuda, D.H.; Hoffman, J.R.; Stout, J.E. Strength and speed/power athletes. In *Body Composition: Health and Performance in Exercise and Sport*; Taylor and Francis Group: Boca Raton, FL, USA, 2017.
9. Silva, A.M.; Santos, D.A.; Matias, C.N. Weight-sensitive sports. In *Body Composition: Health and Performance in Exercise and Sport*; Taylor and Francis Group: Boca Raton, FL, USA, 2017.
10. Malina, R.M.; Geithner, C.A. Body composition of young athletes. *Am. J. Lifestyle Med.* **2011**, *5*, 262–278. [CrossRef]
11. Malina, R.M.; Coelho-e-Silva, M.J. Physical activity, growth, and maturation of youth. In *Body Composition: Health and Performance in Exercise and Sport*; Taylor and Francis Group: Boca Raton, FL, USA, 2017.
12. Sardinha, L.B.; Santos, D.A. Body composition changes with training. In *Body Composition: Health and Performance in Exercise and Sport*; Taylor and Francis Group: Boca Raton, FL, USA, 2017.
13. Gorostiaga, E.M.; Granados, C.; Ibáñez, J.; Izquierdo, M. Differences in physical fitness and throwing velocity among elite and amateur male handball players. *Int. J. Sports Med.* **2005**, *26*, 225–232. [CrossRef]
14. Massuça, L.; Fragoso, I. Study of Portuguese handball players of different playing status. A morphological and biosocial perspective. *Biol. Sport* **2011**, *28*, 37–44. [CrossRef]
15. Massuça, L.; Fragoso, I.; Teles, J. Attributes of top elite team-handball players. *J. Strength Cond. Res.* **2014**, *28*, 178–186. [CrossRef]
16. Hasan, A.A.; Reilly, T.; Cable, N.T.; Ramadan, J. Anthropometric profiles of elite Asian female handball players. *J. Sports Med. Phys. Fit.* **2007**, *47*, 197–202.
17. Hasan, A.A.A.; Rahaman, J.A.; Cable, N.T.; Reilly, T. Anthropometric profile of elite male handball players in Asia. *Biol. Sport* **2007**, *24*, 3–12.
18. Srhoj, V.; Marinovic, M.; Rogulj, N. Position specific morphological characteristics of top-level male handball players. *Coll. Antropol.* **2002**, *26*, 219–227.
19. Hermassi, S.; Laudner, K.; Schwesig, R. Playing level and position differences in body characteristics and physical fitness performance among male team handball players. *Front. Bioeng. Biotech.* **2019**, *7*, 149. [CrossRef]
20. Bayios, I.A.; Bergeles, N.K.; Apostolidis, N.G.; Noutsos, K.S.; Koskolou, D. Anthropometric, body composition and somatotype differences of Greek elite female basketball, volleyball and handball players. *J. Sports Med. Phys. Fit.* **2006**, *46*, 271–280.
21. Malina, R.M.; Battista, R.A.; Siegel, S.R. Anthropometry of adult athletes: Concepts, methods and applications. In *Nutritional Assessment of Athletes*; CRC Press: Boca Raton, FL, USA, 2002; pp. 135–175.
22. Alonso-Fernández, D.; Lima-Correa, F.; Gutierrez-Sánchez, A.; Abadía-García de Vicuña, O. Effects of a high-intensity interval training protocol based on functional exercises on performance and body composition in handball female players. *J. Hum. Sport Exerc.* **2017**, *12*, 1186–1198. [CrossRef]

23. Cavedon, V.; Zancanaro, C.; Milanese, C. Anthropometric prediction of DXA-measured body composition in female team handball players. *Peer J.* **2018**, *6*, e5913. [CrossRef] [PubMed]
24. Milanese, C.; Piscitelli, F.; Lampis, C.; Zancanaro, C. Anthropometry and body composition of female handball players according to competitive level or the playing position. *Sports Sci.* **2011**, *29*, 1301–1309. [CrossRef]
25. Gacesa, J.P.; Barak, O.; Jakovljevic, D.K.; Klaönja, A.; Gali, V.; Drapöin, M.; Luka, D.; Grujic, N. Body mass index and body fat content in elite athletes. *Exerc. Quality Life* **2011**, *3*, 43–48.
26. Ghobadi, H.; Rajabi, H.; Farzad, B.; Bayati, M.; Jeffreys, I. Anthropometry of world-class elite handball players according to playing position: Reports from Men's Handball World Championship 2013. *J. Hum. Kinet.* **2013**, *39*, 213–220. [CrossRef]
27. Chaouachi, A.; Brughelli, M.; Levin, G.; Boudhina, N.B.; Cronin, J.; Chamari, K. Anthropometric, physiological and performance characteristics of elite team-handball players. *J. Sports Sci.* **2009**, *27*, 151–157. [CrossRef]
28. Sibila, M.; Pori, P. Position-related differences in selected morphological body characteristics of top-level handball players. *Coll. Antropol.* **2009**, *33*, 1079–1086.
29. Krüger, K.; Pilat, C.; Uckert, K.; Frech, T.; Mooren, F.C. Physical performance profile of handball players is related to playing position and playing class. *J. Strength Cond. Res.* **2014**, *28*, 117–125. [CrossRef]
30. Schwesig, R.; Hermassi, S.; Fieseler, G.; Erlenbusch, L.; Noack, F.; Delank, K.-S.; Shephard, R.J.; Chelly, M.-S. Anthropometric and physical performance characteristics of professional handball players: Influence of playing position. *J. Sports Med. Phys. Fit.* **2017**, *57*, 1471–1478.
31. Muratovic, A.; Vujovic, D.; Hadzic, R. Comparative study of anthropometric measurement and body composition between elite handball and basketball players. *Monten. J. Sports Sci. Med.* **2014**, *3*, 19–22.
32. Masanovic, B. Comparative study of morphological characteristics and body composition between different team players from Serbian Junior National League: Soccer, handball, basketball and volleyball. *Int. J. Morphol.* **2019**, *37*, 612–619. [CrossRef]

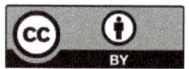

© 2020 by the authors. Licensee MDPI, Basel, Switzerland. This article is an open access article distributed under the terms and conditions of the Creative Commons Attribution (CC BY) license (http://creativecommons.org/licenses/by/4.0/).

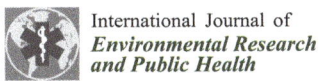

Article

Lower Percentage of Fat Mass among Tai Chi Chuan Practitioners

Silvia Stagi [1,*], Azzurra Doneddu [2], Gabriele Mulliri [2], Giovanna Ghiani [2], Valeria Succa [1], Antonio Crisafulli [2] and Elisabetta Marini [1,*]

1. Department of Life and Environmental Sciences, University of Cagliari, Cittadella Universitaria, Monserrato, 09042 Cagliari, Italy; valerias@unica.it
2. Department of Medical Sciences and Public Health, University of Cagliari, 09124 Cagliari, Italy; didi-zazzy@hotmail.it (A.D.); jabutele84@gmail.com (G.M.); giovanna.ghiani@tiscali.it (G.G.); crisaful@unica.it (A.C.)
* Correspondence: silviastagi@unica.it or silviastagi89@gmail.com (S.S.); emarini@unica.it (E.M.); Tel.: +39-070-675-6612 (S.S.); +39-070-675-6607 (E.M.)

Received: 8 January 2020; Accepted: 11 February 2020; Published: 14 February 2020

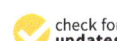

Abstract: The aim of the study was to analyze total and regional body composition in Tai Chi Chuan (TCC) middle-aged and elderly practitioners. A cross-sectional study on 139 Italian subjects was realized: 34 TCC practitioners (14 men, 20 women; 62.8 ± 7.4 years) and 105 sedentary volunteers (49 men, 56 women; 62.8 ± 6.4 years). Anthropometric measurements (height, weight, arm, waist, and calf circumferences), hand-grip strength, and physical capacity values were collected. Total and regional (arm, leg, and trunk) body composition was analyzed by means of *specific* bioelectrical impedance vector analysis (*specific* BIVA). TCC practitioners of both sexes were characterized by a normal nutritional status, normal levels of physical capacity, and normal values of hand-grip strength. Compared to controls, they showed lower percentages of fat mass (lower *specific* resistance) in the total body, the arm, and the trunk, and higher muscle mass (higher phase angle) in the trunk, but lower muscle mass in the arm. Sexual dimorphism was characterized by higher muscle mass (total body, arm, and trunk) and lower %FM (arm) in men; sex differences were less accentuated among TCC practitioners than in the control. TCC middle-aged and elderly practitioners appear to be less affected by the process of physiological aging and the associated fat mass changes, compared to sedentary people.

Keywords: ageing; Tai Chi Chuan; *specific* bioelectrical impedance vector analysis (BIVA); body composition

1. Introduction

Aging is associated with body composition variations: muscle mass progressively declines, while fat mass (FM) initially increases, especially in the visceral region, and then levels off or decreases [1]. These variations may lead to sarcopenia, a condition characterized by both low skeletal muscle mass and low skeletal muscle strength or quality, and to sarcopenic obesity, due to the coexistence of sarcopenia and fat excess or fat infiltration into muscle [2]. Sarcopenic and sarcopenic obese elderly have a lower independence and an increased risk of morbidity and mortality [2].

Physical activity has been shown to contribute substantially to the maintenance of the individual physiological and psychological well-being in all phases of life [3]. In the elderly, physical exercise can slow down or even reverse the trend towards sarcopenia [4,5]. However, which kind of physical activity could provide the more beneficial effects is still unclear and needs to be studied in depth [3]. Furthermore, body composition changes in different body districts were still poorly studied in the elderly. Instead, regional body composition gives relevant information. In particular, it allows better understanding of the role of physical activity in different conditions, such as sarcopenia and obesity [6].

Tai Chi Chuan (TCC) is an ancient Chinese martial art. The practice consists of the repetition of a sequence of slow and harmonious movements, focused on balance and based on respiration techniques. This discipline is particularly adequate for elderly people, who find difficult to perform rapid movements, and has been recommended to improve quality of life and to prevent or retard sarcopenic obesity [4]. TCC practice may help improve coordination and balance [7], retard bone loss [8], maintain cardiorespiratory fitness and flexibility [9]. It also contributes to promote social and psychological health [10], and cognitive function [11].

The effect of TCC on total and regional body composition has been poorly studied and the literature shows a still unclear pattern. Dual-energy X-ray absorptiometry (DXA) has been used to assess bone mass density in postmenopausal TCC women [8], whereas anthropometric techniques [9,12], equations based on bioimpedance measures [12–16], or air displacement [17] have been applied to analyze fat and fat-free mass. The studies on regional body composition have been based on skinfold thickness distribution only [12]. *Specific* bioelectrical impedance vector analysis (*specific* BIVA; [18]) has never been used. *Specific* BIVA is based on the analysis of bioelectrical values (resistance, R; reactance, Xc; Ω), standardized by body height and transversal cross-sections, in order to minimize the effect of conductor dimensions, that is the effect of anthropometric differences. Bioelectrical vectors can be projected on the Cartesian plane, where they are defined by their length (impedance: $(R^2 + Xc^2)^{0.5}$) and inclination angle (phase angle: $\arctan Xc/R \, 180/\pi$). *Specific* BIVA has been validated against DXA in a sample of US adults [19], showing high sensitivity and specificity in the evaluation of %FM (the longer the vector, the higher the %FM). It has also shown to be highly correlated with DXA results in elderly subjects [20,21] and young athletes [22]. Furthermore, phase angle, a variable considered a proxy of muscle mass [23], has shown to be positively correlated with intracellular/extracellular water ratio (ICW/ECW), when compared to dilution techniques [22,24]. Indeed, *specific* BIVA has been proposed as a promising technique for body composition assessment in athletes [25], and has been already applied in different contexts (e.g., cavers: [26]; various athletes: [22]; soccer players: [27]).

The aim of the present research was to analyze total body and regional body composition in TCC middle-aged and elderly practitioners by means of *specific* bioelectrical impedance vector analysis.

2. Materials and Methods

This observational study was realized on a cross-sectional sample of TCC practitioners and an age-matched group of sedentary subjects. The measurement process flow chart is shown in Figure 1.

2.1. Subjects

The sample was composed of 34 middle-aged and elderly TCC volunteers (14 men and 20 women) aged 62.8 ± 7.4 years, recruited from the A.S.D. Tai Chi Chuan school of Cagliari and La Porta d'Oriente of Quartu S.Elena (Italy). At the time of the measurement, the subjects had already been practicing Tai Chi Chuan for an average of six years and were training three times a week or more. Four of them participated in other sports too (swimming, walking, yoga, cycling). All the subjects declared to eat a balanced diet, with a great intake of fruits and vegetables.

The control group was composed of 105 volunteers (49 men, 56 women) of the same mean age (62.8 ± 6.4 years), and living in the same geographical area, selected for not practicing physical exercise.

Criteria of exclusion were physical handicaps, pathologies that might influence the measurements, metallic prostheses, pacemakers, or limb amputations.

Data was deposited in the University of Cagliari repository: http://hdl.handle.net/11584/269226.

The research was approved by the Independent Ethical Committee of the A.O.U. of Cagliari (PG/2017/1700). Each participant was informed about the purposes and methods of the research and signed consent to participate.

Measurement Process Flow Cha

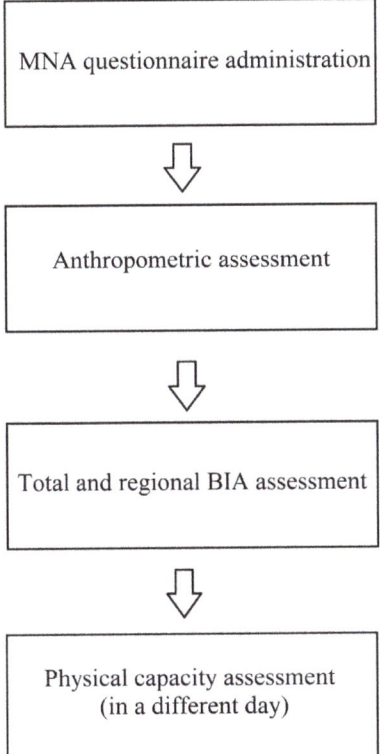

Figure 1. Measurement process flow chart.

2.2. Measurements

2.2.1. Anthropometry

Anthropometric measurements (height, cm; weight, kg; waist circumference, cm; arm and calf circumferences of both sides) were taken using international standard procedures [28]. The length (cm) of each regional district was also recorded: arm length, defined as the acromion-stylion distance; leg length, as the distance between the great trochanter and the malleolus; trunk length, as the distance between injector electrodes.

Body mass index BMI was calculated by the formula: weight/height^2 (kg/m^2). Underweight, normal weight, overweight and obesity, and visceral obesity were defined according to BMI [29].

2.2.2. Bioimpedance

Whole body and regional bioelectrical impedance measurements (resistance, R, and reactance, Xc, at 50 kHz and 800 µA) were taken using a single-frequency phase sensitive impedance analyzer (BIA 101, Akern, Firenze, Italy).

Following the European Society for Clinical Nutrition and Metabolism Working Group guidelines [30], the measurements were taken in the morning and the volunteers were asked to avoid drinking and eating (3 h before the test; alcohol 24 h), exercising (12 h before the test), and to void their bladder before the examination. The device was checked before each session with a calibrated circuit whose impedance values are known: R = 380 Ω, Xc = 47 Ω (±2% error). The intra-observer technical error of measurement (TEM) and the %TEM were calculated in a subsample of 25 subjects (R: TEM = 3.5 ohm, TEM% = 0.6%), that are within the admitted variability of the device. The accuracy of *specific* BIVA in evaluating %FM has been showed by Buffa et al. [19] using DXA as a reference (receiving operator curves, ROC areas: 0.84–0.92), while Marini et al. [22] showed the agreement with dilution techniques in the evaluation of ICW/ECW.

Bioimpedance measurements were taken with the subject lying supine, on the right side of the total body and the trunk, the right arm and leg, using two pairs of detector and injector electrodes. For total body measurements, on the hand, the injector was placed at the distal extremity of the third metacarpal, and the detector on the dorsal surface of the wrist, at level of the styloid process; on the foot, the injector was placed at the base of the second and third metatarsals, and the detector on the dorsal surface, at the median point of the tibial tarsal joint. Regional bioelectrical measurements were taken using the following procedure. Arm: on the shoulder, the injector was placed at the acromion process level and the detector at 5 cm distance, following the axillary line [31]; on the hand, the same position of the total body was used. Leg: on the hip, the injector was placed anterior to the iliac crest and the detector at a distance of 5 cm [32]; on the foot, the same position of the total body was used. Trunk: the electrodes already positioned on the shoulder and hip for the regional measures were used.

Specific bioelectrical impedance vector analysis [18] was used to estimate body composition. Resistance and reactance were multiplied by a correction factor (A/L). For the total body, the A value was estimated as 0.45 arm area + 0.10 trunk area + 0.45 calf area (cm^2); arm, trunk, and calf area were calculated as $C^2 4\pi$, where C (cm) is the circumference of the segment. The length was calculated as L = 1.1H, where H is the height in cm. In the regional approach, A/L for the arm, leg, and trunk were calculated considering the cross section of the mid arm, calf, and wrist (A) and the arm, leg, and trunk length (L), respectively.

Specific impedance (Zsp) was calculated as $(Rsp^2 + Xcsp^2)^{0.5}$ (Ω cm) and phase angle as arctan Xc/R180/π (degree).

2.2.3. Hand-Grip Strength

Hand-grip strength was taken using a Sahean hand dynamometer (Hydraulic Hand Dynamometer Saehan Corporation, MSD buba Belgium). The volunteers were asked to hold the dynamometer with the elbow flexed at 90° and to squeeze it with maximum isometric effort for a few seconds, three times with a 1 min interval between each attempt. Only the highest strength value was taken into account. According to Dodds et al. [33], 27 kg for men and 16 kg for women were considered the diagnostic threshold for assessing probable sarcopenia.

2.2.4. Mini-Nutritional Assessment

The Mini Nutritional Assessment (MNA®; [34]) is a recommended multidimensional method to evaluate nutritional status in the elderly, and was applied to the subgroup of subjects over 60 years old only. It is an 18 item questionnaire considering: dietary habits, living conditions, anthropometry, cognitive and disability status. A normal nutrition score is 24 or higher, a score between 17 and 23.5 designates risk of malnutrition, and a score lower than 17 indicates a condition of malnutrition.

2.2.5. Physical Capacity Assessment

Participants underwent a cardiopulmonary test (CPX) with a gas analyzer (ULTIMA CPX, MedGraphics St. Paul, MN, USA), while pedaling on a mechanically braked cycle ergometer (CUSTO Med, Ottobrunn, Germany). The test consisted of a linear increase of workload (10 W/min), starting at 20 W, at a pedaling frequency of 60 rpm, until exhaustion, which was considered the point when the subject was unable to maintain a pedaling rate of at least 50 rpm. During the CPX, the following variables were gathered: oxygen uptake ($\dot{V}O_2$), carbon dioxide production ($\dot{V}CO_2$), respiratory exchange ratio (RER, calculated as $\dot{V}CO_2/\dot{V}O_2$), pulmonary ventilation (VE), and heart rate (HR). The oxygen pulse ($\dot{V}O_2/HR$), a parameter related to stroke volume and cardiac performance [35], was also calculated. Workloads reached at anaerobic threshold (WAT) and at maximum (Wmax) were taken into consideration. AT was calculated using the V-slope method, while $\dot{V}O_2$ at Wmax ($\dot{V}O_{2max}$) was calculated as the average $\dot{V}O_2$ during the final 30 s of the incremental test. Achievement of $\dot{V}O_{2max}$ was considered as the attainment of at least two of the following criteria: (1) a plateau in $\dot{V}O_2$ despite increasing workload (<80 mL·min^{-1}); (2) RER above 1.10; and (3) HR ± 10 beats·min^{-1} of predicted maximum HR calculated as 220-age [36].

2.3. Statistical Analysis

The comparison between anthropometric and bioelectrical measurements in the TCC group and controls, considering sex, was realized using a two-way ANOVA. Cohen's d [37] for independent samples was calculated to measure the effect size in the comparison between TCC practitioners and controls.

Confidence ellipses, representing the area around the sample mean within which the "true mean" is expected to lie with a probability of 95%, and Hotelling's T^2 test were used to compare total body composition characteristics in the TCC and control samples, and between sexes.

The SPSS program was used to calculate univariate and bivariate statistics. *Specific* BIVA was applied using an ad hoc software available online (www.specificbiva.unica.it).

3. Results

Men and women practicing Tai Chi Chuan showed in mean a normal weight condition, according to BMI, and were below the threshold for visceral adiposity, according to waist circumference (Table 1). A good nutritional status was observed also in the individuals aged more than 60 years (MNA: men, 27.3 ± 1.0; women, 27.5 ± 0.6); no subjects were at risk of malnutrition. Compared to the age-matched control sample, TCC men and women showed higher height, lower circumferences, and lower BMI. They also showed lower total body and arm *specific* resistance, higher phase angle in the trunk, and lower phase angle in the arm (Table 1, Figures 2 and 3). According to *specific* BIVA, these values indicate lower %FM in the total body and the arm, and higher ICW/ECW and muscle mass in the trunk, but not in the arm. Furthermore, among the controls there was a high prevalence of individuals at risk of malnutrition (18%). Cohen's d showed large or medium size effects on anthropometric (with the exception of stature) and on total body and arm bioelectrical comparisons (with the exception of total body phase angles), while the effect was small on leg and trunk bioelectrical measurements, hand-grip strength, and age.

Table 1. Anthropometry, total and regional body composition in the Tai Chi Chuan group. Two-way ANOVA for the comparison between sexes and with the control sample of healthy Italian adults.

Total Body Composition	Tai Chi Chuan				Control				F		
	Men ($n = 14$)		Women ($n = 20$)		Men ($n = 49$)		Women ($n = 56$)		p_{sex}	p_{sport}	$p_{sex \bullet sport}$
	Mean	s.d.	Mean	s.d.	Mean	s.d.	Mean	s.d.			
Age (y)	63.4	7.9	62.5	7.1	62.9	6.6	62.8	6.4	0.713	0.948	0.763
Height (cm)	172.2	5.1	155.5	6.7	166.1	6.2	153.2	6.7	0.000	0.001	0.151
Weight (kg)	70.1	7.2	54.1	7.4	77.8	11.8	64.0	11.5	0.000	0.000	0.615
BMI (kg/m^2)	23.7	2.5	22.4	3.0	28.2	4.1	27.3	4.7	0.186	0.000	0.824
Waist (cm)	87.2	9.0	74.0	6.9	97.4	11.3	85.2	12.1	0.000	0.000	0.822
Arm (cm)	28.6	2.1	26.0	2.2	30.3	3.1	29.0	3.2	0.000	0.000	0.297
Calf (cm)	35.2	2.0	33.0	2.4	36.8	3.3	34.9	3.7	0.002	0.009	0.876
Rsp (ohm·cm)	352.7	45.6	380.4	54.2	454.9	56.3	553.2	50.5	0.010	0.001	0.677
Xcsp (ohm·cm)	39.7	6.5	39.2	7.4	53.4	8.9	58.8	9.1	0.794	0.001	0.955
Zsp (ohm·cm)	355.0	45.6	382.5	54.3	391.12	59.4	429.0	71.8	0.011	0.001	0.680
Phase angle sp (°)	6.5	1.0	5.9	1.0	6.7	1.0	6.1	0.8	0.001	0.275	0.756
Regional Body Composition	Men ($n = 14$)		Women ($n = 20$)		Men ($n = 27$)		Women ($n = 33$)		p_{sex}	p_{sport}	$p_{sex \bullet sport}$
Arm: R sp (ohm·cm)	248.8	31.7	285.4	47.9	266.9	44.7	330.0	61.9	0.000	0.005	0.230
Arm: Xc sp (ohm·cm)	25.4	4.8	24.7	5.2	31.8	7.65	31.2	8.0	0.687	0.000	0.993
Arm: Z sp sp (ohm·cm)	250.1	31.8	286.4	48.1	268.8	45.03	331.6	62.0	0.000	0.005	0.235
Arm: phase angle sp (°)	5.8	1.0	5.0	0.6	6.8	1.1	5.4	1.1	0.000	0.002	0.287
Leg: R sp (ohm·cm)	254.6	17.4	287.0	34.2	255.2	44.4	297.9	58.52	0.000	0.562	0.601
Leg: Xc sp (ohm·cm)	27.3	3.6	29.6	8.0	31.3	9.6	31.7	9.9	0.476	0.116	0.621
Leg: Z sp sp (ohm·cm)	256.1	17.4	288.7	33.7	257.2	45.0	299.7	58.9	0.000	0.545	0.619
Leg: phase angle sp (°)	6.1	0.8	6.0	2.2	6.9	1.4	6.03	1.3	0.135	0.229	0.241
Trunk: R sp (ohm·cm)	492.9	142.5	436.5	132.4	520.0	196.8	506.7	159.3	0.523	0.305	0.791
Trunk: Xc sp (ohm·cm)	68.1	24.1	44.8	14.0	63.8	25.1	49.0	22.6	0.000	0.793	0.538
Trunk: Z sp sp (ohm·cm)	497.7	144.1	438.9	132.9	524.0	198.0	509.2	160.4	0.491	0.313	0.783
Trunk: phase angle sp (°)	7.8	1.4	5.9	1.0	7.1	1.4	5.4	1.4	0.000	0.048	0.700
Hand grip (kg)	39.6	8.9	24.3	5.0	38.0	9.4	23.6	5.4	0.000	0.789	0.913

s.d.: standard deviation; BMI: body mass index; Rsp: *specific resistance*; Xcsp: *specific reactance*; Zsp: *specific impedance*.

specific BIVA - Total body

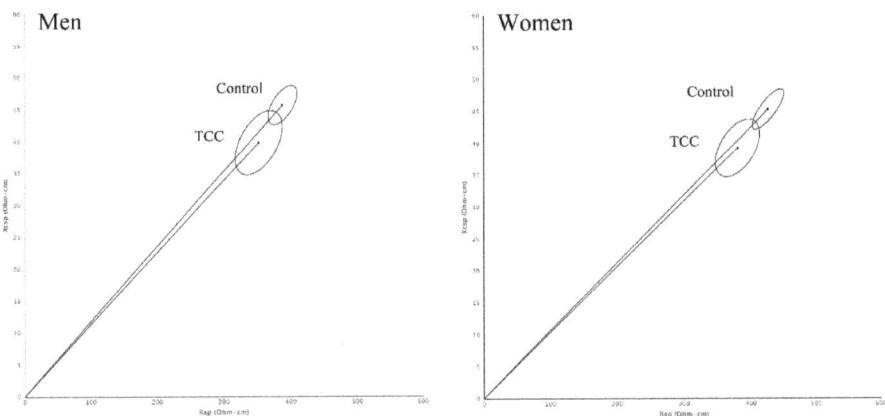

Figure 2. Total body confidence ellipses. Comparison between the Tai Chi Chuan (TCC) group and controls. Men: $T^2 = 6.6$, $p = 0.047$; women: $T^2 = 8$, $p = 0.023$.

specific BIVA - Regional body composition

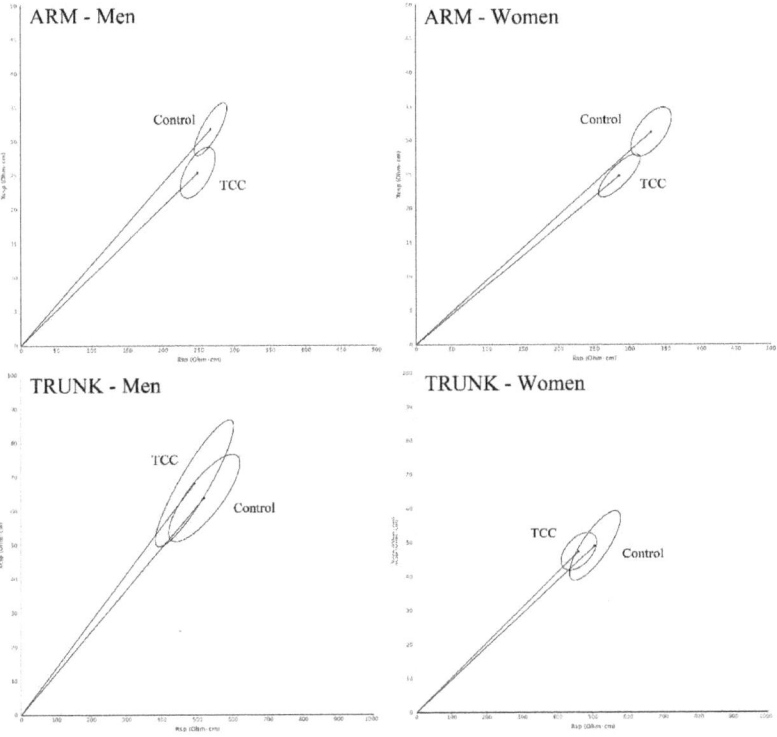

Figure 3. Regional confidence ellipses. Comparison between TCC group and controls. Arm (men: $T^2 = 9.8$, $p = 0.001$; women: $T^2 = 11.2$, $p = 0.007$); trunk (men $T^2 = 2.7$, $p = 0.285$; women $T^2 = 2.2$, $p = 0.340$).

Hand-grip strength (HGS) values were above the cut offs for sarcopenia in both TCC and controls. Table 2 reports values of cardiopulmonary parameters gathered during the CPX test.

Both TCC and control men showed higher values than women in all anthropometric measurements, except for BMI, higher values of hand-grip strength and of total body, arm and trunk phase angles, and lower values of arm *specific* resistance and impedance (Table 1). Sex differences in bioelectrical values were less accentuated among TCC practitioners than in the controls. In fact, bioimpedance mean vectors were significantly different between in the control group only (Figure 4).

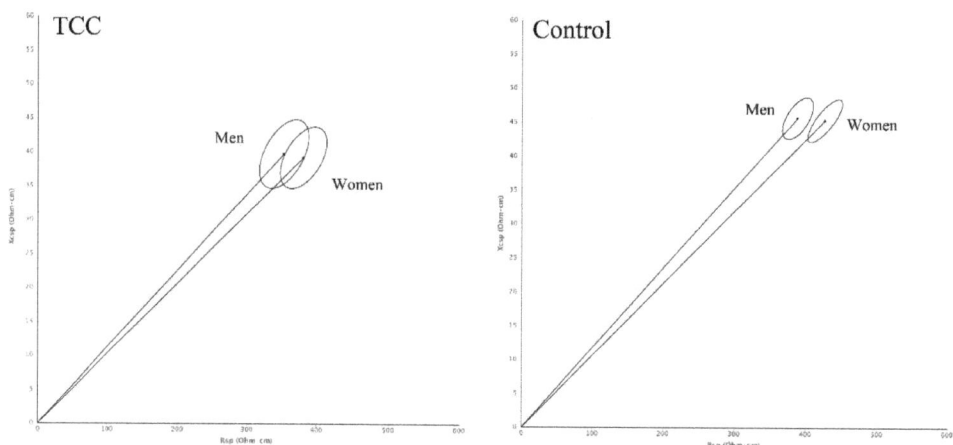

Figure 4. Total body confidence ellipses. Comparison between sexes. TCC: $T^2 = 3, 8, p = 0.177$; controls: $T^2 = 20.1, p = 0.000$.

Table 2. Results of the cardiopulmonary test (CPX) test for the whole group (top table), and for women (middle table) and men subgroups (bottom panel).

	Workload (w)	$\dot{V}O_2$ (mL/kg·min^{-1})	$\dot{V}O_2$ (mL·min^{-1})	$\dot{V}CO_2$ (mL·min^{-1})	RER	VE (L·min^{-1})	HR (bpm)	OP (mL·bpm^{-1})
Average Result for the Whole Group								
Rest	0	4.05 ± 0.79	257.5 ± 57.5	249.1 ± 73.5	0.96 ± 0.16	9.1 ± 2.8	77.6 ± 13.7	3.4 ± 1.1
WAT	90.7 ± 40.0	18.03 ± 5.41	1153.4 ± 409.8	1303.6 ± 522.6	1.12 ± 0.13	35.8 ± 12.4	130.9 ± 24.2	8.8 ± 2.5
Wmax	119.4 ± 49.4	22.76 ± 6.63	1449.3 ± 473.3	1824.3 ± 669.5	1.25 ± 0.13	54.9 ± 18.9	150.3 ± 25.6	9.7 ± 2.8
Average Results for Women Subgroup								
Rest	0	4.08 ± 0.90	233.5 ± 52.7	228.9 ± 86.7	0.96 ± 0.21	8.2 ± 2.9	80.0 ± 12.5	2.9 ± 0.8
WAT	73.1 ± 30.8	18.91 ± 4.09	976.12 ± 267.3	1075.1 ± 286.9	1.11 ± 0.16	29.4 ± 7.9	131.1 ± 19.7	7.4 ± 1.5
Wmax	92.7 ± 32.5	19.75 ± 3.90	1142.8 ± 278.6	1429.3 ± 361.3	1.25 ± 0.42	43.0 ± 12.4	148.3 ± 18.2	7.7 ± 1.6
Average Results for Men Subgroup								
Rest	0	4.14 ± 0.84	291.0 ± 52.4	287.4 ± 47.2	0.99 ± 0.11	10.7 ± 2.1	73.5 ± 15.0	4.1 ± 1.1
WAT	95.4 ± 33.7	16.99 ± 4.79	1194.2 ± 311.5	1375.9 ± 435.4	1.14 ± 0.11	39.3 ± 11.8	122.0 ± 27.1	9.8 ± 2.1
Wmax	128.6 ± 44.8	22.81 ± 6.09	1583.6 ± 309.0	1995.4 ± 566.9	1.24 ± 0.15	61.5 ± 18.7	140.7 ± 28.0	11.4 ± 1.7

WAT = workload at anaerobic threshold; Wmax = maximum workload; $\dot{V}O_2$ = oxygen uptake indexed by body weight; $\dot{V}O_2$ = oxygen uptake; $\dot{V}CO_2$ = carbon dioxide production; RER = respiratory exchange ratio; VE = pulmonary ventilation; HR = heart rate; OP = oxygen pulse.

4. Discussions

The present research showed that TCC practitioners of both sexes, including the older ones, were overall characterized by a normal nutritional status, normal levels of physical capacity, and normal values of hand-grip strength. With respect to a sample of sedentary people of similar age, they showed lower percentages of fat in the total body, the arm, and the trunk (as indicated by the lower specific vector length and waist circumferences), and higher muscle mass in the trunk (as indicated by the higher phase angle), but lower muscle mass in the arm, and similar hand-grip strength. Sexual dimorphism was characterized by higher muscle mass (total body, arm, and trunk) and hand-grip strength, and lower %FM (arm) in men; sex differences were less accentuated among TCC practitioners than in the control.

These results suggest a positive effect of TCC practice on body composition, particularly on fat mass. Consistently with our results, the literature focused on body composition in TCC suggest a major effect of TCC on fat mass. Lan et al. [9] observed a lower percentage of body fat among TCC practitioners. Longitudinal studies on the effect of a 10/12-week Tai Chi program showed a reduction of %FM [13,15], or of body fat [14,17]. The analysis of regional body composition and anthropometry confirmed the effect of TCC on %FM. The lower %FM values (lower specific vector length) among TCC practitioners with respect to controls mainly concerned the arm and the trunk, where a lower waist circumference, indicative of lower visceral fat accumulation, was also detected. These results are indicative of a healthy body composition, considering the role of visceral fat in the development of metabolic disorders and cardiovascular diseases [38]. It should also be noted that such phenotype is unexpected, considering the increase of abdominal adiposity commonly associated with physiological aging [39]. The body composition of the legs, instead, was not significantly different from the control. Conversely, Yu et al. [12] detected lower values of subcutaneous adipose tissue in the thighs of TCC practitioners than in the control.

Overall, our results also suggest a weak effect of TCC on muscle mass, as indicated by the similar hand-grip strength and similar or even lower phase angle of TCC practitioners with respect to the control group. Similarly, Yu et al. [12] and Lai et al. [16] failed to detect differences in the comparison with a sample of swimmers, nor respect to the control [12], and Kelly and Gilman [4] observed that TCC was not as effective at building muscle compared to other types of physical exercise. However, other studies showed an improvement of skeletal muscle mass [13,14], of muscle strength [13], and of functional performance [40,41], and suggested that TCC would have a similar effect as walking on parameters related to aerobic metabolism [9,15].

The regional approach of this study also allowed a detailed analysis of sex differences. The observed larger muscle mass in men and the higher %FM in the women, particularly in the arm and leg, are coherent with the known pattern of sexual dimorphism [6]. Furthermore, the higher waist circumference values of men are consistent with their generally greater central fat distribution. However, mean waist values were below the threshold for visceral obesity in both sexes, consistently with the results on low visceral adiposity reported among TCC subjects in this study and by other authors [12]. Furthermore, sex differences were less accentuated among TCC practitioners than in the control. This finding is not consistent with the low degree of sexual dimorphism detected in young subjects practicing different kinds of physical activities [42].

On the whole, the results of this study suggest that TCC practitioners do not strictly follow the trend towards the increase of fat mass, particularly of visceral adiposity, the reduction of hand-grip strength, and the worsening of nutritional status generally observed among middle-aged and elderly people [1]. Hence, TCC practitioners appear to be less affected by the process of physiological aging and the associated fat mass and functional changes. The healthy lifestyle commonly adopted by TCC practitioners could also contribute to such pattern.

This study has points of strength. In fact, this is the first study on total body and regional body composition in middle-aged and elderly athletes of both sexes using, phase angle, and *specific* BIVA, that is a procedure particularly promising for body composition analysis in sport [25]. The main limitation of the study is related to the sample size of TCC practitioners, which is not so large due to the peculiarity of the age range and the still limited diffusion of the discipline in Western countries. However, the information on regional body composition, that is scant in middle-aged and elderly athletes, can be insightful for future research.

5. Conclusions

The present research showed that TCC practitioners were characterized by good nutritional status (normal values of BMI, MNA, and low levels of fat mass in the total body, in the arm, and in the trunk) and had normal values of hand-grip strength. The effect on muscle mass was less evident. These results confirm the positive effect of TCC practice on body composition and functionality. Considering the suitableness of the practice in late adulthood over other disciplines, TCC represents a safe and effective way to help improve nutritional status and physical function.

From a methodological point of view, *specific* BIVA appears a suitable technique to screen and monitor total body and regional body composition in middle-aged and elderly subjects, in order to evaluate their nutritional status and risk of morbidity.

Author Contributions: Conceptualization, S.S. and E.M.; Data curation, S.S., A.D., G.G., A.C., and E.M.; Formal analysis, S.S., G.M., V.S., and E.M.; Investigation, S.S., A.D., G.M., G.G., A.C., and E.M.; Supervision, E.M.; Visualization, S.S.; Writing—original draft, S.S., A.C., and E.M.; Writing—review and editing, S.S., A.D., G.M., G.G., V.S., A.C., and E.M. All authors have read and agreed to the published version of the manuscript.

Funding: This research received no external funding.

Acknowledgments: We are most grateful to all the TCC volunteers of the A.S.D. Tai Chi Chuan school of Cagliari (Italy) and La porta d'Oriente school of Quartu (Italy). Silvia Stagi gratefully acknowledges Sardinia Regional Government for the financial support of her PhD scholarship (P.O.R. Sardegna F.S.E. Operational Programme of the Autonomous Region of Sardinia, European Social Fund 2014-2020-Axis III Education and training, Thematic goal 10, Priority of investment 10ii), Specific goal 10.5, Action partnership agreement 10.5.12.

Conflicts of Interest: The authors declare no conflict of interest.

References

1. Buffa, R.; Floris, G.U.; Putzu, P.F.; Marini, E. Body composition variations in ageing. *Coll. Antropol. Zabreg* **2011**, *35*, 259–265.
2. Cruz-Jentoft, A.J.; Bahat, G.; Bauer, J.; Boirie, Y.; Bruyère, O.; Cederholm, T.; Cooper, C.; Landi, F.; Rolland, Y.; Sayer, A.A.; et al. Sarcopenia: Revised European consensus on definition and diagnosis. *Age Ageing* **2019**, *48*, 16–31. [CrossRef]
3. Koolhaas, C.M.; Dhana, K.; Van Rooij, F.J.A.; Schoufour, J.; Hofman, A.; Franco, O.H. Physical activity type and health-related quality of life among middle-aged and elderly adults: The Rotterdam study. *J. Nutr. Health Aging* **2018**, *22*, 246–253. [CrossRef]
4. Kelly, O.J.; Gilman, J.C. Can unconventional exercise be helpful in the treatment, management and prevention of osteosarcopenic obesity? *Curr. Aging Sci.* **2017**, *10*, 106–121. [CrossRef]
5. Fien, S.; Climstein, M.; Quilter, C.; Buckley, G.; Henwood, T.; Grigg, J.; Keogh, J.W.L. Anthropometric, physical function and general health markers of masters athletes: A cross-sectional study. *Peer J.* **2017**, *5*, e3768. [CrossRef] [PubMed]
6. Hinton, B.J.; Fan, B.; Ng, B.K.; Shepherd, J.A. Dual energy X-Ray Absorptiometry body composition reference values of limbs and trunk from NHANES 1999-2004 with additional visualization methods. *PLoS ONE* **2017**, *12*, 1–17. [CrossRef] [PubMed]
7. Wong, A.M.K.; Pei, Y.C.; Lan, C.; Huang, S.C.; Lin, Y.C.; Chou, S.W. Is Tai Chi Chuan Effective in Improving Lower Limb Response Time to Prevent Backward Falls in the Elderly? *Age* **2009**, *31*, 163–170. [CrossRef] [PubMed]
8. Qin, L.; Choy, W.; Leung, K.; Leung, P.C.; Au, S.; Hung, W.; Dambacher, M.; Chan, K. Beneficial Effects of Regular Tai Chi Exercise on Musculoskeletal System. *J. Bone Miner. Metab.* **2005**, *23*, 186–190. [CrossRef]
9. Lan, C.; Lai, J.S.; Wong, M.K.; Yu, M.L. Cardiorespiratory Function, Flexibility, and Body Composition among Geriatric Tai Chi Chuan Practitioners. *Arch. Phys. Med. Rehabil.* **1996**, *77*, 612–616. [CrossRef]

10. Chan, A.W.K.; Yu, D.S.F.; Choi, K.C. Effects of Tai Chi Qigong on Psychosocial Well-Being Among Hidden Elderly, Using Elderly Neighborhood Volunteer Approach: A Pilot Randomized Controlled Trial. *Clin. Interv. Aging* **2017**, *12*, 85–96. [CrossRef]
11. Lim, K.H.L.; Pysklywec, A.; Plante, M.; Demers, L. The Effectiveness of Tai Chi for Short-Term Cognitive Function Improvement in the Early Stages of Dementia in the Elderly: A Systematic Literature Review. *Clin. Interv. Aging* **2019**, *14*, 827–839. [CrossRef] [PubMed]
12. Yu, T.-Y.; Pei, Y.-C.; Lau, Y.-C.; Chen, C.-K.; Hsu, H.-C.; Wong, A.M.K. Comparison of the Effects of Swimming and Tai Chi Chuan on Body Fat Composition in Elderly People. *Chang Gung Med. J.* **2007**, *30*, 128–134. [PubMed]
13. Barbat-Artigas, S.; Filion, M.E.; Dupontgand, S.; Karelis, A.D.; Aubertin-Leheudre, M. Effects of Tai Chi Training in Dynapenic and Nondynapenic Postmenopausal Women. *Menopause* **2011**, *18*, 974–979. [CrossRef] [PubMed]
14. Hsu, W.H.; Hsu, R.W.W.; Lin, Z.R.; Fan, C.H. Effects of Circuit Exercise and Tai Chi on Body Composition in Middle-Aged and Older Women. *Geriatr. Gerontol. Int.* **2015**, *15*, 282–288. [CrossRef] [PubMed]
15. Hui, S.S.; Xie, Y.J.; Woo, J.; Kwok, T.C.Y. Practicing Tai Chi had lower energy metabolism than walking but similar health benefits in terms of aerobic fitness, resting energy expenditure, body composition and self-perceived physical health. *Complement. Ther. Med.* **2016**, *27*, 43–50. [CrossRef] [PubMed]
16. Lai, H.M.; Liu, M.S.Y.; Lin, T.J.; Tsai, Y.L.; Chien, E.J. Higher Dheas Levels Associated with Long-Term Practicing of Tai Chi. *Chin. J. Physiol.* **2017**, *60*, 124–130. [CrossRef]
17. Dechamps, A.; Gatta, B.; Bourdel-Marchasson, I.; Tabarin, A.; Roger, P. Pilot Study of a 10-Week Multidisciplinary Tai Chi Intervention in Sedentary Obese Women. *Clin. J. Sport Med.* **2009**, *19*, 49–53. [CrossRef]
18. Buffa, R.; Mereu, E.; Comandini, O.; Ibanez, M.E.; Marini, E. Bioelectrical Impedance Vector Analysis (BIVA) for the Assessment of Two-Compartment Body Composition. *Eur. J. Clin. Nutr.* **2014**, *68*, 1234. [CrossRef]
19. Buffa, R.; Saragat, B.; Cabras, S.; Rinaldi, A.C.; Marini, E. Accuracy of Specific BIVA for the Assessment of Body Composition in the United States Population. *PLoS ONE* **2013**, *8*, e58533. [CrossRef]
20. Marini, E.; Sergi, G.; Succa, V.; Saragat, B.; Sarti, S.; Coin, A.; Manzato, E.; Buffa, R. Efficacy of Specific Bioelectrical Impedance Vector Analysis (BIVA) for Assessing Body Composition in the Elderly. *J. Nutr. Health Aging* **2013**, *17*, 515–521. [CrossRef]
21. Saragat, B.; Buffa, R.; Mereu, E.; De Rui, M.; Coin, A.; Sergi, G.; Marini, E. Specific bioelectrical impedance vector reference values for assessing body composition in the Italian elderly. *Exp. Gerontol.* **2014**, *50*, 52–56. [CrossRef] [PubMed]
22. Marini, E.; Campa, F.; Buffa, R.; Stagi, S.; Matias, C.N.; Toselli, S.; Sardinha, L.B.; Silva, A.M. Phase Angle and Bioelectrical Impedance Vector Analysis in the Evaluation of Body Composition in Athletes. *Clin. Nutr.* **2019**. [CrossRef] [PubMed]
23. Norman, K.; Stobäus, N.; Pirlich, M.; Bosy-Westphal, A. Bioelectrical phase angle and impedance vector analysis–clinical relevance and applicability of impedance parameters. *Clin. Nutr.* **2012**, *31*, 854–861. [CrossRef] [PubMed]
24. Campa, F.; Matias, C.N.; Marini, E.; Heymsfield, S.B.; Toselli, S.; Sardinha, L.B.; Silva, A.M. Identifying athlete body-fluid changes during a competitive season with bioelectrical impedance vector analysis. *Int. J. Sports Physiol. Perform.* **2019**, *1*, 1–21. [CrossRef]
25. Castizo-Olier, J.; Irurtia, A.; Jemni, M.; Carrasco-Marginet, M.; Fernández-García, R.; Rodríguez, F.A. Bioelectrical Impedance Vector Analysis (BIVA) in Sport and Exercise: Systematic Review and Future Perspectives. *PLoS ONE* **2018**, *13*, e0197957. [CrossRef]
26. Antoni, G.; Marini, E.; Curreli, N.; Tuveri, V.; Comandini, O.; Cabras, S.; Gabba, S.; Madeddu, C.; Crisafulli, A.; Rinaldi, A.C. Energy expenditure in caving. *PLoS ONE* **2017**, *12*, e0170853. [CrossRef]
27. Toselli, S.; Marini, E.; Maietta Latessa, P.; Benedetti, L.; Campa, F. Maturity Related Differences in Body Composition Assessed by Classic and Specific Bioimpedance Vector Analysis among Male Elite Youth Soccer Players. *Int. J. Environ. Res. Public Health* **2020**, *22*, 729. [CrossRef]
28. Lohman, T.G.; Roche, A.F.; Martorell, R. *Anthropometric Standardization Reference Manual*; Human Kinetics Books Champaign: Champaign, IL, USA, 1988.
29. World Health Organization. *Obesity: Preventing and Managing the Global Epidemic. Report of a WHO Consultation*; World Health Organization Technical Report Series; WHO: Geneva, Switzerland, 2000; Volume 894, pp. 1–253.

30. Kyle, U.G.; Bosaeus, I.; De Lorenzo, A.D.; Deurenberg, P.; Elia, M.; Manuel Gómez, J.; Lilienthal Heitmann, B.; Kent-Smith, L.; Melchior, J.C.; Pirlich, M.; et al. Bioelectrical impedance analysis—Part II: Utilization in clinical practice. *Clin. Nutr.* **2004**, *23*, 1430–1453. [CrossRef]
31. Baumgartner, R.N.; Chumlea, W.C.; Roche, A.F. Bioelectric Impedance Phase Angle and Body Composition. *Am. J. Clin. Nutr.* **1988**, *48*, 16–23. [CrossRef]
32. Fuller, N.J.; Elia, M. Potential Use of Bioelectrical Impedance of the "whole Body" and of Body Segments for the Assessment of Body Composition: Comparison with Densitometry and Anthropometry. *Eur. J. Clin. Nutr.* **1989**, *43*, 779–791.
33. Dodds, R.M.; Syddall, H.E.; Cooper, R.; Benzeval, M.; Deary, I.J.; Dennison, E.M.; Der, G.; Gale, C.R.; Inskip, H.M.; Jagger, C.; et al. Grip Strength across the Life Course: Normative Data from Twelve British Studies. *PLoS ONE* **2014**, *9*, e113637. [CrossRef] [PubMed]
34. Guigoz, Y. The Mini Nutritional Assessment (MNA®) Review of the Literature-What Does It Tell Us? *J. Nutr. Health Aging* **2006**, *10*, 466.
35. Crisafulli, A.; Piras, F.; Chiappori, P.; Votelli, S.; Caria, M.A.; Lobina, A.; Millia, R.; Tocco, F.; Concu, A.; Melis, F. Estimating stroke volume from oxygen pulse during exercise. *Physiol. Meas.* **2007**, *28*, 1201. [CrossRef] [PubMed]
36. Howley, E.T.; Bassett, D.R.; Welch, H. Criteria for maximal oxygen uptake: Review and commentary. *Med. Sci. Sports Exerc.* **1995**, *27*, 1292–1301. [CrossRef]
37. Cohen, J. *Statistical Power Analysis for the Behavioral Sciences*; Routledge: London, UK, 2013.
38. Neeland, I.J.; Ross, R.; Després, J.P.; Matsuzawa, Y.; Yamashita, S.; Shai, I.; Seidell, J.; Magni, P.; Santos, R.D.; Arsenault, B.; et al. Visceral and ectopic fat, atherosclerosis, and cardiometabolic disease: A position statement. *Lancet Diabetes Endocrinol.* **2019**, *7*, 715–725. [CrossRef]
39. Bosy-Westphal, A.; Booke, C.A.; Blöcker, T.; Kossel, E.; Goele, K.; Later, W.; Heller, M.; Glüer, C.C.; Müller, M.J. Measurement site for waist circumference affects its accuracy as an index of visceral and abdominal subcutaneous fat in a Caucasian population. *J. Nutr.* **2010**, *140*, 954–996. [CrossRef]
40. Manor, B.; Lough, M.; Gagnon, M.M.; Cupples, A.; Wayne, P.M.; Lipsitz, L.A. Functional benefits of tai chi training in senior housing facilities. *J. Am. Geriatr. Soc.* **2014**, *62*, 1484–1489. [CrossRef]
41. Lan, C.; Lai, J.S.; Chen, S.Y.; Wong, M.K. 12-month Tai Chi training in the elderly: Its effect on health fitness. *Med. Sci. Sports Exerc.* **1998**, *30*, 345–351. [CrossRef]
42. Buffa, R.; Marini, E.; Floris, G. Variation in sexual dimorphism in relation to physical activity. *Am. J. Hum. Biol.* **2001**, *13*, 341–348. [CrossRef]

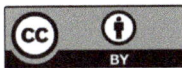

© 2020 by the authors. Licensee MDPI, Basel, Switzerland. This article is an open access article distributed under the terms and conditions of the Creative Commons Attribution (CC BY) license (http://creativecommons.org/licenses/by/4.0/).

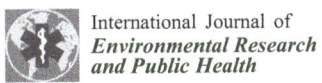
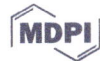

Article

Comparison of the Effect of Different Resistance Training Frequencies on Phase Angle and Handgrip Strength in Obese Women: A Randomized Controlled Trial

Stefania Toselli [1], Georgian Badicu [2,*], Laura Bragonzoni [1], Federico Spiga [1], Paolo Mazzuca [3] and Francesco Campa [1,4]

1. Department of Biomedical and Neuromotor Sciences, University of Bologna, 40126 Bologna, Italy; stefania.toselli@unibo.it (S.T.); laura.bragonzoni4@unibo.it (L.B.); Federico2907@gmail.com (F.S.); francesco.campa3@unibo.it (F.C.)
2. Department of Physical Education and Special Motricity, University Transilvania of Brasov, 500068 Brasov, Romania
3. Unit of Internal Medicine, Diabetes and Metabolic Disease Center, Romagna Health District, 47921 Rimini, Italy; Paolo.mazzuca4@unibo.it
4. Department for Life Quality Studies, University of Bologna, 47921 Rimini, Italy
* Correspondence: georgian.badicu@unitbv.ro; Tel.: +40-769-219-271

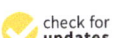

Received: 18 January 2020; Accepted: 11 February 2020; Published: 12 February 2020

Abstract: Phase angle (PA) is a strong predictor of sarcopenia, fragility, and risk of mortality in obese people, while an optimal muscular function and handgrip strength (HS) are required to perform different daily activities. Although there is a general agreement that resistance training improves health status in obese people, the optimal weekly training frequency for PA and physical performance parameters is not clear. This study aimed to compare the effects of different weekly resistance training frequencies performed over a 24 week exercise program on PA and HS in obese people. Forty-two women (56.2 ± 9.1 years, body mass index (BMI) 37.1 ± 4.9 kg/m^2) were randomly allocated to one of two groups: a group with a high weekly training frequency of three times a week (HIGH, n = 21) and a group that performed only one weekly session (LOW, n = 21). The groups trained with an identical exercise intensity and volume per session for 6 months. Before and after the intervention period, the participants were assessed for anthropometric measures, bioimpedance analysis, and HS. There was a significant group × time interaction ($p < 0.05$) for waist circumference, bioimpedance reactance divided by body height (Xc/H), PA, and HS measures. In addition, only the HIGH group increased Xc/H, PA, and HS after the intervention period ($p < 0.05$), even after adjusting for weight loss and menopausal status. Physical exercise performed three times a week promotes better adaptations in PA and HS when compared with the same program performed once a week in obese women.

Keywords: bioimpedance; BIVA; body composition; R-Xc graph

1. Introduction

In recent years, obesity has become widely recognized as a growing public issue requiring urgent action, especially in high-risk groups. Currently, more than 1.5 million people are obese or overweight, reaching about 25% of the population in Canada and 35% in the United States [1,2]. Moreover, in most countries of northern Europe, including the UK and Scandinavian countries, as well as southern European countries, the rate of obesity has more than doubled over the past 30 years [3–5]. Obesity is associated with increased morbidity, and disability, from cardiovascular disease, diabetes, cancer, hypertension, osteoarthritis, and musculoskeletal disorders [6]. Although bariatric surgery remains the most effective treatment to reduce and maintain weight loss, as well as improve comorbidities and mortality, physical activity is recommended as the first step to achieving weight loss and reducing obesity-related comorbidities in subjects with severe obesity [7–9].

The bioimpedance vector analysis (BIVA) is used in clinical and sports fields to study the change in body fluids and nutritional state [10–13]. It represents the raw bioimpedance parameters (resistance (R) and reactance (Xc)) as a point on the R–Xc graph in which both length and slope are considered. The vector slope represented by the bioelectrical phase angle (PA) is an indicator of cell membrane integrity and extracellular/intracellular(ECW/ICW) ratio [14,15]. Recent studies on obese people have taken into consideration PA and its relationship to different health status measurements, suggesting it as a biomarker to quantify inflammation, which might help in identifying high-risk patients [16,17]. In particular, it has been shown that obese women with a low PA tertile have high fat mass with high levels of glucose and higher cardiovascular risk factors [18]. On the other hand, in relation to muscle function, improvements in PA are also associated with increases in strength, in particular that of hand grip (HS) [19,20]. In this regard, HS and muscle strength, indicators of muscle quality, have shown to be more significant than muscle mass in estimating mortality risk [21].

Previous studies have shown that the PA can be modulated by exercise. These studies, which have offered resistance training as physical activity, have been used for training protocols with a frequency of two or three times a week [22–25]. The World Health Organization (WHO) recommends that all adults should engage in a minimum of 150 to 300 minutes of moderate-intensity physical activity or at least 75 minutes of vigorous-intensity exercise throughout the week, involving the major muscle groups [26].

To the best of our knowledge, no study compared the effects of different training frequencies on BIVA patterns and muscular function in obese people. Therefore, the aim of this study was to evaluate the effects of a resistance training program of one or three times a week on PA and HS in obese women.

2. Methods

2.1. Experimental Approach to the Problem

A randomized controlled trial was carried out over a period of 28 weeks. The first 2 weeks and the last 2 weeks were used for measurements and evaluation. The participants were randomly divided into one of two groups: a group with a high weekly frequency of three times a week (HIGH) and a group where participants attended the program with a low weekly rate of one workout per week (LOW). A blinded researcher was responsible for generating random numbers (random.org) for group placement. All measures were taken in the hospital department, while the training program was performed in a contracted sports center (from January to June 2017). Our study was designed, implemented, and reported per the CONSORT statement [27]. This study was registered at www.clinicaltrials.gov (registration code: NCT03410329).

2.2. Participants

An a priori power analysis was conducted to determine the sample size for the study (G*Power 3.1.9.2, Germany). The primary outcomes investigated in this research were phase angle, flexibility, and handgrip strength. The following design specifications were considered: $\alpha = 0.05$; $(1-\beta) = 0.8$; effect size $f = 0.25$; test family = F test and statistical test = ANOVA repeated measures. The sample size estimated according to these specifications was 34 subjects, 17 in each group. Thus, we selected 60 women patients referred to the Lifestyle program from the Department of Endocrinology of the "Infermi" hospital of Rimini, who volunteered to participate in this study. The inclusion criteria for participation in the treatment program were as follows: body mass index (BMI) greater than or equal to 30. We did not accept candidates who smoked, had cardiovascular disease or any other major illness, or were taking medications that could have affected the results.

All participants gave written informed consent after a detailed description of the study procedures was provided. The Project was conducted in accordance with the guidelines of the declaration of Helsinki and was approved by the local Bioethics Committee (approval code: 12012016).

2.3. Procedures

The supervised exercise program was specifically devised to favor a stepwise incremental approach to exercise. After enrollment, patients exercised in a gymnasium where a trained team supervised the individual progressive exercise program (120 min, for 24 weeks). At the beginning of each session, a series of respiratory, proprioceptive, and flexibility exercises were carried out, followed by progressively increasing resistance training. Resistance training consisted of an isotonic machine circuit for major muscle groups (four sets of 8–12 repetitions at 10RM for leg press, leg extension, lat machine, low row, chest press, pectoral machine, and shoulder press, with each set completed in approximately 30sec with 1min rest), with the 10RM level determined during the initial session by the exercise physiologist. Starting workload levels for each piece of equipment were tested by participants and if more than 10 repetitions were achieved, the weight was increased and after a short rest, the participants tried again. Likewise, if less than 8 repetitions were achieved, the weight was decreased and after a short rest, the participants tried again. The last part of each session was devoted to stretching.

The anthropometric traits were weight, height, and waist circumference (WC). All anthropometric measurements were taken according to standard methods [28]. Height was recorded to the nearest 0.1 cm with a stadiometer, and weight was measured to the nearest 0.1 kg with a high-precision mechanical scale. BMI was calculated as the ratio of body weight to height squared (kg/m^2). WC was taken to the nearest 0.1 cm with a tape measure.

Bioelectrical impedance was measured with a phase-sensitive impedance plethysmograph (BIA-101 Anniversary Sport Edition, Akern-RJL Systems, Florence, Italy). The device was used to obtain whole-body R and Xc at a single frequency (50 kHz) and was calibrated every morning, using a calibration circuit procedure of known impedance (R = 380 Ohm, Xc = 47 Ohm, 1% error) supplied by the manufacturer. Standard whole-body tetrapolar measurements were taken according to conventional procedures established in the literature [29]. Participants were instructed to urinate about 30 min before the measures, refrain from ingesting food or drink in the last 4 hours, avoid strenuous physical exercise for at least 24 hours, and refrain from consumption of alcoholic and caffeinated beverages for at least 48 hours. PA was calculated as the arctangent of $Xc/R \times 180°/\pi$. Bioimpedance vector analysis was carried out using the BIVA method, normalizing R and Xc parameters for height (H) in meters [30]. Fat mass percentage (F%) was predicted using the software Bodygram®(AkernSrl., Pontassieve, Florence, Italy).

Left and right handgrip strengths were measured to the nearest 0.5 kg with a mechanical dynamometer (Takei K.K. 5001, Takei Scientific Instruments, Ltd., Niigata City, Japan) in a sitting position by holding the dynamometer at a 90degree flexion of their elbow. Maximal readings of three measurements from both hands were recorded. Dominant handgrip strength (DHS) and total handgrip strength (THS) were measured. THS was as summed from readings of both hands [31].

2.4. Statistical Analyses

Normality was verified with the Shapiro–Wilk test. The main hypothesis was interpreted using analysis of variance for repeated measures (ANOVA two-way) for between- and within-group comparisons. When F-ratio was significant, Bonferroni's post hoc test was used for the identification of specific differences in the variables. Effect size (ES) was calculated as post-training mean minus pre-training mean divided by the pooled standard deviation. The ES values were then classified as follows: 0.20–0.49 was considered small, 0.50–0.79 was considered moderate, and ≥ 0.80 was considered large. Two-way analysis of covariance (ANCOVA) for repeated measures was applied for comparisons, using weight loss and menopausal status as covariates. The paired, one-sample Hotelling's T^{2}test was performed to determine if the changes in the mean group vectors (measured at the first and second time points) were significantly different from zero (null vector). A 95% confidence ellipse excluding the null vector indicated a significant vector displacement. Statistical significance for all analyses was defined as $p < 0.05$. SPSS (SPSS 23.0.0.0; SPSS Inc., Chicago, IL, USA) was used for all statistical calculations.

3. Results

The characteristics of the participants at baseline are shown in Table 1. The flow chart with a schematic representation of participant allocation is presented in Figure 1.

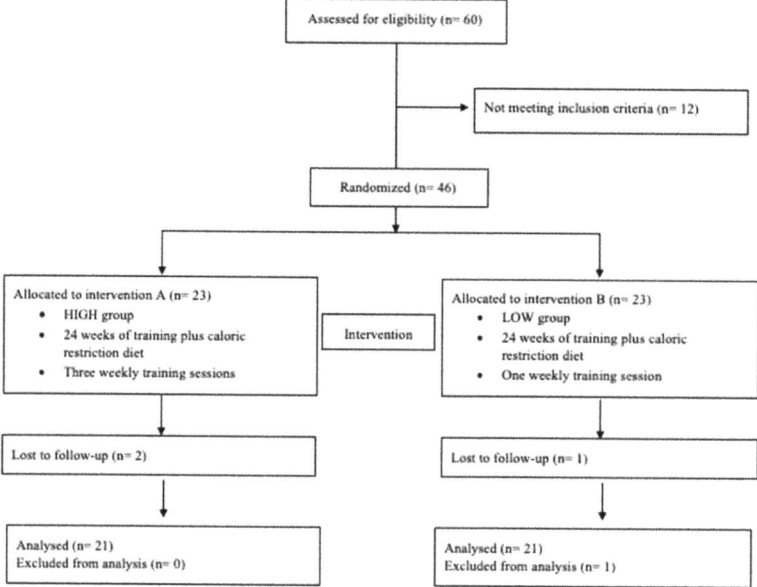

Figure 1. Flow chart.

Twenty-three women had been randomly assigned to a HIGH group (age 53.7 ± 9.3 years, BMI 37.9 ± 4.1 kg/m^2) and 23 to the LOW group (age 58.7 ± 8.5 years, BMI 36.2 ± 5.7 kg/m^2).

No significant differences in age (t = −1.540, p = 0.135) and BMI (t = 0.977, p = 0.337) were found between the two groups before the intervention period.

There was a significant group by time interaction for WC, Xc/H, PA, DHS, and THS. Post hoc revealed that in both groups, body weight, WC, and F% significantly decreased from before to after the intervention period, whereas Xc/H, PA, DHS, and THS increased only in the HIGH group after 24 weeks (Table 2). After adjusting for weight loss and menopausal status, as covariates, the group by time interaction for PA, DHS, and THS remained significant ($p < 0.05$).

Table 1. General characteristics of participants before the intervention period.

Variable	HIGH	LOW
Age (years)	53.7 ± 9.3	58.7 ± 8.5
BMI (kg/m^2)	37.9 ± 4.1	36.2 ± 5.7

Note: Data are expressed as mean and standard deviation. BMI: body mass index.

Table 2. Two-way ANOVA for the comparison between the groups before and after the intervention.

Variable	HIGH (n=21)		LOW (n=21)		ES §	Interaction P-Value	SP
	Before	After	Before	After			
Weight (kg)	96.8 ± 13.1	89.0 ± 12.4 *	88.4 ± 13.7	83.4 ± 10.8 *	−0.57	0.12	0.33
WC (cm)	108.4 ± 12.3	99.3 ± 11.5 *	107.9 ± 11.7	103.1 ± 11.3 *	−0.91	0.01	0.67
F (%)	39.7 ± 3.0	36.4 ± 3.3 *	39.3 ± 3.8	37.1 ± 3.9 *	−0.58	0.12	0.34
R/H (Ω)	299.1 ± 28.4	295.6 ± 28.8	303.3 ± 32.4	309.8 ± 33.8	−0.51	0.16	0.27
Xc/H (Ω)	31.3 ± 3.0	33.7 ± 2.0 *	33.9 ± 6.6	33.8 ± 6.23	0.77	0.04	0.52
PA (degrees)	6.0 ± 0.5	6.5 ± 0.5 *	6.2 ± 0.8	6.4 ± 0.6	0.86	0.02	0.62
DHS (kg)	24.0 ± 5.5	28.1 ± 5.4 *	23.0 ± 5.6	24.0 ± 5.2	1.03	<0.01	0.78
THS (kg)	45.9 ± 52.0	52.0 ± 9.4 *	43.5 ± 10.3	45.6 ± 10.7	0.80	0.03	0.56

Note: Data are expressed as mean and standard deviation. * $P < 0.05$ vs. before, WC: waist circumference, F: fat mass, R/H: resistance divided by body height, Xc/H: reactance divided by body height, PA: phase angle, DHS: dominant handgrip strength, THS: total handgrip strength, SP: statistical power, §: the Hedges' g effect size was used.

In Figure 2 is illustrated the bioelectrical impedance mean vector displacements against the 95%, 75%, and 50% tolerance ellipses of the reference population [32].

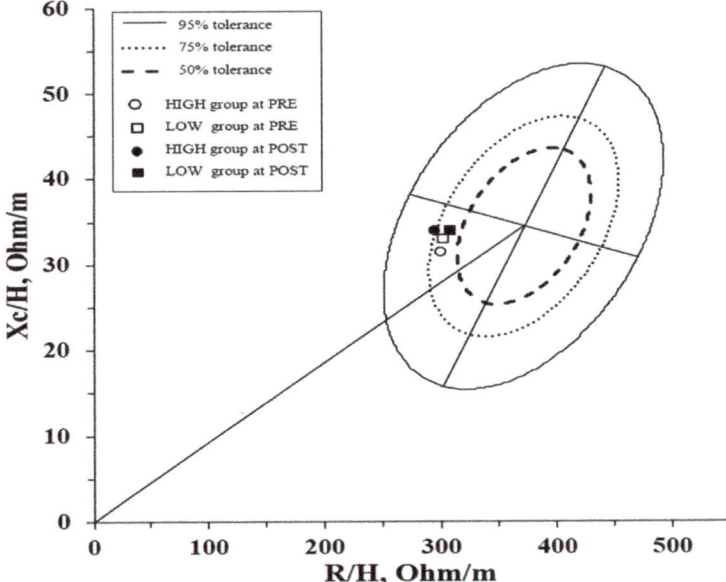

Figure 2. R-Xc graph and vector displacements from before (PRE) to after (POST) the intervention period using the mean R/H and the mean Xc/H plotted on the reference population tolerance ellipses [32]. HIGH: the group with a high-weekly training frequency of three times a week; LOW: the group that performed only one weekly session.

The paired one-sample Hotelling's T^2 test indicated a significant difference in the mean vectors between the first measurement and the second measurement only for the HIGH group (HIGH, $T^2 = 35.9$, $F = 16.7$, $p = < 0.01$, Mahalanobis D = 1.5; LOW, $T^2 = 1.7$, $F = 0.8$, $p = 0.5$, Mahalanobis D = 0.3) (Figure 3).

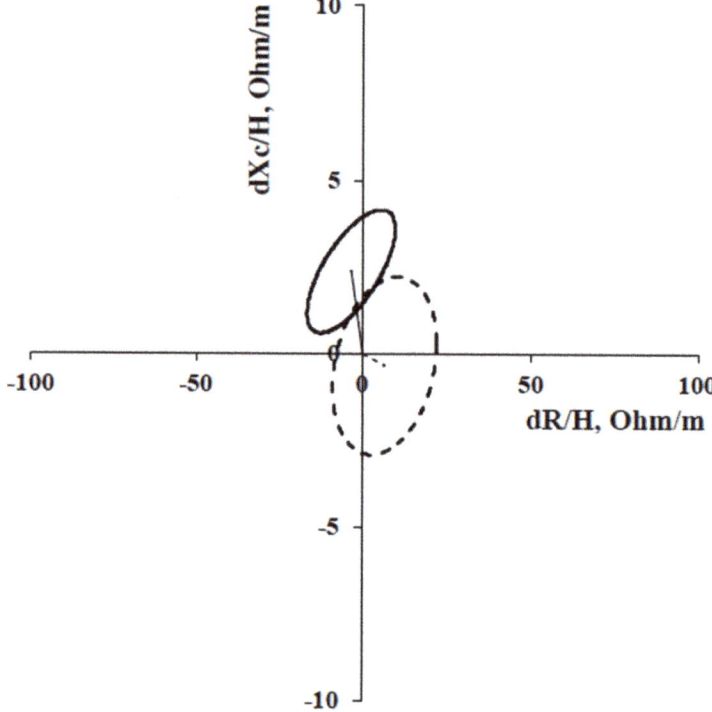

Figure 3. Paired Graph and impedance vector displacements with 95% confidence ellipses from before to after the intervention period. Continuous and dotted lines for the HIGH group and the LOW group, respectively. HIGH: the group with a high-weekly training frequency of three times a week; LOW: the group that performed only one weekly session.

4. Discussion

The aim of this study was to compare the effects of different weekly resistance training frequencies performed over a 24 week exercise program on PA and HS in obese people. Although both groups had an improvement trend after 26 weeks of intervention, the major effects on the examined parameters were measured in the group that performed the training program at a higher weekly frequency. In fact, although body weight, WC, and F% significantly decreased in both group after the intervention period, Xc/H, PA, DHS, and THS increased only in the group that performed the training program at a higher weekly frequency.

In the physical activity prescription, this study was based on the upper limit of the amount recommended by the American College of Sports Medicine in terms of both frequency and volume per session [33] and on the minimum frequency of physical activity suggested by WHO [26]. Our resistance training program has led to weight loss and a reduction in fat mass in participants, and this is in line with the findings of other authors [34,35]. However, there are conflicting reports in the literature on whether or not resistance training induces fat mass loss. Some studies report a statistically insignificant trend or no change in fat mass after a resistance training program [22,36]. These discrepancies in the results may be due to experimental designs that did not include a calorie restriction program or the fact that they considered fat mass in absolute and non-percentage terms with respect to body weight.

The literature is abundant about resistance training studies, but very little is known regarding the effects of different frequencies of weekly training on PA and HS. As demonstrated by our results, the choice of weekly training frequency causes different effects on the examined variables. However, it is well known that aging and a sedentary lifestyle cause a decrease in PA and HS [19,37], therefore even the results obtained by the LOW group, where no significant parameter changes were shown, are still noteworthy. Ribeiro et al. [37] showed improvements in PA following resistance training exercises carried out 3 times a week in obese women. In their study, the results after 8 weeks of training showed a significant reduction in resistance and no change in reactance. In our study, after 24 weeks of resistance training, even if R tended to decrease in the HIGH group, this change did not reach statistical significance. On the other hand, our results showed a significant increase in Xc after the intervention period. Changes in PA are determined by alteration in cellular membrane integrity (Xc) or body fluid (R) or a combination of both. Theoretically, high Xc values are expected from a BIA measurement in healthy membranes with higher integrity. The healthy cell membranes act as capacitors by storing the current and releasing it. In fact, Nescolarde et al. [38] showed that Xc and PA decrease after a muscle injury. Thus, Xc is proportional to cellmembrane integrity, with Xc and PA decrements occurring when the cell membrane is compromised. Our hypothesis states that in our study, the increase in PA was caused by an improvement in cellular membrane integrity, causing increases in Xc and a reduction in the ECW/ICW relationship, which is inversely proportionate to PA [14,15,39]. Furthermore, since R is inversely proportional to body fluid content, it could decrease absolutely following a reduction in body weight, causing a tendency to increase R and to elongate the vector in the R-Xc graph (Figure 2). On the contrary, increase in PA and therefore in the ICW/ECW ratio could cause a reduction in R, resulting in no significant variable change. However, as in our case, nutritional habits during the intervention period have not been monitored by Ribeiro et al. [37] and this may have caused a disparity of changes in Xc and R, which in both cases led to an increase in AP after a resistance training program in obese women. Recently, Norman et al. [40] have shown significant correlations between PA with muscle strength and other physical performance parameters, including the capability to perform daily activities. HS decreases with inactivity and aging [19], therefore the tendency to increase DHS and THS measured in the LOW group can be a noteworthy result. Our view is that high-frequency training is crucial in the development of strength, which plays also an important role in cardiovascular health. On this point, Lee et al. [41] reported that HS is correlated with cardiometabolic risk factors including blood pressure, triglyceride, HDL cholesterol, HbA1c, and fasting glucose.

Despite the encouraging results obtained in this study, some limitations are present and should be considered. First, our results are applicable to BIA equipment using the 50 kHz frequency and to a similar population. In fact, in a recent study by Silva and colleagues [42], a comparison between single (50 kHz) and multi-frequency devices was conducted in a highly active population. The authors found that multi-frequency instruments provided significantly lower values of R and Xc but higher values of PA at 50kHz.Second, although BIA is used in clinical and sports fields to reflect body fluids, nutritional state, and phase angle [29,43–45], it is not a direct measurement method of body composition. In particular, in this study, F% was determined from the bioimpedance raw parameters rather than by a gold standard method. Third, glucose level and cardiovascular risk factors changes were not monitored during the experiment. Lastly, we were not able to monitor physical activity levels outside of the study environment and to track dietary intake throughout the study, though individuals were asked to maintain their usual lifestyle habits. Further evidence on the subject could be collected, contributing to this particular field of research and supporting the work of clinicians working with physical exercise for obese people.

5. Conclusions

Resistance training is effective to induce improvement in body composition, but increases of PA and HS can only be achieved with a high training frequency. From our observations, a high training frequency gave greater benefits for the health status than a training program with only one weekly session. Moreover, BIVA can help to evaluate and monitor health status and effectiveness of physical activity programs. There is considerable scope for researchers and trainers to contribute to reducing the problem of obesity and its related consequences.

Author Contributions: Conceptualization, F.C. and S.T.; methodology, F.C. and L.B.; software, F.C and F.S.; formal analysis, P.M.; investigation, F.C. and L.B.; data curation, F.C and F.S.; writing—original draft preparation, G.B., F.C., F.S., L.B., S.T.; visualization, G.B., F.C.; supervision, S.T., L.B., F.S., P.M.; project administration, F.C. All authors have read and agreed to the published version of the manuscript.

Funding: This research received no external funding.

Acknowledgments: The authors are grateful to all the participants who took part in this study and to the research assistants who contributed to the collection of data and to the supervision of the Lifestyle program.

Conflicts of Interest: The authors declare no conflict of interest.

References

1. Mackey, E.R.; Olson, A.; Di Fazio, M.; Cassidy, O. Obesity Prevention and Screening. *Prim. Care* **2016**, *43*, 39–51. [CrossRef] [PubMed]
2. Smith, K.B.; Smith, M.S. Obesity Statistics. *Prim. Care* **2016**, *43*, 121–135. [CrossRef] [PubMed]
3. Gallus, S.; Odone, A.; Lugo, A.; Bosetti, C.; Colombo, P.; Zuccaro, P.; LaVecchia, C. Overweight and obesity prevalence and determinants in Italy: An update to 2010. *Eur. J. Nutr.* **2016**, *52*, 677–685. [CrossRef] [PubMed]
4. NCD Risk Factor Collaboration (NCD-RisC). Worldwide trends in body-mass index, underweight, overweight, and obesity from 1975 to 2016: A pooled analysis of 2416 population-based measurement studies in 128·9 million children, adolescents, and adults. *Lancet* **2017**, *390*, 2627–2642. [CrossRef]
5. World Health Organization (WHO). Global Database on Body Mass Index. 2011. Available online: http://apps.who.int/bmi/index.jsp (accessed on 12 December 2019).
6. Farrag, N.S.; Cheskin, L.J.; Farag, M.K. A systematic review of childhood obesity in the Middle East and North Africa (MENA) region: Health impact and management. *Adv. Pediatr. Res.* **2017**, *4*, 6. [PubMed]
7. Huck, C.J. Effects of supervised resistance training on fitness and functional strength in patients succeeding bariatric surgery. *J. Strength Cond. Res.* **2015**, *29*, 589–595. [CrossRef]
8. Ma, C.; Avenell, A.; Bolland, M.; Hudson, J.; Stewart, F.; Robertson, C.; Sharma, P.; Fraser, C.; MacLennan, G. Effects of weight loss interventions for adults who are obese on mortality, cardiovascular disease, and cancer: Systematic review and meta-analysis. *BMJ* **2017**, *359*, j4849. [CrossRef]
9. Scott, D.; Harrison, C.L.; Hutchison, S.; de Courten, B.; Stepto, N.K. Exploring factors related to changes in body composition, insulin sensitivity and aerobic capacity in response to a 12-week exercise intervention in overweight and obese women with and without polycystic ovary syndrome. *PLoS ONE* **2017**, *12*, e0182412. [CrossRef]
10. Lukaski, H.C.; Vega Diaz, N.; Talluri, A.; Nescolarde, L. Classification of Hydration in Clinical Conditions: Indirect and Direct Approaches Using Bioimpedance. *Nutrients* **2019**, *11*, 809. [CrossRef]
11. Campa, F.; Matias, C.; Gatterer, H.; Toselli, S.; Koury, J.C.; Andreoli, A.; Melchiorri, G.; Sardinha, L.B.; Silva, A.M. Classic Bioelectrical Impedance Vector Reference Values for Assessing Body Composition in Male and Female Athletes. *Int. J. Environ. Res. Public Health* **2019**, *16*, 5066. [CrossRef]
12. Campa, F.; Silva, A.M.; Iannuzzi, V.; Mascherini, G.; Benedetti, L.; Toselli, S. The role of somatic maturation on bioimpedance patterns and body composition in male elite youth soccer players. *Int. J. Environ. Res. Public Health* **2019**, *16*, 4711. [CrossRef]
13. Campa, F.; Toselli, S. Bioimpedance Vector Analysis of Elite, Subelite, and Low-Level Male Volleyball Players. *Int J. Sports Physiol. Perform.* **2018**, *13*, 1250–1253. [CrossRef] [PubMed]
14. Campa, F.; Matias, C.N.; Marini, E.; Heymsfield, S.B.; Toselli, S.; Sardinha, L.B.; Silva, A.M. Identifying Athlete Body-Fluid Changes During a Competitive Season With Bioelectrical Impedance Vector Analysis. *Int. J. Sports Physiol. Perform.* **2019**. [CrossRef] [PubMed]
15. Marini, E.; Campa, F.; Buffa, R.; Stagi, S.; Matias, C.N.; Toselli, S.; Sardinha, L.B.; Silva, A.M. Phase angle and bioelectrical impedance vector analysis in the evaluation of body composition in athletes. *Clin. Nutr.* **2019**. [CrossRef] [PubMed]
16. Barrea, L.; Muscogiuri, G.; Laudisio, D.; Di Somma, C.; Salzano, C.; Pugliese, G.; de Alteriis, G.; Colao, A.; Savastano, S. Phase Angle: A Possible Biomarker to Quantify Inflammation in Subjects with Obesity and 25(OH)D Deficiency. *Nutrients* **2019**, *11*, 1747. [CrossRef] [PubMed]

17. Tomeleri, C.M.; Cavaglieri, C.R.; de Souza, M.F.; Cavalcante, E.F.; Antunes, M.; Nabbuco, H.C.G.; Venturini, D.; Sabbatini Barbosa, D.; Silva, A.M.; Cyrino, E.S. Phase angle is related with inflammatory and oxidative stress biomarkers in older women. *Exp. Gerontol.* **2018**, *102*, 12–18. [CrossRef] [PubMed]
18. De Luis, D.A.; Aller, R.; Romero, E.; Dueñas, A.; Perez Castrillon, J.L. Relation of phase angle tertiles with blood adipocytokines levels, insulin resistance and cardiovascular risk factors in obese women patients. *Eur. Rev. Med. Pharmacol. Sci.* **2010**, *14*, 521–526.
19. Campa, F.; Silva, A.M.; Toselli, S. Changes in Phase Angle and Handgrip Strength Induced by Suspension Training in Older Women. *Int. J. Sports Med.* **2018**, *39*, 442–449. [CrossRef] [PubMed]
20. Nunes, J.P.; Ribeiro, A.S.; Silva, A.M.; Schoenfeld, B.J.; Dos Santos, L.; Cunha, P.M.; Nascimento, M.A.; Tomeleri, C.M.; Nabuco, H.C.G.; Antunes, M.; et al. Improvements in Phase Angle Are Related With Muscle Quality Index After Resistance Training in Older Women. *J. Aging Phys. Act.* **2019**, *27*, 515–520. [CrossRef]
21. Roberts, H.C.; Denison, H.J.; Martin, H.J.; Patel, H.P.; Syddall, H.; Cooper, C.; Sayer, A.A. A review of the measurement of grip strength in clinical and epidemiological studies: Towards a standardised approach. *Age Ageing* **2011**, *40*, 423–429. [CrossRef]
22. Dos Santos, L.; Cyrino, E.S.; Antunes, M.; Santos, D.A.; Sardinha, L.B. Changes in phase angle and body composition induced by resistance training in older women. *Eur. J. Clin. Nutr.* **2016**, *70*, 1408–1413. [CrossRef] [PubMed]
23. Tomeleri, C.M.; Ribeiro, A.S.; Cavaglieri, C.R.; Deminice, R.; Schoenfeld, B.J.; Schiavoni, D.; Dos Santos, L.; de Souza, M.F.; Antunes, M.; Venturini, D. Correlations between resistance training-induced changes on phase angle and biochemical markers in older women. *Scand. J. Med. Sci. Sports* **2018**, *28*, 2173–2182. [CrossRef] [PubMed]
24. Ribeiro, A.S.; Avelar, A.; Dos Santos, L.; Silva, A.M.; Gobbo, L.A.; Schoenfeld, B.J.; Sardinha, L.B.; Cyrino, E.S. Hypertrophy-type Resistance Training Improves Phase Angle in Young Adult Men and Women. *Int. J. Sports Med.* **2017**, *38*, 35–40. [CrossRef] [PubMed]
25. Souza, M.F.; Tomeleri, C.M.; Ribeiro, A.S.; Schoenfeld, B.J.; Silva, A.M.; Sardinha, L.B.; Cyrino, E.S. Effect of resistance training on phase angle in older women: A randomized controlled trial. *Scand. J. Med. Sci. Sports* **2017**, *27*, 1308–1316. [CrossRef]
26. World Health Organisation (WHO). Global Recomendations on Physical Activity for Health. 2010. Available online: http://www.whqlibdoc.who.int/publications/2010/9789241599979_eng.pdf (accessed on 14 December 2019).
27. Schulz, K.F.; Altman, D.G.; Moher, D.; CONSORT Group. CONSORT 2010 statement: Updated guidelines for reporting parallel group randomised trials. *J. Clin. Epidemiol.* **2010**, 834–840. [CrossRef]
28. Lohman, T.G.; Roche, A.F.; Martorell, R. *Anthropometric Standardization Reference Manual*; Human Kinetics Books: Champaign, IL, USA, 1988.
29. Lukaski, H.; Piccoli, A. Bioelectrical impedance vector analysis for assessment of hydration in physiological states and clinical conditions. In *Handbook of Anthropometry*; Preedy, V., Ed.; Springer: London, UK, 2012; pp. 287–305.
30. Piccoli, A.; Rossi, B.; Pillon, L.; Bucciante, G. A new method for monitoring body fluid variation by bioimpedance analysis: The RXc graph. *Kidney Int.* **1994**, *46*, 534–539. [CrossRef]
31. Choquette, S.; Bouchard, D.R.; Sénéchal, M.; Brochu, M.; Dionne, I.J. Relative strength as a determinant of mobility in elders 67–84 years of age. anuage study: Nutrition as a determinant of successfulaging. *J. Nutr. Health Aging* **2010**, *14*, 190–195. [CrossRef]
32. Piccoli, A.; Nigrelli, S.; caberlotto, A.; Bottazzo, S.; Rossi, B.; Pillon, S.; Maggiore, Q. Bivariate normal values of the bioelectrical impedance vector in adult and elderly populations. *Am. J. Clin. Nutr.* **1995**, *61*, 269–270. [CrossRef]
33. Whaley, M.H.; Brubaker, P.H.; Otto editors, R.M. *ACSM's Guidelines for Exercise Testing and Prescription*. Baltimore; Lippincott Williams & Wilkins: Baltimore, MD, USA, 2006.
34. Straight, C.R.; Dorfman, L.R.; Cottell, K.E.; Krol, J.M.; Lofgren, I.E.; Delmonico, M.J. Effects of resistance training and dietary changes on physical function and body composition in overweight and obese older adults. *J. Phys. Act. Health* **2002**, *9*, 875–883. [CrossRef]
35. Beavers, K.M.; Ambrosius, W.T.; RejeskiBurdette, J.H.; Walkup, M.P.; Sheedy, J.L.; Nesbit, A.B.; Gaukstern, J.E.; Nicklas, B.J.; Marsh, A.P. Effect of Exercise Type During Intentional Weight Loss on Body Composition in Older Adults with Obesity. *Obesity* **2017**, *25*, 1823–1829. [CrossRef]

36. Hansen, D.; Dendale, P.; Berger van Loon, L.J.; Meeusen, R. The effects of exercise training on fat-mass loss in obese patients during energy intake restriction. *Sports Med.* **2007**, *37*, 31–46. [CrossRef] [PubMed]
37. Ribeiro, A.S.; Schoenfeld, B.J.; Dos Santos, L.; Nunes, J.P.; Tomeleri, C.M.; Cunha, P.M.; Sardinha, L.B.; Cyrino, E.S. Resistance Training Improves a Cellular Health Parameter in Obese Older Women: A Randomized Controlled Trial. *J. Strength Cond. Res.* **2018**, *00*, 1–7. [CrossRef] [PubMed]
38. Nescolarde, L.; Yanguas, J.; Lukaski, H.; Alomar, X.; Rosell-Ferrer, J.; Rodas, G. Localizedbioimpedance to assess muscle injury. *Physiol. Meas.* **2013**, *34*, 237–245. [CrossRef] [PubMed]
39. Francisco, R.; Matias, C.N.; Santos, D.A.; Campa, F.; Minderico, C.S.; Rocha, P.; Heymsfield, S.B.; Lukaski, H.; Sardinha, L.B.; Silva, A.M. The Predictive Role of Raw Bioelectrical Impedance Parameters in Water Compartments and Fluid Distribution Assessed by Dilution Techniques in Athletes. *Int. J. Environ. Res. Public Health* **2020**, *17*, 759. [CrossRef] [PubMed]
40. Norman, K.; Stobäus, N.; Pirlich, M.; Bosy-Westphal, A. Bioelectrical phase angle and impedance vector analysis–clinical relevance and applicability of impedance parameters. *Clin. Nutr.* **2012**, *31*, 854–861. [CrossRef]
41. Lee, W.J.; Peng, L.N.; Chiou, S.T.; Chen, L.K. Relative Handgrip Strength Is a Simple Indicator of Cardiometabolic Risk among Middle-Aged and Older People: A Nationwide Population-Based Study in Taiwan. *PLoS ONE* **2016**, *11*, e0160876. [CrossRef]
42. Silva, A.M.; Matias, C.N.; Nunes, C.L.; Santos, D.A.; Marini, E.; Lukaski, H.C.; Sardinha, L.B. Lack of agreement of in vivo raw bioimpedance measurements obtained from two single and multi-frequency bioelectrical impedance devices. *Eur. J. Clin. Nutr.* **2019**, *73*, 1077–1083. [CrossRef]
43. Campa, F.; Gatterer, H.; Lukaski, H.; Toselli, S. Stabilizing Bioimpedance-Vector-Analysis Measures Witha 10-Minute Cold Shower After Running Exercise to Enable Assessment of Body Hydration. *Int. J. Sports Physiol. Perform.* **2019**, *14*, 1006–1009. [CrossRef]
44. Khazem, S.; Itani, L.; Kreidieh, D.; El Masri, D.; Tannir, H.; Citarella, R.; El Ghroch, M. Reduced Lean Body Mass and Cardiometabolic Diseases in Adult Males with Overweight and Obesity: A Pilot Study. *Int. J. Environ. Res. Public Health* **2018**, *15*, 2754. [CrossRef]
45. Toselli, S.; Marini, E.; MaiettaLatessa, P.; Benedetti, L.; Campa, F. Maturity Related Differences in Body Composition Assessed by Classic and Specific Bioimpedance Vector Analysis among Male Elite Youth Soccer Players. *Int. J. Environ. Res. Public Health* **2020**, *17*, 729. [CrossRef]

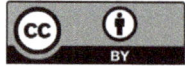

© 2020 by the authors. Licensee MDPI, Basel, Switzerland. This article is an open access article distributed under the terms and conditions of the Creative Commons Attribution (CC BY) license (http://creativecommons.org/licenses/by/4.0/).

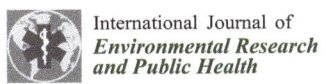 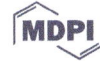

International Journal of
Environmental Research and Public Health

Article

The Effects of Dehydration on Metabolic and Neuromuscular Functionality during Cycling

Francesco Campa [1,2,*], **Alessandro Piras** [2], **Milena Raffi** [2], **Aurelio Trofè** [1], **Monica Perazzolo** [2], **Gabriele Mascherini** [3] **and Stefania Toselli** [2]

1. Department for Life Quality Studies, University of Bologna, 47921 Rimini, Italy; aurelio.trofe2@unibo.it
2. Department of Biomedical and Neuromotor Sciences, University of Bologna, 40126 Bologna, Italy; alessandro.piras3@unibo.it (A.P.); milena.raffi@unibo.it (M.R.); monica.perazzolo2@unibo.it (M.P.); stefania.toselli@unibo.it (S.T.)
3. Department of Experimental and Clinical Medicine, University of Florence, AOUC, 50139 Careggi, Florence, Italy; gabriele.mascherini@unifi.it
* Correspondence: francesco.campa3@unibo.it; Tel.: +39-051-2094195; Fax: +39-051-2094286

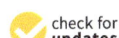

Received: 14 January 2020; Accepted: 10 February 2020; Published: 12 February 2020

Abstract: This study aimed to determine the effects of dehydration on metabolic and neuromuscular functionality performance during a cycling exercise. Ten male subjects (age 23.4 ± 2.7 years; body weight 74.6 ± 10.4 kg; height 177.3 ± 4.6 cm) cycled at 65% VO_{2max} for 60 min followed by a time-to-trial (TT) at 95% VO_{2max}, in two different conditions: dehydration (DEH) and hydration (HYD). The bioelectrical impedance vector analysis (BIVA) and body weight measurements were performed to assess body fluid changes. Heart rate (HR), energy cost, minute ventilation, oxygen uptake, and metabolic power were evaluated during the experiments. In addition, neuromuscular activity of the vastus medialis and biceps femoris muscles were assessed by surface electromyography. After exercise induced dehydration, the bioimpedance vector significantly lengthens along the major axis of the BIVA graph, in conformity with the body weight change (−2%), that indicates a fluid loss. Metabolic and neuromuscular parameters significantly increased during TT at 95% VO_{2max} with respect to constant workload at 65% of VO_{2max}. Dehydration during a one-hour cycling test and subsequent TT caused a significant increase in HR, while neuromuscular function showed a lower muscle activation in dehydration conditions on both constant workload and on TT. Furthermore, a significant difference between HYD and DEH for TT duration was found.

Keywords: bioimpedance; BIVA; body composition; hydration status; phase angle; vector length

1. Introduction

Analyzing and monitoring body composition combined with the search for optimal physical condition and recovery of physiological parameters in high-level athletes have always been topics of study for researchers, trainers, and coaches [1–3]. For decades, the relationship between hydration status and performance has been closely evaluated, with hydration status being directly linked with physical performance. Many studies have reported the consequences of dehydration on physical and mental levels, highlighting humoral changes and cognitive deficits, which not only compromise normal daily activities but can negatively affect sports performance [4–6]. More specifically, it has been shown that the inadequate restoration of fluids during exercise compromises neuromuscular function, increases fatigue perception, reduces technical skills, affecting metabolic and autonomic nervous system parameters [7–10].

The National Athletic Trainers' Association (NATA) recommends using a combination of methods to assess hydration status, including body mass change, urine color or urine specific gravity (USG) after first morning void, as well as thirst level to track hydration status [11]. Studies show that only a loss of 1% to 2% of body mass from sweating is enough to compromise physiological functioning and sport performance during exercise. On the contrary, maintenance of body water during exercise is thought to provide protection from thermal injury, reduce physiological strain and maintain or even improve sport performance [11,12]. Recently, it has been shown that the BIVA method is capable of measuring changes in body composition in the short and long term, even after exercise [13–16]. This method plots the impedance parameters [resistance (R) and reactance (Xc)] standardized for the subject's height on a graph as a single vector [17], where the shortening or lengthening of vectors represents fluid loss or gain respectively [18,19]. R arises from Extracellular Water (ECW) and Intracellular Water (ICW). Conversely, Xc arises from cell membranes and represents the cell membrane's quality of taking an electric load and liberate it in a second moment, after a brief delay; it could be compared to a vessel-capacitance-like property [20].

There is still an incomplete picture regarding the loss of fluids due to exercise and its relationship with physical performance variables. Despite the importance of maintaining a euhydrated state, studies have shown individuals are not adequately replacing fluid during exercise [21]. Although many studies have investigated the physiological responses to dehydration [4–12], to our knowledge, no research has evaluated the impact of dehydration on both metabolic and neuromuscular variables during performance in active males. Therefore, the purpose of our study was to investigate the effects of progressive dehydration on heart rate (HR), oxygen uptake (VO_2), energetic cost, and neuromuscular functionality during both submaximal cycling exercise at a constant work rate and subsequent time-to-trial (TT) performance.

2. Materials and Methods

2.1. Participants

We recruited ten active male subjects (age 23.4 ± 2.7 years; body weight 74.6 ± 10.4 kg; height 177.3 ± 4.6 cm) who volunteered to participate in this study. The following inclusion criteria were used: (1) a minimum of 10 hours of training per week; (2) tested negative for performance-enhancing drugs, and (3) not taking any medications. Subjects were instructed to avoid physical activity in the 48 hours prior to the tests and to refrain from consuming alcohol and caffeine for at least 24 hours. After being informed on the objectives and the research procedures, participants signed the consent document. The study was approved by the Bioethics Committee of the University of Bologna (No. 25027).

2.2. Procedures

The participants visited the laboratory three times. All tests were performed at the same time of the day (9:00–12:00 AM), in a quiet room with stable temperature (21 °C; 52% of humidity). On the first visit, subjects performed an incremental cycling test to exhaustion on an electronically braked cycle ergometer (LODE Excalibur, Quinton Instrument, Groningen, the Netherlands) to determine the VO_{2max}. The expired gas analysis was performed with the Quark CPET device (Cosmed, Pavona, RM, Italy) while subjects cycled at 30 W for 3 min as a warm-up, followed by an instantaneous increase of 1 W every 2s at a cadence between 70–80 rpm [22] The maximal exercise test lasted until VO_2 plateau was obtained or at least one of the two additional criteria: (i) a plateau of heart rate despite an increased velocity or (ii) exercise cessation due to substantial fatigue. VO_2 plateau was defined as an increase in $VO_2 \leq 50$ ml min^{-1} during the last 30s despite increased power [23]. Heart rate (HR) was collected using a Polar RS400 downloadable HR monitor (Polar Electro, Lachine, QC). All data collected and analyzed at visit one was used to individualize the load (at 65 and 95% of VO_{2max}) of each participant.

During the second and third visits, separated by 1 week, the athletes were tested in a randomized, counterbalanced, crossover design (Figure 1); subjects returned to the laboratory and cycled at 65% VO_{2max} for 60 min followed by a TT at 95% VO_{2max}, in two different conditions: dehydration (DEH) and hydration (HYD). During the dehydration, subjects completed the trial without ingesting fluids [12,24]. Instead, during the hydration condition, the athletes drank 1 L of water subdivided in 4 steps interspersed by 15 min each other, removing the metabolimeter mask and consuming 0.250 mL of water [25].

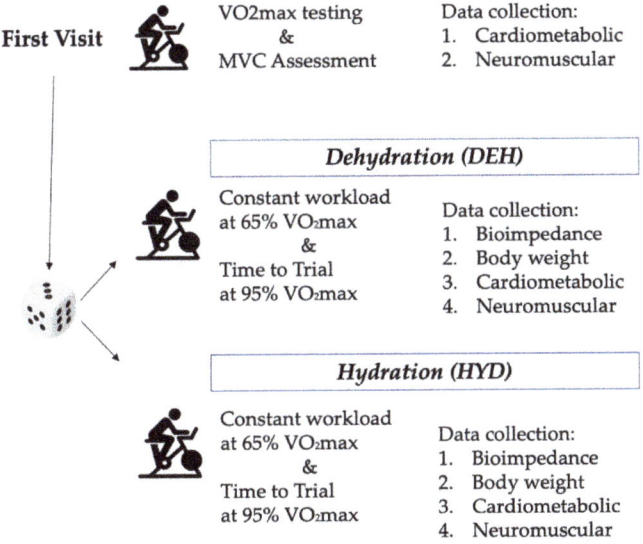

Figure 1. Graphical overview of the testing protocol with the timeline of events.

At the early morning, before eating breakfast, subjects were weighed (SECA model, Chino, California, USA) 874 with precision to 0.01 kg); then, two hours prior to the cycling, they ingested a meal of 790 kcal; 144 g carbohydrate, 35 g fat, 19 g protein. Additionally, they drank as they normally would the night before and drank 300 mL of water 90 and 45 min before the trial to ensure they were well hydrated before cycling [12]. After the TT, subjects were weighed again to determine their body mass loss over the trial. In addition, to assess fluid loss, bioelectric impedance was measured before cycling (T1) and after 10-minute of shower (T2) according to the procedures reported by Campa et al. [26]. The impedance measurements were performed with a bioimpedance analyzer (BIA 101 Anniversary, Akern, Florence, Italy) using a phase-sensitive device with alternating current at a frequency of 50 kHz. The accuracy of the bioimpedance instrument was validated before each test session following the manufacturer's instructions. Bioimpedance values were analyzed according to the BIVA method [17]. Bioelectrical phase angle was calculated as the arc tangent of $Xc/R \times 180°/\pi$, while the vector length as the hypotenuses of individual impedance values.

Electromyographic (EMG) data were acquired by a Free-EMG (BTS Bioengineering Corp, MA, USA) using Ag/Ag Cl disposable electrodes 32×32 mm in a bipolar configuration (RAM Apparecchi Medicali s.r.l., GE, Italy) Electrodes had an active area of 0.8 cm^2 with an inter-electrode distance of about 2 cm. The skin was shaved and cleaned with ethanol before placing the electrodes to improve the contact with the skin. Electrodes were positioned on the muscular belly of the following muscles of the right leg: vastus medialis (RVM) and biceps femoris (RBF). After placing the electrodes, we acquired the maximum voluntary contraction (MVC) in which each subject had to perform, for 5 s, an isometric contraction against a maximum load using isotonic machines (Technogym, Cesena, FC, Italy). Data was recorded at a sample rate of 1000 Hz and stored for analysis. All raw EMG signals were band pass filtered (20–450 Hz), positively rectified and resampled at 500 Hz. The EMG signals were normalized to the peak of the MVC. Onset and offset times were determined using the double threshold method [27]. The first threshold occurred when the value of the signal exceeded 3SD above the baseline signal, and the second threshold required the signal to remain above this value for at least

30 ms [28]. The criteria used for the first threshold was based on a minimum threshold of 3 SD above the resting baseline signal and a minimum burst duration of 100 ms. The normalized root mean square (RMS) values were calculated in a time window of 100 ms using Matlab (The Mathworks Inc., Natick, Massachusetts, USA).

In both cycling trials, the energetic cost (EC) was calculated considering data when a metabolic steady state was reached by all subjects [29,30]. The breath-by-breath net oxygen uptake (VO_{2NET}, expressed in ml/min/kg), calculated by subtracting the resting VO_2 (assumed equal to 3.6 ml/min/kg) from VO_2 values, and the respiratory exchange ratio (RER) were used to determine the instantaneous metabolic power (expressed in W/kg) as VO_{2NET} [(4.94 · RER + 16.04)/60] [30].

2.3. Statistical Analysis

Descriptive statistics including means ± SD and data distribution were calculated for all outcome variables. The normal distribution of the data was checked using the Shapiro–Wilk test; thus, the following parametric tests were used: A 2 (condition: hydration/dehydration) × 2 (Time: T1/T2 for bioimpedance and constant workload/Time-to-trial for metabolic and neuromuscular variables) for repeated measure ANOVA was performed. Effect sizes were calculated using partial eta squared (ηp^2). The paired one-sample Hotelling's T^2-test was performed to determine if the changes in the mean group vectors (measured between T1 vs. T2) were significantly different from zero (null vector). A 95% confidence ellipse excluding the null vector indicated a significant vector displacement. Data was analyzed with IBM SPSS Statistics version 24.0 (IBM, Chicago, IL, USA), BIVA software [31], and Bodygram TM software (Akern, Florence, Italy). For all tests, statistical significance was set at $p < 0.05$.

3. Results

3.1. Bioimpedance d-Data

Table 1 shows the changes in the bioelectric values. R/H, Xc/H (where H represents height measured in meters) and vector length significantly changed ($p < 0.05$) in T2 compared to T1 in the DEH condition. On the contrary, when the athletes performed the trial in the HYD condition, the same values did not change.

Table 1. Bioimpedance parameters before and after the exercise in both tests.

		T1	T2	ANOVA	
		Mean ± SD	Mean ± SD	Time Effect	Time × Condition
R/H (Ω/m)	HYD	259.9 ± 36.4	260.4 ± 36.9	$F = 79.1; p = <0.001;$ $\eta^2_p = 0.82$	$F = 67.8; p = <0.001;$ $\eta^2_p = 0.79$
	DEH	255.6 ± 35.8	267.4 ± 36.1 *		
Xc/H (Ω/m)	HYD	35.2 ± 5.4	35.3 ± 5.4	$F = 56.3; p = <0.001;$ $\eta^2_p = 0.76$	$F = 50.1; p = <0.001;$ $\eta^2_p = 0.73$
	DEH	34.7 ± 6.9	36.9 ± 4.9 *		
Vector length (Ω/m)	HYD	262.3 ± 36.7	262.8 ± 37.2	$F = 82.8; p = <0.001;$ $\eta^2_p = 0.82$	$F = 71.1; p = <0.001;$ $\eta^2_p = 0.79$
	DEH	257.9 ± 36.1	269.9 ± 36.4 *		
Phase angle (°)	HYD	7.7 ± 0.5	7.8 ± 0.4	$F = 3.7; p = 0.07;$ $\eta^2_p = 0.17$	$F = 3.8; p = 0.67;$ $\eta^2_p = 0.17$
	DEH	7.7 ± 0.4	7.9 ± 0.4		

Note: HYD: hydration condition; DEH: dehydration condition; * = $p < 0.05$ vs. T1.

The averages of body weight of athletes in T0 were 74.7 ± 10.4 kg and 74.9 ± 10.3 kg in HYD and DHE conditions, respectively. After both trials body weight showed a significant decrease by measuring 74.5 ± 10.5 kg in HYD ($p = 0.005$) and 73.5 ± 10.3 kg in DEH ($p < 0.001$). When the athletes performed the DEH trial, their body weight decreased by 1.76% ± 0.39%, while when they performed the HYD trial their body weight decreased by 0.3% ± 0.27%.

Figure 2 shows the vector displacements (on the left side) and the Hotelling's T^2 test results (on the right side) for DEH and HYD conditions, panel A and B, respectively.

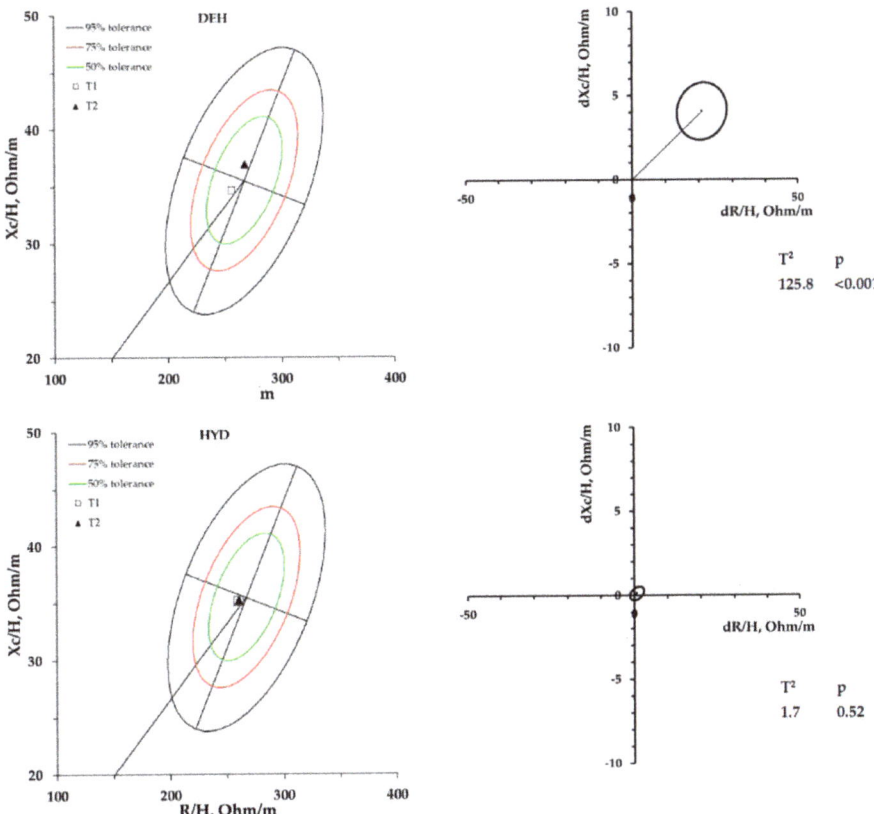

Figure 2. On the left side mean impedance vectors, plotted on the 50%, 75%, and 95% tolerance ellipses of the male athlete's endurance reference population [32] are displayed both for DEH and HYD trial. On the right side, mean vector displacements and results of the Hotelling's T^2 test.

3.2. Cardiometabolic Data

Table 2 shows the comparisons of exercise duration, power output and cardiometabolic parameters between HYD and DEH on both exercise condition. We found significant differences on time main effect ($p < 0.001$) for all parameters, in which mean values were higher during TT with respect to constant workload at 65% of VO_{2max}. Moreover, we found a condition mean effect for duration ($F_{1,8} = 8.24$; $p = 0.021$; $n_p^2 = 0.51$; 95%CI = 5.3–48.9) and for HR ($F_{1,8} = 55.21$; $p < 0.001$; $n_p^2 = 0.87$; 95%CI = 2.9–5.5). Post-hoc analysis showed significant differences between HYD and DEH for duration on TT and for HR during both constant workload and TT (Table 2).

Table 2. Comparison (mean ± SD) of the exercise duration, power output, and cardiometabolic parameters between hydration status on both exercise conditions.

Variable	Constant Workload (65% VO$_2$max)					Time-to-Trial (95% VO$_2$max)				
	HYD	DEH	Mean Diff	p	d	HYD	DEH	Mean Diff	p	d
Duration (min)	-	-	-	-	-	3.19 ± 0.60	2.39 ± 0.61	0.80	* 0.027	1.32
VO$_2$ (ml/Kg/min)	31.41 ± 4.28	31.70 ± 4.88	−0.29	0.616	−0.06	43.79 ± 6.51	43.59 ± 8.89	0.21	0.904	0.03
RER	0.93 ± 0.06	0.94 ± 0.04	−0.01	0.400	−0.26	1.10 ± 0.10	1.07 ± 0.07	0.04	0.344	0.43
EC (W/Kg)	9.55 ± 1.40	9.68 ± 1.64	−0.14	0.436	−0.09	14.26 ± 2.41	14.21 ± 3.11	0.05	0.925	0.02
HR (bpm)	136.22 ± 8.75	139.53 ± 8.12	−3.31	* 0.005	−0.39	166.56 ± 8.91	171.65 ± 7.89	−5.09	* 0.002	−0.60
Power (Watt)	147.56 ± 29.64	147.56 ± 29.64	0.00	-	-	280.67 ± 56.24	280.67 ± 56.24	0.00	-	-

Note: HYD: hydration condition; DEH: dehydration condition; RER: respiratory exchange ratio; EC: energetic cost; HR: hear rate; p-value and Cohen's d; *= significant differences between hydration status on each exercise condition ($p < 0.05$).

3.3. Neuromuscular Data

Table 3 shows the comparison of the normalized RMS values of RVM and RBF muscles between the two-hydration status on both exercise condition. During cycling, significant differences were observed for time and condition main effect on both RVM (Time: $F_{1,7} = 96.45$; $p < 0.001$; $n_p^2 = 0.93$; 95%CI = 10.8–17.8; Condition: $F_{1,7} = 13.16$; $p = 0.008$; $n_p^2 = 0.65$; 95%CI = 2.7–13.2) and RBF muscles (Time: $F_{1,7} = 33.46$; $p = 0.001$; $n_p^2 = 0.83$; 95%CI = 4.0–9.6; Condition: $F_{1,7} = 28.30$; $p = 0.001$; $n_p^2 = 0.80$; 95%CI = 2.8–7.5). RVM and RBF showed higher sEMG activity during the HYD condition on both constant workload at 65% of VO$_{2max}$ and on Time-to-Trial at 95% of VO$_{2max}$ (Table 3).

Table 3. Comparison (mean) of the muscle activation between hydration status on both exercise condition.

	Constant Workload (65% VO$_{2max}$)					Time-to-Trial (95% VO$_{2max}$)				
	HYD	DEH	Mean Diff	p	d	HYD	DEH	Mean Diff	p	d
RVM-RMS (%MVC)	41.96 ± 10.39	34.92 ± 6.53	7.4	0.011 *	0.81	57.30 ± 10.98	48.29 ± 6.13	9.00	0.014 *	1.01
RBF-RMS (% MVC)	20.40 ± 3.88	14.91 ± 2.55	5.49	0.003 *	1.67	26.97 ± 4.41	22.05 ± 4.04	4.92	0.021 *	1.16

Note: HYD: hydration; DEH: dehydration; RVM: right vastus medialis; RBF: right biceps femoris; MVC: maximum voluntary contraction; RMS: root mean square; p-value and Cohen's d; *= significant differences between hydration status on each exercise condition ($p < 0.05$).

4. Discussion

The aim of the present study was to investigate the effects of dehydration on metabolic and neuromuscular functionality and TT performance during a cycling exercise. This study demonstrated that physiological parameters along with HR and neuromuscular function were altered during a moderate intensity exercise and subsequently TT performance when subjects did not restore fluid loss. Additionally, all metabolic and neuromuscular parameters investigated significantly increased during TT with respect to constant workload at 65% of VO$_{2max}$.

Fluid loss and therefore dehydration during the DEH session was evaluated by BIVA, which identified a significant vector displacement along the major axis of the ellipses; on the contrary, when the athletes restored the fluids lost during the HYD trial, no vector displacement was detected Lengthening of vectors in R-Xc graph represent a decrease in body fluids [16,18]. This evaluation was also supported by the body weight change measured after the DEH trial. Our results showed that although the bioimpedance vectors lengthen as a result of body fluid loss, the slope and phase angle does not change, implying that the ICW/ECW ratio remains unchanged. In this regard, different studies have shown how the phase angle which determines the vector slope of the R-Xc graph, is directly proportionate to the ICW/ECW ratio [33–35]. Similar results have been found by Gatterer et al. [16] in regard to dehydration after a running test. No significant difference was observed for metabolic parameters (e.g., VO$_2$, RER and EC) between the two trials in both phases of the cycling exercise. However, TT duration and HR variation observed during the cycling performance at 65% and 95%VO$_{2max}$ was significantly different between the two conditions; in fact, a higher HR and a shorter TT performance during DEH session was observed. Our hypothesis was that HR increases during dehydration because of the blood flow redistribution, which causes a high body temperature and a consequent decrease in the stroke and blood volume and consequently compensatory increase in HR. In line with these results, previous studies have documented the resultant tachycardia and diminished stroke volume during dehydration. Our results are similar to those obtained by Logan-Sprenger et al. [12] in an experiment in which 9 subjects who completed two cycling trials lasting 60 minutes at 65% VO_{2max} followed by a TT; as in our study, the subjects showed an increase in HR during dehydration condition compared to when the subjects were hydrated. Furthermore, VO_2 kinetics, RER, and EC showed tendentially higher values during DEH, although not statistically significant. Probably, a greater percentage of fluid loss is necessary to have significant effects on cardiometabolic parameters during a cycling exercise carried out below the ventilatory threshold (65% VO_{2max}).

The RVM and RBF muscle activity was significantly reduced during the two parts of the DEH test, suggesting that fluid loss compromises the muscle power expression during dehydration. The effects of dehydration on muscle performance have been studied using different protocols and measurement techniques. Studies vary in the percentage of lost fluids achieved from 1.7% to 5.8% of body mass reduction [36–39]. After a literature review, [40] concluded that dehydration consistently attenuates muscle power by approximately 3%. The origin of these reductions has been speculated to reside on alterations in cardiovascular, metabolic or buffering functions. In fact, heat stress, with or without dehydration, compromises blood flow to active muscles and skin during strenuous exercise as the systemic circulation [41].

In a meta-analysis conducted by Goulet [42], it was showed that levels of exercise induced dehydration, similar to those in the present study, did not reduce cycling TT performance. Additionally, in response to a similar hydration status (progressive loss to 2% body weight loss), no significant differences were reported when trained men completed a 40 km cycling TT performance as measured by power output and mean finish time [43]. These records of data suggest the influence of dehydration may, in part, be protocol specific. In our study, athletes cycled for 60 min at 65% VO_{2max} and performed a 95% VO_{2max} TT in two different tests. During the HYD session, in order to restore the fluids lost during exercise, the athletes ingested 0.5 ml of water every 15 min to maintain a body weight similar to that recorded at the baseline. However, to the best of our knowledge, this is the first experiment to use this experimental protocol to ensure a well-hydration status of the athletes during the exercise, and therefore, it is not possible to compare our results with other researches. One of the most common potential limitations is the inherent difficulty in blinding subjects to the fact that they are dehydrating versus rehydrating during a given trial. Another possible limitation in the present study is the participant sample, which may compromise detectable differences among the two hydration conditions in the examined parameters. Nonetheless, other studies evaluating exercise performance and dehydration/rehydration have used samples ranging from n = 6 to 11 [37,44,45].

A strong point of this study is demonstrating how BIVA can be used to monitor the changes in fluids by identifying dehydration. In addition, new evidence regarding the effects of dehydration on physical performance have been provided and these should also be considered in non-athletes because health could be compromised during sports practice.

From the discussion above it is clear that more research is needed to address several remaining questions regarding the potential impact of dehydration on sports performance. Valid and reliable protocols should be developed and used in future studies to ensure that tests are able to detect the effects of fluid loss on central and peripheral parameters. Lastly, future studies should also include female participants to study the impacts of dehydration on both metabolic and neuromuscular variables in subjects of different gender.

5. Conclusions

Neuromuscular and metabolic function were altered during a cycling performance when subjects dehydrated versus maintaining a well-hydration status through drinking. The practical application of this study demonstrated that athletes exercising in a dehydrated state significantly decreased physical performances; therefore, attention needs to be paid to strategies to maintain a good-hydration status during exercise. In addition, this study confirms the ability of BIVA to assess body fluid changes even in sports practice.

Author Contributions: Conceptualization, F.C., A.P., M.R. and S.T.; data curation, F.C.; formal analysis, F.C. and A.P.; investigation, F.C., A.P., A.T. and M.P.; methodology, F.C., A.P. and G.M.; supervision, A.P. and S.T.; writing—original draft, F.C.; writing—review and editing, A.P., G.M. and S.T. All authors have read and agreed to the published version of the manuscript.

Acknowledgments: The authors thank the subjects whose participation made this study possible.

Conflicts of Interest: The authors declare no conflict of interest.

References

1. Campa, F.; Semprini, G.; Júdice, P.B.; Messina, G.; Toselli, S. Anthropometry, Physical and Movement Features, and Repeated-sprint Ability in Soccer Players. *Int. J. Sports Med.* **2019**, *40*, 100–109. [CrossRef]
2. Piras, A.; Cortesi, M.; Campa, F.; Perazzolo, M.; Gatta, G. Recovery Time Profiling After Short-, Middle- and Long-Distance Swimming Performance. *J. Strength. Cond. Res.* **2019**, *33*, 1408–1415. [CrossRef]
3. Piras, A.; Gatta, G. Evaluation of the Effectiveness of Compression Garments on Autonomic Nervous System Recovery After Exercise. *J. Strength Cond. Res.* **2017**, *31*, 1636–1643. [CrossRef]
4. Masento, N.A.; Golightly, M.; Field, D.T.; Butler, L.T.; van Reekum, C.M. Effects of Hydration Status on Cognitive Performance and Mood. *Br. J. Nutr.* **2014**, *111*, 1841–1852. [CrossRef] [PubMed]
5. Pethick, W.A.; Murray, H.J.; McFadyen, P.; Brodie, R.; Gaul, C.A.; Stellingwerff, T. Effects of Hydration Status during Heat Acclimation on Plasma Volume and Performance. *Scand. J. Med. Sci. Sports* **2019**, *29*, 189–199. [CrossRef] [PubMed]
6. Zhang, N.; Du, S.M.; Zhang, J.F.; Ma, G.S. Effects of Dehydration and Rehydration on Cognitive Performance and Mood among Male College Students in Cangzhou, China: A Self-Controlled Trial. *Int. J. Environ. Res. Public Health* **2019**, *6*, 1891. [CrossRef]
7. Barley, O.R.; Chapman, D.W.; Blazevich, A.J.; Abbiss, C.R. Acute Dehydration Impairs Endurance Without Modulating Neuromuscular Function. *Front Physiol.* **2018**, *9*, 1562. [CrossRef] [PubMed]
8. Castro-Sepulveda, M.; Cerda-Kohler, H.; Perez-Luco, C.; Monsalves, M.; Andrade, D.C.; Zbinden-Foncea, H.; Báez-San Martín, E.; Ramírez-Campillo, R. Hydration Status after Exercise Affect Resting Metabolic Rate and Heart Rate Variability. *Nutr. Hosp.* **2014**, *31*, 1273–1277.
9. Georgescu, V.P.; de Souza Junior, T.P.; Behrens, C.; Barros, M.P.; Bueno, C.A.; Utter, A.C.; McAnulty, L.S.; McAnulty, S.R. Effect of Exercise-Induced Dehydration on Circulatory Markers of Oxidative Damage and Antioxidant Capacity. *Appl. Physiol. Nutr. Metab.* **2017**, *42*, 694–699. [CrossRef]
10. Nuccio, R.P.; Barnes, K.A.; Carter, J.M.; Baker, L.B. Fluid Balance in Team Sport Athletes and the Effect of Hypohydration on Cognitive, Technical, and Physical Performance. *Sports Med.* **2017**, *47*, 1951–1982. [CrossRef]
11. McDermott, B.P.; Anderson, S.A.; Armstrong, L.; Casa, D.G.; Cheuvront, S.N.; Cooper, L.; Kenney, W.L.; O'Connor, F.G.; Roberts, W.O. National Athletic Trainers' Association Position Statement: Fluid Replacement for the Physically Active. *J. Athl. Train.* **2017**, *2017 52*, 877–895. [CrossRef]
12. Logan-Sprenger, H.M.; Heigenhauser, G.F.; Jones, G.L.; Spriet, L.L. The Effect of Dehydration on Muscle Metabolism and Time Trial Performance during Prolonged Cycling in Males. *Physiol. Rep.* **2015**, *3*, e12483. [CrossRef] [PubMed]
13. Campa, F.; Silva, A.M.; Iannuzzi, V.; Mascherini, G.; Benedetti, L.; Toselli, S. The role of somatic maturation on bioimpedance patterns and body composition in male elite youth soccer players. *Int. J. Environ. Res. Public Health* **2019**, *16*, 4711. [CrossRef] [PubMed]
14. Campa, F.; Silva, A.M.; Toselli, S. Changes in Phase Angle and Handgrip Strength Induced by Suspension Training in Older Women. *Int. J. Sports Med.* **2018**, *39*, 442–449. [CrossRef]
15. Campa, F.; Toselli, S. Bioimpedance Vector Analysis of Elite, Subelite, and Low-Level Male Volleyball Players. *Int. J. Sports Physiol. Perform.* **2018**, *13*, 1250–1253. [CrossRef]
16. Gatterer, H.; Schenk, K.; Laninschegg, L.; Lukaski, H.; Burtscher, M. Bioimpedance Identifies Body Fluid Loss after Exercise in the Heat: A Pilot Study with Body Cooling. *PLoS ONE* **2014**, *9*, e109729. [CrossRef]

17. Piccoli, A.; Rossi, B.; Pillon, L.; Bucciante, G. A New Method for Monitoring Body Fluid Variation by Bioimpedance Analysis: The RXc Graph. *Kidney Int.* **1994**, *46*, 534–539. [CrossRef]
18. Campa, F.; Matias, C.N.; Marini, E.; Heymsfield, S.B.; Toselli, S.; Sardinha, L.B.; Silva, A.M. Identifying Athlete Body-Fluid Changes During a Competitive Season With Bioelectrical Impedance Vector Analysis. *Int. J. Sports Physiol. Perform.* **2019**. [CrossRef]
19. Marini, E.; Campa, F.; Buffa, R.; Stagi, S.; Matias, C.N.; Toselli, S.; Sardinha, L.B.; Silva, A.M. Phase angle and bioelectrical impedance vector analysis in the evaluation of body composition in athletes. *Clin. Nutr.* **2020**, *39*, 447–454. [CrossRef]
20. Lukaski, H.C.; Piccoli, A. Bioelectrical impedance vector analysis for assessment of hydration in physiological states and clinical conditions. In *Handbook of Anthropometry*; Preedy, V., Ed.; Springer: Berlin, Germany, 2012; pp. 287–305.
21. Muth, T.; Pritchett, R.; Pritchett, K.; Depaepe, J.; Blank, R. Hydration Status and Perception of Fluid Loss in Male and Female University Rugby Union Players. *Int. J. Exerc. Sci.* **2019**, *12*, 859–870.
22. Piras, A.; Persiani, M.; Damiani, N.; Perazzolo, M.; Raffi, M. Peripheral heart action (PHA) training as a valid substitute to high intensity interval training to improve resting cardiovascular changes and autonomic adaptation. *Eur. J. Appl. Physiol.* **2015**, *11*, 763–773. [CrossRef] [PubMed]
23. Astorino, T.A.; Willey, J.; Kinnahan, J.; Larsson, S.M.; Welch, H.; Dalleck, L.C. Elucidating determinants of the plateau in oxygen consumption at VO2max. *Br. J. Sports Med.* **2005**, *39*, 655–660. [CrossRef] [PubMed]
24. Holland, J.; Skinner, T.L.; Irwin, C.G.; Leveritt, M.D.; Goulet, E.D.B. The Influence of Drinking Fluid on Endurance Cycling Performance: A Meta-Analysis. *Sports Med.* **2017**, *47*, 2269–2284. [CrossRef]
25. Backes, T.P.; Fitzgerald, K. Fluid Consumption, Exercise, and Cognitive Performance. *Biol. Sport* **2016**, *33*, 291–296. [CrossRef] [PubMed]
26. Campa, F.; Gatterer, H.; Lukaski, H.; Toselli, S. Stabilizing Bioimpedance-Vector-Analysis Measures With a 10-Minute Cold Shower After Running Exercise to Enable Assessment of Body Hydration. *Int. J. Sports Physiol. Perform.* **2019**, *14*, 1006–1009. [CrossRef]
27. Lee, T.Q.; Yang, B.Y.; Sandusky, M.D.; McMahon, P.J. The effects of tibial rotation on the patellofemoral joint: assessment of the changes in in situ strain in the peripatellar retinaculum and the patellofemoral contact pressures and areas. *J. Rehabil. Res. Dev.* **2001**, *38*, 463–469.
28. Kamen, G.; Gabriel, D.A. EMG signal processing. In *Essentials of Electromyography*; Human Kinetics: Champaign, IL, USA, 2010; pp. 105–154.
29. Piras, A.; Campa, F.; Toselli, S.; Di Michele, R.; Raffi, M. Physiological responses to partial-body cryotherapy performed during a concurrent strength and endurance session. *Appl. Physiol. Nutr. Metab.* **2019**, *44*, 59–65. [CrossRef]
30. Piras, A.; Raffi, M.; Atmatzidis, C.; Merni, F.; Di Michele, R. The energy cost of running with the ball in soccer. *Int. J. Sports Med.* **2017**, *38*, 877-822. [CrossRef]
31. Piccoli, A.; Pastori, G. BIVA Software. 2002. Available online: www.renalgate.it/formule_calcolatori/BIVAguide.pdf (accessed on 30 December 2019).
32. Campa, F.; Matias, C.; Gatterer, H.; Toselli, S.; Koury, J.C.; Andreoli, A.; Melchiorri, G.; Sardinha, L.B.; Silva, A.M. Classic Bioelectrical Impedance Vector Reference Values for Assessing Body Composition in Male and Female Athletes. *Int. J. Environ. Res. Public Health* **2019**, *16*, 5066. [CrossRef]
33. Gonzalez, M.C.; Barbosa-Silva, T.G.; Bielemann, R.M.; Gallagher, D.; Heymsfield, S.B. Phase angle and its determinants in healthy subjects: influence of body composition. *Am. J Clin. Nutr.* **2016**, *103*, 712e6. [CrossRef]
34. Francisco, R.; Matias, C.N.; Santos, D.A.; Campa, F.; Minderico, C.S.; Rocha, P.; Heymsfield, S.B.; Lukaski, H.; Sardinha, L.B.; Silva, A.M. The Predictive Role of Raw Bioelectrical Impedance Parameters in Water Compartments and Fluid Distribution Assessed by Dilution Techniques in Athletes. *Int. J. Environ. Res. Public. Health* **2020**, *17*, 759. [CrossRef]
35. Toselli, S.; Marini, E.; Maietta Latessa, P.; Benedetti, L.; Campa, F. Maturity Related Differences in Body Composition Assessed by Classic and Specific Bioimpedance Vector Analysis among Male Elite Youth Soccer Players. *Int. J. Environ. Res. Public Health* **2020**, *17*, 729. [CrossRef]
36. Bowtell, J.L.; Avenell, G.; Hunter, S.P.; Mileva, K.N. Effect of Hypohydration on Peripheral and Corticospinal Excitability and Voluntary Activation. *PLoS ONE* **2013**, *8*, e77004. [CrossRef] [PubMed]

37. Minshull, C.; James, L. The Effects of Hypohydration and Fatigue on Neuromuscular Activation Performance. *Appl. Physiol. Nutr. Metab.* **2013**, *38*, 21–26. [CrossRef] [PubMed]
38. Pallares, J.G.; Martinez-Abellan, A.; Lopez-Gullon, J.M.; Morán-Navarro, R.; De la Cruz-Sánchez, E.; Mora-Rodríguez, R. Muscle Contraction Velocity, Strength and Power Output Changes Following Different Degrees of Hypohydration in Competitive Olympic Combat Sports. *J. Int. Soc. Sports Nutr.* **2016**, *13*, 10. [CrossRef] [PubMed]
39. Schoffstall, J.E.; Branch, J.D.; Leutholtz, B.C.; Swain, D.E. Effects of Dehydration and Rehydration on the One-Repetition Maximum Bench Press of Weight-Trained Males. *J. Strength Cond. Res.* **2001**, *15*, 102–108. [PubMed]
40. Judelson, D.A.; Maresh, C.M.; Anderson, J.M.; Adams, W.M.; Armstrong, L.E.; Baker, L.B.; Burke, L.; Cheuvront, S.; Chiampas, G.; González-Alonso, J.; et al. Hydration and muscular performance: does fluid balance affect strength, power and high-intensity endurance? *Sports Med.* **2007**, *37*, 907–921. [CrossRef]
41. Crandall, C.G.; Gonzalez-Alonso, J. Cardiovascular Function. In the Heat-Stressed Human. *Acta Physiol.* **2010**, *199*, 407–423. [CrossRef]
42. Goulet, E. Effect of Exercise-Induced Dehydration on Endurance Performance: Evaluating the Impact of Exercise Protocols on Outcomes Using a Meta-Analytic Procedure. *Br. J. Sports Med.* **2013**, *47*, 679–686. [CrossRef]
43. Berkulo, M.A.; Bol, S.; Levels, K.; Lamberts, R.P.; Daanen, H.A.M.; Noakes, T.D. Ad-Libitum Drinking and Performance during a 40-Km Cycling Time Trial in the Heat. European. *J. Sports Sci.* **2016**, *16*, 213–220.
44. Buono, M.J.; Wall, A.J. Effect of Hypohydration on Core Temperature during Exercise in Temperate and Hot Environments. *Eur. J. Appl. Physiol.* **2000**, *440*, 476–480. [CrossRef] [PubMed]
45. Laitano, O.; Kalsi, K.K.; Pearson, J.; Lotlikar, M.; Reischak-Oliveira, A.; González-Alonso, J. Effects of Graded Exercise-Induced Dehydration and Rehydration on Circulatory Markers of Oxidative Stress across the Resting and Exercising Human Leg. European. *J. Appl. Physiol.* **2012**, *112*, 1937–1944. [CrossRef] [PubMed]

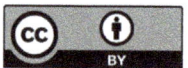

© 2020 by the authors. Licensee MDPI, Basel, Switzerland. This article is an open access article distributed under the terms and conditions of the Creative Commons Attribution (CC BY) license (http://creativecommons.org/licenses/by/4.0/).

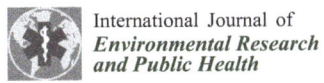

Article

Effects of a Bout of Intense Exercise on Some Executive Functions

Marinella Coco [1,2,*], Andrea Buscemi [3,4], Claudia Savia Guerrera [1], Donatella Di Corrado [5], Paolo Cavallari [6], Agata Zappalà [1], Santo Di Nuovo [7], Rosalba Parenti [1], Tiziana Maci [8], Grazia Razza [8], Maria Cristina Petralia [7], Vincenzo Perciavalle [5] and Valentina Perciavalle [7]

1 Department of Biomedical and Biotechnological Sciences, University of Catania, 95123 Catania, Italy; claguerre@hotmail.it (C.S.G.); azappala@unict.it (A.Z.); Parenti@unict.it (R.P.)
2 Motor Activity Research Center (CRAM) University of Catania, 95123 Catania, Italy
3 Horus Social Cooperative, Department of Research, 97100 Ragusa, Italy; andreabuscemi@virgilio.it
4 Department of Research, Italian Center Studies of Osteopathy, 95100 Catania, Italy
5 Department of Human and Social Sciences, School of Sport Sciences, Kore University, 94100 Enna, Italy; didinawoody@gmail.com (D.D.C.); perciava@libero.it (V.P.)
6 Department of Pathophysiology and Transplantation, Human Physiology Section, University of Milan, 20122 Milan, Italy; paolo.cavallari@unimi.it
7 Department of Educational Sciences, 95100 Catania, Italy; s.dinuovo@unict.it (S.D.N.); m.cristinapetralia@gmail.com (M.C.P.); valentinaperciavalle@hotmail.it (V.P.)
8 Independent Researcher, 95100 Catania, Italy; tizianamaci@libero.it (T.M.); grazia.r@live.it (G.R.)
* Correspondence: marinella.coco@gmail.com

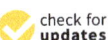

Received: 21 December 2019; Accepted: 24 January 2020; Published: 31 January 2020

Abstract: The present study examined the effects of an exhaustive exercise on executive functions by using the Stroop Color Word Test (SCWT), Trail Making Test (TMT), A and B, and simple Reaction Time (RT). Thirty adults agreed to participate; 15 participants had a mean age of 24.7 years ± 3.2 Standard Deviation (SD, Standard Deviation) (group YOUNG), while the remaining 15 had a mean age of 58.9 years ± 2.6 SD (group OLD). Each subject performed the cognitive tasks at rest and blood lactate was measured (pre); each subject executed the acute exhaustive exercise and, immediately after the conclusion, executed the cognitive tasks and blood lactate was again measured (end). Cognitive tests were repeated and blood lactate measured 15 min after its conclusion of the exhaustive exercise (post). We observed: (1) a significant positive correlation between blood lactate levels and RT levels; (2) a significant negative relationship between levels of blood lactate and the SCWT mean score; (3) no significant correlation between blood lactate levels and TMT scores (time and errors), both A and B; (4) variations in blood lactate levels, due to exhaustive exercise, and parallel deterioration in the execution of RT and SCWT are significantly more pronounced in the group YOUNG than in the group OLD. The present study supports the possibility that high levels of blood lactate induced by an exhaustive exercise could adversely affect the executive functions pertaining to the prefrontal cortex.

Keywords: executive functions; young sport; blood lactate; exhaustive exercise; fatigue; elderly sport

1. Introduction

The effects of acute physical exercise on the cognitive performances of an adult individual are still under discussion [1–18]. The existing literature tends to highlight a positive relationship if the exercise is of sub-maximal intensity, while the effects seem to be negative for exhaustive exercises [19–26].

Within cognitive processes, there are few studies on the effects of an exhaustive exercise on executive functions. [27–32]. This term indicates a set of cognitive processes that allow us to plan, regulate, control, and evaluate behaviors that are useful for achieving a goal [17]. Executive functions include planning, problem solving, flexibility, inhibition, multitasking, and working memory [18]. A negative effect of high blood lactate levels induced by an exhaustive exercise or with an intravenous infusion of a lactate solution has been found for attentional processes [3,5,6,8,10,19]. Regarding the working memory, a negative effect of exhaustive exercise on both non-spatial working memory and motor working memory was found [9]. Concerning other executive functions, a study that used a combination of a Spatial Delayed-Response task and a Go/No-Go task found no correlation between blood lactate levels and cognitive functions [12].

The purpose of the present study was to examine the effects of an exhaustive exercise on executive functions by using the Stroop Color Word Test (SCWT), correlated with cognitive flexibility and resistance to interference from external stimuli [25], and Trail Making Test (TMT), associated with visual attention and task switching [28]. Simple Reaction Time (RT), as basic measure of processing speed [33], was also evaluated.

2. Materials and Methods

2.1. Participants

In this study, 30 adults agreed to participate; 15 participants had a mean age of 24.7 years ± 3.2 SD (group YOUNG), while the remaining 15 had a mean age of 58.9 years ± 2.6 SD (group OLD). All participants had practiced amateur sports for at least one year and had medical authorization to practice non-competitive sports. Table 1 illustrates the anthropometric characteristics of the participants. The T-test showed that there were no statistically significant differences in height, weight, and Body Mass Index (BMI).

The study was approved by the Ethical committee of the University of Milan (number 15/16). All participants were informed about the trials of the study and the anonymity of their answers before providing their written consent to participate, in accordance with the Declaration of Helsinki.

Table 1. The anthropometric characteristics of the participants

Subject	YOUNG				OLD			
	Age (years)	Height (cm)	Weight (kg)	BMI *	Age (years)	Height (cm)	Weight (kg)	BMI
1	28	169	71	24.86	60	168	73	25.86
2	24	178	77	24.30	55	171	73	24.96
3	27	168	69	24.45	58	166	70	25.40
4	20	170	71	24.57	65	173	71	23.72
5	29	175	74	24.16	59	178	80	25.25
6	22	174	79	26.09	60	174	78	25.76
7	23	181	83	25.34	58	162	65	24.77
8	28	171	78	26.67	59	174	79	26.09
9	25	166	69	25.04	61	169	72	25.21
10	23	177	80	25.54	57	171	76	25.99
11	21	173	78	26.06	55	171	69	23.60
12	20	170	73	25.26	59	170	73	25.26
13	25	176	74	23.89	60	168	70	24.80
14	27	168	70	24.80	61	167	70	25.10
15	29	173	71	23.72	56	176	72	23.24
Mean	24.73	172.60	74.47	24.98	58.87	170.53	72.73	25.00
SD **	3.17	4.26	4.42	0.85	2.59	4.12	4.06	0.87

* BMI = Body Mass Index; ** SD = Standard Deviation.

2.2. Experimental Design

The tests were executed between 9 am and 1 pm, with participants who had eaten breakfast before 8 am [5]. Each subject performed the cognitive tasks at rest and blood lactate was measured (pre). Each subject executed the acute exhaustive exercise and, immediately after the conclusion, performed the cognitive tasks and blood lactate was again measured (end). Finally, cognitive tests were repeated and blood lactate measured 15 min after the exhaustive exercise (post). The overall duration of the cognitive tests did not exceed 6 min.

2.3. Exercise

The participants performed a maximal multistage discontinuous incremental cycling test on a mechanically braked cycloergometer (Monark, Sweden), at a pedaling rate of 60 rpm, while an electrocardiogram was monitored. Each subject started with unloaded cycling during 3 min, and the load was increased by 30 W every 3 min until volitional exhaustion or the required pedaling frequency of 60 rpm could not be maintained [17].

2.4. Blood Lactate

Blood lactate was measured before as well as at the end and 15 min after the conclusion of the exercise, using a "Lactate Pro 2" portable lactate analyzer (Arkray Inc., Kyoto, Japan), since this automated lactate analyzer has a good reliability [1].

2.5. Simple Reaction Time

The procedure for measuring RT was the same one as the one that was used previously [3]. The subject must press the bar-space of the computer to appearing on the screen of the symbol target "star." This is a RT task that demands an intense simple attention; in order to avoid settling habituation, the target presentation was randomized with intervals comprised between 1 and 3 s.

2.6. Stroop Colour Word Test

In the present study the golden version of the SCWT was used [25]. The test comprises three parts. In the first part, the subject reads a list of 50 names printed with black ink. In the second part, the subject observes 50 circles of different colors and must indicate their color. In the third part, the subject receives a list of 50 words with the names of the colors written with an incongruent color ink; the subject must indicate the color of the ink, ignoring the written word. The number of correct answers in 45 s in the third part is considered to be representative of the "interference" component of the SCWT.

2.7. Trial Making Test

TMT was chosen for evaluating information processing speed and executive functioning [28]. The TMT consists of two parts. In TMT-A, the subject had to draw lines sequentially connecting 25 numbered circles distributed on a sheet of paper. In TMT-B, the subject must alternate between numbers and letters distributed on the sheet. The score on each part represents the number of seconds required to complete the task and the number of errors.

2.8. Statistical Analysis

Data was collected and averaged, and then compared with the paired t test (2-tailed) or 1-way repeated measures analysis of variance (ANOVA; Friedman test), followed by Dunn's Multiple Comparison Test. Correlation analysis was carried out using one-tailed Pearson's correlation. Significance was set at $p < 0.05$. All descriptive statistics are reported as mean ± SD. All analyses were performed by using GraphPad Prism version 6.03 for Windows (GraphPad Software, San Diego, CA, USA).

3. Results

As can be seen in Figure 1, in both YOUNG and OLD groups the blood lactate increased significantly at the end of the exhaustive exercise, and returned to the pre-exercise values 10 min after its end. In particular, in the group YOUNG, blood lactate levels increased from 1.63 mmol/L (±0.57 SD) before the exercise, to 9.58 mmol/L (±2.08 SD) at its end, and returned to pre-exercise values after 15 min (2.1 mmol/L ± 0.48 SD).

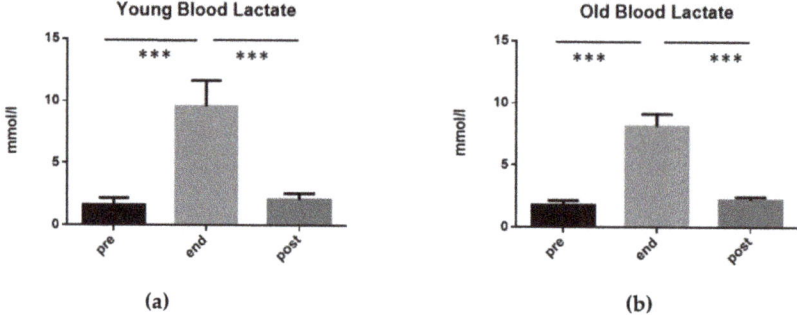

Figure 1. Blood lactate values of the 15 subjects of group YOUNG (**a**) and of the 15 subjects of group OLD (**b**) performing an exhaustive exercise. In both cases, blood lactate mean values measured before the exercise (pre), at its conclusion (end), as well as 15 min after its end (post) are illustrated. Symbols from ANOVA with Dunn's multiple comparison test: *** $p < 0.001$.

However, the level reached by blood lactate at the end of the exercise in the group YOUNG was significantly lower with respect to the value measured in the same moment in the group OLD (t-test: $p < 0.05$).

In Figure 2, it can be seen that, in both YOUNG and OLD groups, the RT augmented significantly at the end of the exhaustive exercise, and returned to the pre-exercise values 15 min after its end. In particular, in the group YOUNG, RT increased from 237.7 ms (±17.40 SD) before the exercise, to 265.6 ms (±19.14 SD) at its end, and returned to pre-exercise values after 15 min (241.6 ms ± 17.15 SD). In the group OLD, RT increased from 254.7 ms (±11.30 SD) before the exercise, to 284.60 ms (±12.80 SD) at its end, and returned to pre-exercise values after 15 min (264.40 ms ± 8.58 SD).

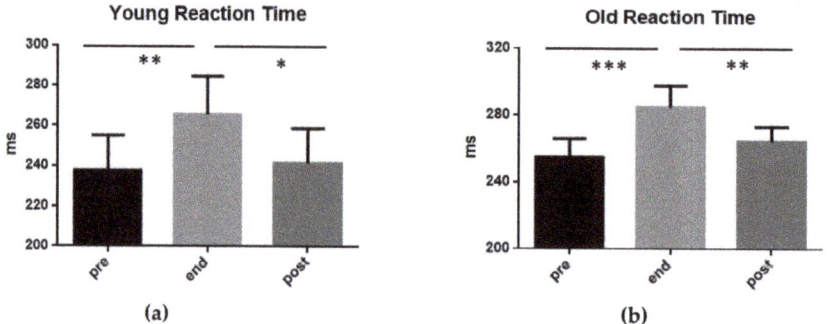

Figure 2. Values of RT exhibited by the 15 subjects of group YOUNG (**a**) and by the 15 subjects of group OLD (**b**) performing an exhaustive exercise. In both cases, RT mean value measured before the exercise (pre), at its conclusion (end), as well as 15 min after its end (post) are displayed. Symbols from ANOVA with Dunn's multiple comparison test: * $p < 0.05$, ** $p < 0.01$, *** $p < 0.001$.

It is interesting to note that the mean values of RT measured in the group YOUNG were significantly inferior to that of the group OLD before the exercise (t-test: $p < 0.01$), at its end (t-test: $p < 0.01$) and 15 min after its completion (t-test: $p < 0.001$).

In Figure 3, it can be observed that, in both YOUNG and OLD groups, the performances at SCWT worsened significantly at the end of the exhaustive exercise, and returned to the pre-exercise values 15 min after its end. In particular, in the group YOUNG, the SCWT mean score decreased from 38.0 (±1.96 SD) before the exercise, to 35.33 (±1.54 SD) at its end, and returned to pre-exercise values after 15 min (37.80 ± 1.41 SD). In the group OLD, SCWT mean score reduced from 38.9 (±1.19 SD) before the exercise, to 33.67 (±1.45 SD) at its end, and returned to pre-exercise values after 15 min (35.13 ± 0.99 SD).

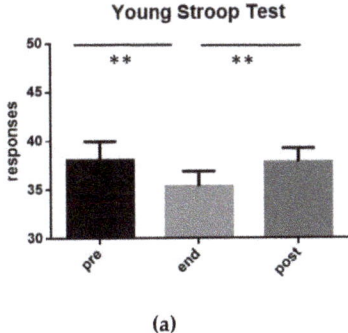
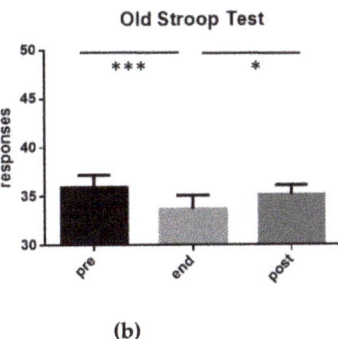

(a) (b)

Figure 3. Values of SCWT mean score exhibited by the 15 subjects of group YOUNG (a) and by the 15 subjects of group OLD (b) performing an exhaustive exercise. In both cases, SCWT mean score measured before the exercise (pre), at its conclusion (end), as well as 15 min after its end (post) are shown. Symbols from ANOVA with Dunn's multiple comparison test: * $p < 0.05$, ** $p < 0.01$, *** $p < 0.001$.

It is worth noting that the mean values of SCWT mean score measured in the group YOUNG were significantly higher than that of the group OLD before the exercise (t-test: $p < 0.01$), at its end (t-test: $p < 0.01$) and 15 min after its completion (t-test: $p < 0.001$).

In Figure 4, there are shown, for both YOUNG and OLD groups, the performances (time and errors) at TMT-A before the exhaustive exercise (pre), at the conclusion (end) and 15 min after its end (post). As can be seen, the only statistically significant variation (t-test: $p < 0.05$) was observed in the YOUNG group where a reduction of the test execution time was detected at the end of the exercise compared to the pre-exercise values.

It should be noted that the time taken by the YOUNG group for the execution of the TMT-A was significantly lower than for the OLD group, both at the end of the exercise (t-test: $p < 0.001$) and after 15 min prior to its end (t-test: $p < 0.001$). Similarly, the number of errors made by the YOUNG group during the execution of the TMT-A was significantly lower than the OLD group both at the end of the exercise (t-test: $p < 0.01$) and after 15 min prior to its completion (t-test: $p < 0.01$).

Figure 5 shows for both YOUNG and OLD groups, the performances (time and errors) at TMT-B before the exhaustive exercise (pre), at the conclusion (end), and 15 min after its end (post). As can be seen, the only statistically significant variation (t-test: $p < 0.001$) was observed in the YOUNG group where a reduction of the execution time was detected at 15 min after its end of the exercise compared to the pre-exercise values.

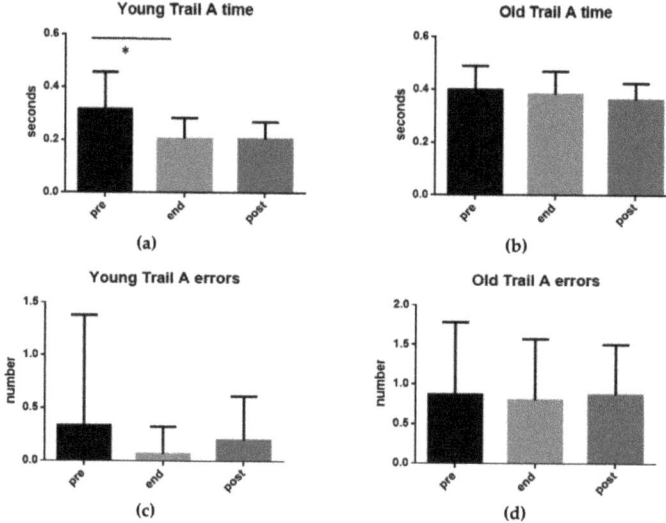

Figure 4. TMT-A. Execution time (**a,b**) and number of errors (**c,d**) found in the 15 subjects of group YOUNG (**a,c**) and in the 15 subjects of group OLD (**b,d**) performing an exhaustive exercise. Mean values measured before the exercise (pre), at its conclusion (end), as well as 15 min after its end (post) are shown. Symbols from ANOVA with Dunn's multiple comparison test: * $p < 0.05$.

It should be noted that the time taken by the YOUNG group for the execution of the TMT-B was significantly lower than the OLD group both at the end of the exercise (t-test: $p < 0.01$) and after 15 min from its end (t-test: $p < 0.001$). Similarly, the number of errors made by the YOUNG group during the execution of the TMT-A was significantly lower than the OLD group both before the exercise (t-test: $p < 0.01$) and during the last 15 min before its end (t-test: $p < 0.001$).

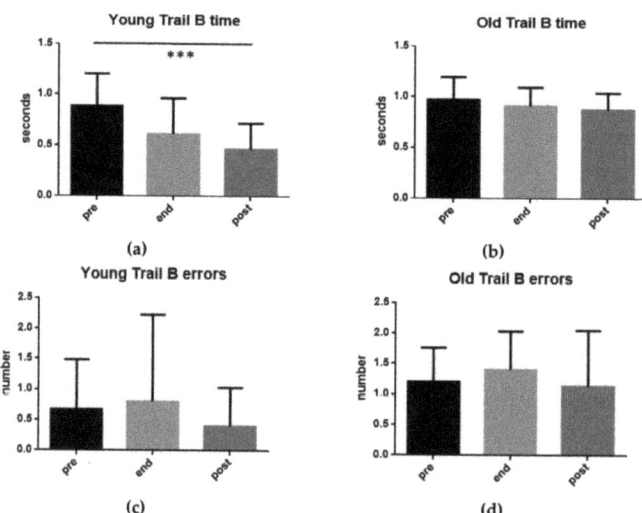

Figure 5. TMT-B. Execution time (**a,b**) and number of errors (**c,d**) found in the 15 subjects of group YOUNG (**a,c**) and in the 15 subjects of group OLD (**b,d**) performing an exhaustive exercise. Mean values measured before the exercise (pre), at its conclusion (end), as well as 15 min after its end (post) are shown. Symbols from ANOVA with Dunn's multiple comparison test: * $p < 0.001$.

Finally, the correlations between blood lactate levels and the performance of the participants in the various tests were analyzed and results are summarized in Figure 6.

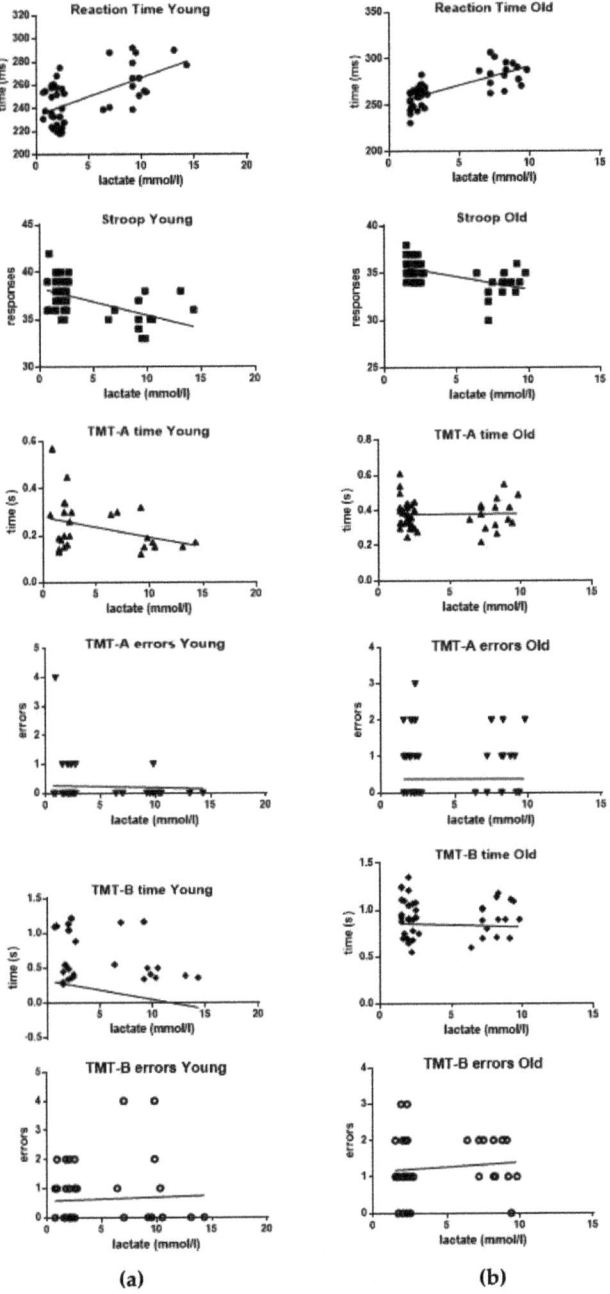

Figure 6. Correlations between blood lactate levels and performances at RT, SCWT, TMT-A and TMT-B in the 15 subjects of group YOUNG (**a**) and in the 15 subjects of group OLD (**b**).

First of all, the statistical analysis showed a strong positive correlation between blood lactate levels and RT values, both in the group YOUNG (R square = 0.3445; $p < 0.001$) and in the group OLD (R square = 0.5288; $p < 0.001$).

A significant negative correlation was also found between blood lactate levels and SCWT mean score, both in the group YOUNG (R square = 0.2963; $p < 0.001$) and in the group OLD (R square = 0.2878; $p < 0.001$).

Regarding the possible correlations between blood lactate levels and TMT-A and TMT-B tests, only a slight negative correlation between lactate and time was found for TMT-A in the group YOUNG (R square = 0.0915; $p = 0.044$). No other statistically significant correlation was detected in both YOUNG and OLD groups.

4. Discussion

The results of this study can be summarized as follows:

1) A significant positive correlation was observed between the levels of lactate in the blood and the levels of RT;
2) A significant negative relationship was observed between blood lactate levels and the average SCWT score;
3) No significant correlations between blood lactate levels and TMT scores (time and errors), both A and B were observed;
4) The comparison between the group YOUNG and the group OLD showed that the variations in blood lactate levels, due to exhaustive exercise, and parallel deterioration in the execution of RT and SCWT are significantly more pronounced in the former than in the latter.

The effects of acute physical exercise on the cognitive performances of an adult individual are still under discussion. The existing literature tends to highlight a positive relationship if the exercise is of sub-maximal intensity while the effects seem to be negative for exhaustive exercises [2–7,9–11,14,15,18–21,24,27,30].

The present study confirm results previously observed for working memory [20], since the increases in blood lactate levels, deriving from exhaustive exercise, are associated with a worsening of executive functions [34–36].

However, in this study, not all the domains that fall within the executive functions were systematically analyzed. In fact, having used only RT, SCWT, and TMT were essentially explored processing speed, cognitive flexibility, resistance to interference from external stimuli, visual attention, and task switching.

Therefore, high levels of blood lactate are associated with a deterioration of processing speed, cognitive flexibility, and resistance to interference, with no significant influences on visual attention and task switching. These results support the idea that the tasks for executive functions may show differential results in different conditions of health and functional stages or levels of physical activity, even in normal subjects. Therefore, it is possible to conclude that, under physiological conditions, executive functions are not cognitive abilities stable over time, but rather are capable of quantitatively changing in relation with psycho-physical modifications.

Why an exhaustive exercise influences only certain executive functions is unclear. One possibility is that the high blood lactate levels, induced by the exercise, may affect some areas of the cortex and not others. In this way, functions supported by the prefrontal cortex, as processing speed [26], cognitive flexibility [34], and resistance to interference [12] seem to be affected, while those supported by more posterior cortical areas, such as visual attention [22] and task switching [29], are not.

This possibility seems to be in agreement with what reported by Sudo et al. [27] which found that exhaustive exercise did not alter the performance in a Go/No-Go task and in a Spatial Delayed-Response task.

Sudo and coworkers [27], in their study, conclude that an exhaustive exercise would be able to influence the executive functions, studied through a Go/No-Go task and in a Spatial Delayed-Response task, for changes in oxygenation of the cerebral cortex and not for the increase in blood lactate; in this way a direct action of lactate on brain tissue is excluded,

The possibility that the effects of exhaustive exercise on cognitive processes may also depend on metabolic, vascular, or thermal phenomena cannot be excluded.

However, a negative effect on attentional processes of high blood lactate levels induced with an intravenous infusion of a lactate solution was found [3] and a negative correlation between CSF lactate levels and cognitive capabilities was observed [37–40]. Moreover, lactate receptors were found in the brain [16] and a role as a neural regulator for lactate was proposed [23].

Among the limitations of the present study, it is necessary to report the training level of each group of subjects that might influence the final results.

5. Conclusions

In conclusion, the present study supports the possibility that high levels of blood lactate induced by an exhaustive exercise could adversely affect the executive functions pertaining to the prefrontal cortex. These influences, even if reduced in quantity, remain present even in older people.

Author Contributions: Conceptualization, M.C., A.B., C.S.G., P.C. and V.P.; Data curation, M.C., A.B., D.D.C., A.Z., V.P. (Vincenzo Perciavalle) and V.P. (Valentina Perciavalle); Formal analysis, M.C., A.B., C.S.G., D.D.C., A.Z., T.M., M.C.P., V.P. (Vincenzo Perciavalle) and V.P. (Valentina Perciavalle); Methodology, M.C., P.C. and V.P. (Vincenzo Perciavalle); Supervision, A.Z., R.P., T.M. and G.R.; Visualization, R.P.; Writing—original draft, M.C., A.B., C.S.G., D.D.C. and V.P. (Vincenzo Perciavalle); Writing—review & editing, M.C., S.D.N. and V.P. (Valentina Perciavalle). All authors have read and agreed to the published version of the manuscript.

Funding: This research received no external funding.

Acknowledgments: The authors would like to thank Giuseppe Marchesano for his availability.

Conflicts of Interest: The authors declare no conflict of interest.

References

1. Buckley, J.D.; Bourdon, P.C.; Woolford, S.M. Effect of measuring blood lactate concentrations using different automated lactate analysers on blood lactate transition thresholds. *J. Sci. Med. Sport* **2003**, *6*, 408–421. [CrossRef]
2. Chang, Y.K.; Labban, J.D.; Gapin, J.I.; Etnier, J.L. The effects of acute exercise on cognitive performance: A meta-analysis. *Brain Res.* **2012**, *1453*, 87–101. [CrossRef] [PubMed]
3. Coco, M.; Di Corrado, D.; Calogero, R.A.; Perciavalle, V.; Maci, T.; Perciavalle, V. Attentional processes and blood lactate levels. *Brain Res.* **2009**, *1302*, 205–211. [CrossRef] [PubMed]
4. Coco, M.; Di Corrado, D.; Ramaci, T.; Di Nuovo, S.; Perciavalle, V.; Puglisi, A.; Cavallari, P.; Bellomo, M.; Buscemi, A. Role of lactic acid on cognitive functions. *Phys. Sportsmed.* **2019**, *3*, 329–335. [CrossRef]
5. Coco, M.; Perciavalle, V.; Cavallari, P.; Perciavalle, V. Effects of an Exhaustive Exercise on Motor Skill Learning and on the Excitability of Primary Motor Cortex and Supplementary Motor Area. *Medicine (Baltimore)* **2016**, *95*, e2978. [CrossRef]
6. Dalla Vecchia, L.; Traversi, E.; Porta, A.; Lucini, D.; Pagani, M. On site assessment of cardiac function and neural regulation in amateur half marathon runners. *Open Heart* **2014**, *1*, e000005. [CrossRef]
7. Dalla Vecchia, L.A.; Barbic, F.; De Maria, B.; Cozzolino, D.; Gatti, R.; Dipaola, F.; Brunetta, E.; Zamuner, A.R.; Porta, A.; Furlan, R. Can strenuous exercise harm the heart? Insights from a study of cardiovascular neural regulation in amateur triathletes. *PLoS One* **2019**, *5*, e0216567. [CrossRef]
8. Diamond, A. Executive functions. *Annu. Rev. Psychol.* **2013**, *64*, 135–168. [CrossRef]
9. Duncan, M.J.; Clarke, N.D.; Cox, M.; Smith, M. The influence of cycling intensity upon cognitive response during inferred practice and competition conditions. *J. Sports Sci.* **2017**, *19*, 1865–1871. [CrossRef]
10. Itagi, A.B.H.; Patil, N.A.; Kotian, R.K.; Reddy, S.K.; Abhyankar, S.; Parveen, R.S. (Accepted/In press). Physical Exhaustion Induced Variations in Event-Related Potentials and Cognitive Task Performance in Young Adults. *Ann. Neurosci.* **2018**, *25*, 299–304. [CrossRef]

11. Kleinloog, J.P.D.; Mensink, R.P.; Ivanov, D.; Adam, J.J.; Uluda, K.; Joris, P.J. Aerobic Exercise Training Improves Cerebral Blood Flow and Executive Function: A Randomized, Controlled Cross-Over Trial in Sedentary Older Men. *Front. Aging Neurosci.* **2019**, *11*, 333. [CrossRef] [PubMed]
12. Laurent, J.S.; Watts, R.; Adise, S.; Allgaier, N.; Chaarani, B.; Garavan, H.; Potter, A.; Mackey, S. Associations Among Body Mass Index, Cortical Thickness, and Executive Function in Children. *JAMA Pediatr.* **2019**. [CrossRef]
13. Miller, E.K.; Cohen, J.D. An integrative theory of prefrontal cortex function. *Annu. Rev. Neurosci.* **2001**, *24*, 167–202. [CrossRef] [PubMed]
14. Moghetti, P.; Bacchi, E.; Brangani, C.; Donà, S.; Negri, C. Metabolic Effects of Exercise. *Front. Horm. Res.* **2016**, *47*, 44–57. [PubMed]
15. Moreira, A.; Aoki, M.S.; Franchini, E.; da Silva Machado, D.G.; Paludo, A.C.; Okano, A.H. Mental fatigue impairs technical performance and alters neuroendocrine and autonomic responses in elite young basketball players. *Physiol. Behav.* **2018**, *196*, 112–118. [CrossRef]
16. Morland, C.; Lauritzen, K.H.; Puchades, M.; Holm-Hansen, S.; Andersson, K.; Gjedde, A.; Attramadal, H.; Storm-Mathisen, J.; Bergersen, L.H. The lactate receptor, G-protein-coupled receptor 81/hydroxycarboxylic acid receptor 1: Expression and action in brain. *J. Neurosci. Res.* **2015**, *7*, 1045–1055. [CrossRef]
17. Perciavalle, V.; Alagona, G.; De Maria, G.; Rapisarda, G.; Costanzo, E.; Perciavalle, V.; Coco, M. Somatosensory evoked potentials and blood lactate levels. *Neurol. Sci.* **2015**, *9*, 1597–1601. [CrossRef]
18. Perciavalle, V.; Alagona, G.; Maci, T.; Petralia, M.C.; Costanzo, E.; Perciavalle, V.; Coco, M. Attentional processes during submaximal exercises. *Somatosens. Mot. Res.* **2014**, *1*, 1–6. [CrossRef]
19. Perciavalle, V.; Blandini, M.; Fecarotta, P.; Buscemi, A.; Di Corrado, D.; Bertolo, L.; Fichera, F.; Coco, M. The role of deep breathing on stress. *Neurol. Sci.* **2017**, *3*, 451–458. [CrossRef]
20. Perciavalle, V.; Maci, T.; Perciavalle, V.; Massimino, S.; Coco, M. Working memory and blood lactate levels. *Neurol. Sci.* **2015**, *11*, 2129–2136. [CrossRef]
21. Perciavalle, V.; Marchetta, N.S.; Giustiniani, S.; Borbone, C.; Perciavalle, V.; Petralia, M.C.; Buscemi, A.; Coco, M. Attentive processes, blood lactate and CrossFit®. *Phys. Sportsmed.* **2016**, *4*, 403–406. [CrossRef] [PubMed]
22. Praß, M.; de Haan, B. Multi-target attention and visual short-term memory capacity are closely linked in the intraparietal sulcus. *Hum. Brain Mapp.* **2019**, *12*, 3589–3605. [CrossRef] [PubMed]
23. Proia, P.; Di Liegro, C.M.; Schiera, G.; Fricano, A.; Di Liegro, I. Lactate as a Metabolite and a Regulator in the Central Nervous System. *Int. J. Mol. Sci.* **2016**, *9*, 1450. [CrossRef] [PubMed]
24. Schwarck, S.; Schmicker, M.; Dordevic, M.; Rehfeld, K.; Müller, N.; Müller, P. Inter-Individual Differences in Cognitive Response to a Single Bout of Physical Exercise-A Randomized Controlled Cross-Over Study. *J. Clin. Med.* **2019**, *8*, 1101. [CrossRef]
25. Strauss, E.; Sherman, E.; Spreen, O. *A Compendium of Neuropsychological Tests: Administration, Norms, and Commentary*; Oxford University Press: New York, NY, USA, 2006.
26. Strömmer, J.M.; Davis, S.W.; Henson, R.N.; Tyler, L.K.; Cam-CAN; Campbell, K.L. Physical Activity Predicts Population-Level Age-Related Differences in Frontal White Matter. *J. Gerontol. Biol. Sci. Med. Sci.* **2020**, *75*, 236–243. [CrossRef]
27. Sudo, M.; Komiyama, T.; Aoyagi, R.; Nagamatsu, T.; Higaki, Y.; Ando, S. Executive function after exhaustive exercise. *Eur. J. Appl. Physiol.* **2017**, *10*, 2029–2038. [CrossRef]
28. Tombaugh, T.N. Trail Making Test A and B: normative data stratified by age and education. *Arch. Clin. Neuropsychol.* **2004**, *2*, 203–214. [CrossRef]
29. Uehara, S.; Mizuguchi, N.; Hirose, S.; Yamamoto, S.; Naito, E. Involvement of human left frontoparietal cortices in neural processes associated with task-switching between two sequences of skilled finger movements. *Brain Res.* **2019**, *1*, 1722–146365. [CrossRef]
30. Vrijkotte, S.; Meeusen, R.; Vandervaeren, C.; Buyse, L.; Cutsem, J.V.; Pattyn, N.; Roelands, B. Mental Fatigue and Physical and Cognitive Performance During a 2-Bout Exercise Test. *Int. J. Sports Physiol. Perform.* **2018**, *4*, 510–516. [CrossRef]
31. Petralia, M.C.; Perciavalle, V.; Basile, M.S.; Alagona, G.; Monaca, A.; Buscemi, A.; Coco, M. The rise of lactic acid, from a pharmacist's laboratory to entry into the central nervous system. *Sport Sci. Health* **2018**, *14*, 455. [CrossRef]

32. Coco, M.; Platania, S.; Castellano, S.; Sagone, E.; Ramaci, T.; Petralia, M.C.; Agati, M.; Massimino, S.; Di Corrado, D.; Guarnera, M.; et al. Memory, personality and blood lactate during a judo competition. *Sport Sci. Health* **2018**, *14*, 547–553. [CrossRef]
33. Coco, M.; Guerrera, C.S.; Di Corrado, D.; Ramaci, T.; Maci, T.; Pellerone, M.; Santisi, G.; Minissale, C.; Di Nuovo, S.; Perciavalle, V.; et al. Personality traits and athletic young adults. *Sport Sci. Health* **2019**, *15*, 435–441. [CrossRef]
34. Calabrese, V.; Dattilo, S.; Petralia, A.; Parenti, R.; Pennisi, M.; Koverech, G.; Calabrese, V.; Graziano, A.; Monte, I.; Maiolino, L.; et al. Analytical approaches to the diagnosis and treatment of aging and aging-related disease: Redox status and proteomics. *Free Radic. Res.* **2015**, *49*, 511–524. [CrossRef] [PubMed]
35. Serapide, M.F.; Zappalà, A.; Parenti, R.; Pantò, M.R.; Cicirata, F. Laterality of the pontocerebellar projections in the rat. *Eur. J. Neurosci.* **2002**, *15*, 1551–1556. [CrossRef] [PubMed]
36. Cicirata, F.; Parenti, R.; Spinella, F.; Giglio, S.; Tuorto, F.; Zuffardi, O.; Gulisano, M. Genomic organization and chromosomal localization of the mouse Connexin36 (mCx36) gene. *Gene* **2000**, *251*, 123–130. [CrossRef]
37. Wang, H.; Tan, X.; Xu, J.; Li, H.; Wang, M.; Chen, S.; Yang, X.; Liu, Y.; Wang, F. Negative correlation between CSF lactate levels and MoCA scores in male Chinese subjects. *Psychiatry Res.* **2017**, *255*, 49–51. [CrossRef] [PubMed]
38. Wang, M.; Chua, S.C.; Bouhadir, L.; Treadwell, E.L.; Gibbs, E.; McGee, T.M. Point-of-care measurement of fetal blood lactate - Time to trust a new device. *Aust. N. Z. J. Obstet. Gynaecol.* **2018**, *1*, 72–78. [CrossRef]
39. Woods, D.L.; Wyma, J.M.; Yund, E.W.; Herron, T.J.; Reed, B. Factors influencing the latency of simple reaction time. *Front. Hum. Neurosci.* **2015**, *9*, 131. [CrossRef]
40. Zaehringer, J.; Falquez, R.; Schubert, A.L.; Nees, F.; Barnow, S. Neural correlates of reappraisal considering working memory capacity and cognitive flexibility. *Brain Imaging Behav.* **2018**, *6*, 1529–1543. [CrossRef]

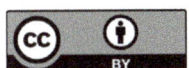

© 2020 by the authors. Licensee MDPI, Basel, Switzerland. This article is an open access article distributed under the terms and conditions of the Creative Commons Attribution (CC BY) license (http://creativecommons.org/licenses/by/4.0/).

Article

The Predictive Role of Raw Bioelectrical Impedance Parameters in Water Compartments and Fluid Distribution Assessed by Dilution Techniques in Athletes

Ruben Francisco [1], Catarina N. Matias [1], Diana A. Santos [1], Francesco Campa [2,3,*], Claudia S. Minderico [1], Paulo Rocha [1], Steven B. Heymsfield [4], Henry Lukaski [5], Luís B. Sardinha [1] and Analiza M. Silva [1]

1. Exercise and Health Laboratory, CIPER, Faculdade Motricidade Humana, Universidade de Lisboa, 1499-002 Lisbon, Portugal; ruben92francisco@gmail.com (R.F.); cmatias@fmh.ulisboa.pt (C.N.M.); dianasantos@fmh.utl.pt (D.A.S.); cminderico@gmail.com (C.S.M.); procha@fmh.ulisboa.pt (P.R.); lbsardinha55@gmail.com (L.B.S.); analiza.monica@gmail.com (A.M.S.)
2. Departments of Biomedical and Neuromotor Sciences, University of Bologna, 40121 Bologna, Italy
3. Department for Life Quality Studies, University of Bologna, 47921 Rimini, Italy
4. Pennington Biomedical Research Foundation, Baton Rouge, Louisiana, LO 70808, USA; Steven.Heymsfield@pbrc.edu
5. Department of Kinesiology and Public Health Education, Hyslop Sports Center, University of North Dakota, Grand Forks, ND 58202, USA; henry.lukaski@und.edu
* Correspondence: francesco.campa3@unibo.it; Tel.: +39-345-0031-080

Received: 20 December 2019; Accepted: 23 January 2020; Published: 24 January 2020

Abstract: The aims of this study were to analyze the usefulness of raw bioelectrical impedance (BI) parameters in assessing water compartments and fluid distribution in athletes. A total of 202 men and 71 female athletes were analyzed. Total body water (TBW) and extracellular water (ECW) were determined by dilution techniques, while intracellular water (ICW) was calculated. Fluid distribution was calculated as the ECW/ICW ratio (E:I). Phase angle (PhA), resistance (R) and reactance (Xc) were obtained through BI spectroscopy using frequency 50kHz. Fat (FM) and fat-free mass (FFM) were assessed by dual-energy X-ray absorptiometry. After adjusting for height, FM, FFM, age and sports category we observed that: PhA predicted ICW (females: β = 1.62, $p < 0.01$; males: β = 2.70, $p < 0.01$) and E:I (males and females: β = −0.08; $p < 0.01$); R explained TBW (females: β = −0.03; $p < 0.01$; males: β = −0.06; $p < 0.01$) and ECW (females: β = −0.02, $p < 0.01$; males: β = −0.03, $p < 0.01$) and ICW (females: β = −0.01, $p < 0.053$; males: β = −0.03 $p < 0.01$); and Xc predicted ECW (females: β = −0.06, $p < 0.01$; males: β = −0.12, $p < 0.01$). A higher PhA is a good predictor of a larger ICW pool and a lower E:I, regardless of body composition, age, height, and sports category. Lower R is associated with higher water pools whereas ECW expansion is explained by lower Xc. Raw BI parameters are useful predictors of total and extracellular pools, cellular hydration and fluid distribution in athletes.

Keywords: phase angle; resistance; reactance; bioimpedance; health

1. Introduction

Assessing fluid balance to monitor the hydration status in athletes has received substantial interest over the last years for maximizing performance [1–3].

Bioelectrical impedance analysis (BIA) has been widely used as a rapid, safe and non-invasive method for monitoring active adults performing recreational exercise and elite athletes [4–6] and in estimating body composition and nutritional status in healthy non-athletes and adults with clinical conditions [7–9]. Alternating current is introduced into the body by bioimpedance electronic devices at single or multiple frequencies. Passive bioelectrical measurements can be related to physiological or body composition parameters.

In addition, this test is important because it enables the use of resistance (R), reactance (Xc) and phase angle (PhA) as indices of biological variables. The resistance (R) arises from body fluids, i.e., extra and intracellular fluids behave as resistive components and resistance is inversely proportional to fluid volume and Reactance (Xc) arises from cell membranes [8]. PhA has been studied as an indicator of nutritional status and disease prognosis, mortality and cellular vitality [10,11]. Its assessment may be valuable for coaches, physicians, nutritionists, and exercise physiologists to provide specific recommendations to improve athletic performance and to avoid compromising health status.

For example, from the wide range of conditioning factors of an athlete's career, muscle injuries can be decisive in limiting participation in training or competitions. Muscle injuries cause marked reductions in R, Xc and PhA [12]; these changes indicated cell membrane disruption and may suggest alteration of fluid compartments. Further, in disease status, the PhA is sensitive to electrical changes in tissues [13]. In a recent study the authors verified that PhA was negatively correlated with fluid retention evaluated using the extracellular water (ECW): total body water (TBW) ratio in patients with advanced cancer [14]. Bioimpedance analysis also has been the focus of previous studies involving patients with hemodialysis [15] and acute heart failure [16].

Thus, because of its relevance, it is pertinent to understand the role of PhA and raw bioelectrical impedance (BI) parameters on water compartments and fluid distribution for potentially provide strategies to promote an adequate fluid balance and cellular hydration.

To our knowledge, only one study analyzed the relation between raw BI variables and fluid compartments in athletes [17]. Marini and colleagues [17] observed that higher values of PhA were related to lower values of the E:I ratio, commonly used as an indicator of fluid distribution. However, the authors did not explore the magnitude of the correlation between raw BI parameters and the water compartments considering the potential impact of body composition. Indeed, the PhA is associated with fat free mass (FFM) and fat mass (FM) and therefore, these variables should be accounted for when exploring the association between this BI marker and fluid-related compartments [10]. However, this analysis is yet to be determined.

Moreover, simple methods are required to assess water compartments and fluid distribution in athletes. Raw BI measure may provide relevant information related to reference methods, i.e., dilution techniques. Therefore, the aim of this study was to investigate the usefulness of raw bioelectrical impedance spectroscopy (BIS) parameters (R, Xc and PhA) at frequency 50kHz on water compartments and fluid distribution, assessed through dilution techniques, in athletes, adjusting for the potential effect of confounding variables such as height, age, body composition, and sports category.

2. Material and Methods

2.1. Participants

A total of 202 males (21.5 ± 4.5y) and 71 females (20.4 ± 5.2y) participated in this observational cross-sectional study. The inclusion criteria were: 1) Tanner stage V or greater [18]; 2) >10 hours of sport specific training per week; 3) have negative anti-doping results, and 4) currently not taking any medication or dietary supplements. Prior to participation, all athletes (parental or guardian) gave their written informed consent, with all procedures approved by the Ethics Committee of the Faculty of Human Kinetics, Technical University of Lisbon and conducted in accordance with the declaration of Helsinki

2.2. Anthropometric Measurements

Height and weight were measured while the subject wore a swimsuit and standardized procedures were used [19].

2.3. Fat Mass (FM) and Fat-Free Nass (FFM)

Whole body FFM and FM were determined by dual-energy X-ray absorptiometry (Hologic Explorer W, QDR for Windows version 12.4, Waltham, MA, USA). In our laboratory, in ten healthy adults, the test-retest CV for FFM and FM are 0.8% and 1.7%, respectively. The technical error of measurement (t.e.m.) is 0.4kg.

2.4. Hydration Status

After a fasting baseline urine sample was collected, the specific gravity (USG) was determined using a refractometer (Urisys 1100, Roche Diagnostics, Portugal) to ensure that all athletes were euhydrated (USG < 1.010) [20]. The coefficient of variation (CV) of the urine specific gravity procedure in our laboratory based on 10 adults is 0.1% [21].

2.5. Total Body Water

Total body water (TBW) was measured by deuterium dilution using a Hydra stable isotope ratio mass spectrometer (PDZ, Europa Scientific, UK). After a 12h fast, the first urine sample was collected. Each participant was given an oral dose of 0.1g of 99.9% ^2H_2O per kg of body weight (Sigma-Aldrich; St. Louis, MO). After a 4 h equilibration period, during which no food or beverage was consumed, a urine sample was collected. Urine and diluted dose samples were prepared for $^1H/^2H$ analysis using the equilibration technique of Prosser and Scrimgeour [22], using procedures described elsewhere [23]. The CV based on 10 repeated measures for TBW with the stable isotope ratio mass spectrometry in this laboratory is 0.3% [21].

2.6. Extracellular Water

Through dilution of sodium bromide (NaBr) was determined extracellular water (ECW). After collection of a saliva sample, each participant was asked to drink 0.030 g of 99.0% NaBr (Sigma-Aldrich; St. Louis, MO) per kg of body weight, diluted in 50 mL of distilled-deionized water, using procedures described elsewhere [23]. Saliva samples were collected into salivettes. Then, the samples were centrifuged and frozen for posterior analyses. The CV in our laboratory based on 10 repeated measures for ECW using high-performance liquid chromatography is 0.4% [23].

2.7. Intracellular Water

Intracellular water (ICW) was determined as the difference between TBW and ECW using the dilution techniques (ICW = TBW − ECW).

2.8. Raw BIA Parameters

Whole body PhA, R and Xc were obtained using bioelectrical impedance spectroscopy (BIS) analyzer (model 4200, Xitron Technologies, San Diego, CA) at frequency of 50kHz. Measurements were performed after a 10-minute period of rest with the participant in a supine position with a leg opening of 45° compared to the median line of the body and the upper limbs positioned 30° away from trunk. Four electrodes were placed on the dorsal surfaces of right foot and ankle and right wrist and hand, as described elsewhere [24]. The biological reliability determined in six participants in our laboratory for R and Xc at 50kHz was 0.6 and 1.5%, respectively [25].

2.9. Statistical Analysis

Descriptive analysis including means ± standard deviations were calculated. Normality was evaluated using Shapiro–Wilk test. Since the data showed a normal distribution a person's correlation was performed between independent (PhA, R and Xc), and dependent variables (ICW, ECW, TBW and E:I ratio) and an independent sample t test was used to compare males and females. Multiple regression analysis was used to assess the association between each of the dependent variables and each independent variable using the unstandardized beta coefficient and adjusting for the confounding variables height, sports category, FFM, FM and age. The variable "sports category" was created to differentiate athletes from modalities of (1) 'endurance' where athletes of swimming, pentathlon, triathlon and sailing were included, (2) 'velocity/power' that encompassed modalities of judo, karate, taekwondo and athletics and (3) 'team sports' which included basketball, handball, volleyball, rugby and soccer.

Significance level was set at $P < 0.05$. The data was analyzed with IBM SPSS Statistics program (TM 24.0 for MacOS). If more than one variable was a predictor in the model, a calculated to evaluate multicollinearity, and values below five were considered not to have multicollinearity issues.

3. Results

Table 1 shows the main characteristics of the athletes included in the sample and identifies the differences between males and females.

Table 1. Body composition, water compartments and raw bioelectrical impedance (BI) parameters at 50 kHz frequency.

Variable	WOMEN (N = 71)			MEN (N = 202)		
	Minimum	Mean ± SD	Maximum	Minimum	Mean ± SD	Maximum
Age (y)	15	20.4 ± 5.2	35	15	21.5 ± 4.5	38
Body Mass (kg)	48.5	63.9 ± 8.8	81.9	56.5	77.6 ± 13.0 §	130.3
Height (cm)	152.2	170.8 ± 8.0	195.0	164.4	181.4 ± 9.2 §	204.7
BMI (kg/m^2)	17.7	21.9 ± 2.1	26.0	18.6	23.7 ± 4.1 §	58.7
FM (kg)	8.3	15.6 ± 4.3	26.5	4.8	11.2 ± 5.8 §	45.2
FFM (kg)	35.4	48.0 ± 6.1	60.4	49.5	65.6 ± 8.7 §	91.7
Resistance (Ω)	435.1	561.2 ± 65.9	720.1	305.6	456.0 ± 56.5 §	582.1
Reactance (Ω)	48.8	67.3 ± 8.5	87.1	43.5	62.9 ± 7.9 §	85.2
Impedance (Ω)	438.1	565.1 ± 68.3	724.4	120.6	459.5 ± 62.1 §	587.9
R/H ((Ω/m)	246.0	329.0 ± 39.6	432.5	164.6	251.8 ± 31.8 §	319.7
Xc/H (Ω/m)	27.4	39.5 ± 5.4	52.9	23.4	34.8 ± 4.9 §	46.9
Z/H (Ω/m)	247.7	331.4 ± 39.9	435.7	166.3	254.5 ± 32.2 §	321.9
Phase Angle (°)	5.8	6.9 ± 0.6	8.7	5.8	7.9 ± 0.7 §	10.0
Intracellular Water (kg)	14.4	20.5 ± 3.5	29.9	18.1	30.3 ± 6.2 §	56.5
Extracellular Water (kg)	11.0	14.9 ± 1.9	19.25	12.7	19.3 ± 2.9 §	29.0
Total Body Water (kg)	25.6	35.4 ± 4.9	45.9	34.5	49.5 ± 7.8 §	76.3
ECW/ICW ratio	0.5	0.7 ± 0.1	0.9	0.3	0.6 ± 0.1 §	0.9

Abbreviations: BMI, body-mass index; FM, fat mass; FFM, free fat mass; E:I, extracellular:intracellular water ratio; R/H, resistance standardized for height; Xc/H, reactance standardized for height; Z/H, vector length standardized for height; SD, standard deviation. § $P < 0.01$ (independent sample t test).

Body mass and height were higher in the male group ($p < 0.01$). Male sample present higher values of FFM ($p < 0.01$). Whereas the female sample presents FM values significantly greater than the males ($p < 0.01$). R, Xc, R/H and Xc/H were higher in the female group ($p < 0.01$), while the PhA was higher in the male group ($p < 0.01$). Men presented higher ICW, ECW and TBW values ($p < 0.01$), while women had higher E:I ratio values ($p < 0.01$).

The association between the raw BIA parameters and the water compartments (ICW, ECW and TBW) and fluid distribution (E:I ratio) is presented in Table 2.

For PhA, the strongest correlation was shown with E:I ratio. The PhA was inversely related with E:I ratio in females ($r = -0.52$, $p < 0.01$) and males ($r = -0.55$, $p < 0.01$). While R/H was negatively associated with TBW ($r = -0.84$, $p < 0.01$ for females and $r = -0.87$, $p < 0.01$ for males). For Xc, an association was found with ECW ($r = -0.76$, $p < 0.01$ for females and $r = -0.68$, $p < 0.01$ for males). Additionally, for FFM we observed the strongest correlation with TBW for males ($r = 0.91$, $p < 0.01$) and females ($r = 0.92$, $p < 0.01$). For FM, the strongest correlation was observed with TBW for men ($r = 0.64$, $p < 0.01$) and with ECW in women ($r = 0.55$, $p < 0.01$).

As described in Table 3, the PhA was a significant predictor of ICW for both sexes ($\beta = 1.62$; $p < 0.01$ for females and $\beta = 2.70$; $p < 0.01$ for males), regardless of height, sports category, FFM, FM and age. PhA explained alone (without adjustment to covariables) 12% and 17% of the ICW values, respectively for females and males.

Table 2. Pearson correlation coefficients (r) between raw bioelectrical impedance parameters and fluid volumes and distribution.

Variable	ICW			ECW			TBW			E:I		
	Total N = 273	Women N = 71	Men N = 202	Total N = 273	Women N = 71	Men N = 202	Total N = 273	Women N = 71	Men N = 202	Total N = 273	Women N = 71	Men N = 202
PhA°	0.60** p < 0.01	0.34** p = 0.003	0.42** p < 0.01	0.25** p < 0.01	−0.08 p = 0.505	−0.10 p = 0.152	0.53** p < 0.01	0.22 p = 0.071	0.30** p < 0.01	−0.61** p < 0.01	−0.52** p < 0.01	−0.55** p < 0.01
R/H (Ω/m)	−0.84** p < 0.01	−0.75** p < 0.01	−0.78** p < 0.01	−0.81** p < 0.01	−0.79** p < 0.01	−0.69** p < 0.01	−0.91** p < 0.01	−0.84** p < 0.01	−0.87** p < 0.01	0.40** p < 0.01	0.19 p = 0.110	0.27** p = 0.001
Xc/H (Ω/m)	−0.55** p < 0.01	−0.44** p < 0.01	−0.44** p < 0.01	−0.74** p < 0.01	−0.76** p < 0.01	−0.68** p < 0.01	−0.66** p < 0.01	−0.61** p < 0.01	−0.60** p < 0.01	0.01 p = 0.148	−0.17 p = 0.157	−0.12 p = 0.089
FFM	0.89** p < 0.01	0.82** p < 0.01	0.81** p < 0.01	0.84** p < 0.01	0.87** p < 0.01	0.72** p < 0.01	0.95** p < 0.01	0.92** p < 0.01	0.91** p < 0.01	−0.41** p < 0.01	−0.20** p < 0.01	−0.27** p < 0.01
FM	0.20** p < 0.01	0.27* p = 0.03	0.59** p < 0.01	0.16** p < 0.01	0.55** p < 0.01	0.46** p < 0.01	0.21** p < 0.01	0.40** p < 0.01	0.64** p < 0.01	−0.01 p = 0.95	0.21 p = 0.09	−0.21** p < 0.01

Abbreviations: ICW, intracellular water; ECW, extracellular water; TBW, total body water; E:I, extracellular:intracellular water; Z/H, impedance standardized for height (m); Xc/H, reactance standardized for height (m); R/H, resistance standardized for height; PhA, phase angle. ** Correlations were significant at $p < 0.05$; * correlations were significant at $p < 0.01$.

Table 3. Linear and Multiple Regression Analysis Between PhA and ICW, TBW and E:I.

	ICW				TBW				E:I		
Women	β	SE	p	Women	β	SE	p	Women	β	SE	p
PhA (°)	1.62	0.38	<0.01	PhA (°)	1.25	0.38	0.02	PhA (°)	−0.08	0.02	<0.01
Height (cm)	−0.04	0.04	0.427	Height (cm)	−0.04	0.04	0.355	Height (cm)	0.001	0.002	0.792
Sports Category	0.27	0.29	0.354	Sports Category	−0.03	0.29	0.929	Sports Category	−0.02	0.01	0.145
FFM (kg)	0.52	0.06	<0.01	FFM (kg)	0.76	0.06	<0.01	FFM (kg)	−0.01	0.003	0.047
FM (kg)	0.01	0.06	0.984	FM (kg)	0.11	0.06	0.062	FM (kg)	0.01	0.003	0.045
Age	−0.12	0.04	0.009	Age	−0.11	0.04	0.011	Age	0.004	0.002	0.038
Men	β	SE	p	Men	β	SE	p	Men	β	SE	p
PhA (°)	2.70	0.33	<0.01	PhA (°)	2.01	0.29	<0.01	PhA (°)	−0.08	0.01	<0.01
Height (cm)	−0.06	0.03	0.082	Height (cm)	−0.07	0.03	0.017	Height (cm)	0.001	0.001	0.640
Sports Category	−0.03	0.30	0.912	Sports Category	0.51	0.27	0.061	Sports Category	0.01	0.01	0.205
FFM (kg)	0.54	0.04	<0.01	FFM (kg)	0.76	0.03	<0.01	FFM (kg)	−0.002	0.001	0.052
FM (kg)	0.18	0.04	<0.01	FM (kg)	0.20	0.04	<0.01	FM (kg)	−0.002	0.001	0.204
Age	−0.08	0.05	0.080	Age	−0.11	0.04	0.008	Age	0.001	0.001	0.844

Model adjusted for height, sports category, fat free mass, fat mass, and age. Abbreviations: PhA, phase angle; TBW, total-body water; ECW, extracellular water; ICW, intracellular water; FM, fat mass; FFM, fat-free mass; SE, standard error, β, regression coefficient.

PhA was also considered a significant predictor of TBW in males ($\beta = 2.01; p < 0.01$), explaining alone about 9% of TBW values. In both sexes, PhA explained 27% and 30% of E:I, respectively. When adjusted to covariables, the PhA presented a negative β value ($\beta = -0.08; p < 0.01$ for both), which means that it is inversely related to the fluid distribution in females and males.

R explains alone (the unadjusted r^2, i.e., the predictive power of R in explaining the variability of the ICW values without adjusting for confounding variables) about 33% and 45% of the ICW values in females and males, respectively. When adjusted to covariables (Table 4) the R is inversely related to the ICW for females ($\beta = -0.01, p = 0.053$) and males ($\beta = -0.03, p < 0.01$).

In both sexes, R was also considered a significant predictor of ECW ($\beta = -0.02, p < 0.01$ for females and $\beta = -0.03, p < 0.01$ for males) explaining alone 32% and 24% of ECW values, respectively (the unadjusted r^2). When adjusted to covariables the R was considered a significant predictor in females ($\beta = -0.03, p < 0.01$) and males ($\beta = -0.06, p < 0.01$) of TBW values. R explained alone (without adjustment for covariables) about 39% in females and 51% in males.

As described in Table 5, Xc was considered a significant predictor of ECW ($\beta = -0.06, p < 0.01$ for females and $\beta = -0.12, p < 0.01$ for males) and is directly related to the ICW ($\beta = 0.06, p = 0.069$ for females and $\beta = 0.08, p = 0.010$ for males).

The Xc explains without adjustment for confounding variables 35% and 32% of ECW values and 9% and 14% of ICW values in females and males, respectively.

The associations between BI parameters and fluid-related variables assessed through dilution techniques are displayed in Figure 1.

Table 4. Multiple regression analysis between R and ICW, ECW and TBW.

	ICW			ECW			TBW		
Women	β	SE	p	β	SE	p	β	SE	p
R (Ω)	−0.01	0.01	0.053	−0.02	0.003	<0.01	−0.03	0.01	<0.01
Height (cm)	0.01	0.07	0.887	0.12	0.03	<0.01	0.13	0.06	0.037
Sports Category	0.37	0.32	0.248	−0.17	0.12	0.154	0.20	0.27	0.462
FFM (kg)	0.42	0.11	<0.01	0.04	0.04	0.307	0.47	0.09	<0.01
FM (kg)	−0.06	0.06	0.343	0.12	0.02	<0.01	0.06	0.05	0.28
Age	−0.11	0.05	0.021	0.01	0.02	0.740	−0.11	0.04	0.01
Men	β	SE	p	β	SE	p	β	SE	p
R (Ω)	−0.03	0.01	<0.01	−0.03	0.004	<0.01	−0.06	0.01	<0.01
Height (cm)	−0.05	0.05	0.340	0.17	0.03	<0.01	0.12	0.04	0.001
Sports Category	−0.04	0.34	0.898	0.29	0.19	0.127	0.25	0.24	0.287
FFM (kg)	0.45	0.07	<0.01	−0.04	0.04	0.905	0.44	0.05	<0.01
FM (kg)	0.18	0.05	<0.01	0.05	0.03	0.089	0.23	0.03	<0.01
Age	−0.06	0.05	0.238	−0.02	0.03	0.568	−0.08	0.04	0.032

Model adjusted for height, sports category, fat free mass, fat mass, and age Abbreviations: R, resistance; TBW, total-body water; ECW, extracellular water; ICW, intracellular water; FM, fat mass; FFM, fat-free mass; SE, standard error, β, regression coefficient.

Table 5. Linear and multiple regression analysis between Xc and ICW, ECW and TBW.

	ICW				ECW				TBW		
Women	β	SE	p	**Women**	β	SE	p	**Women**	β	SE	p
Xc(Ω)	0.06	0.03	0.069	Xc(Ω)	−0.06	0.01	<0.01	Xc(Ω)	0.001	0.03	0.968
Height (cm)	−0.13	0.05	0.012	Height (cm)	0.04	0.02	0.044	Height (cm)	−0.09	0.05	0.071
Sports Category	0.20	0.32	0.526	Sports Category	−0.24	0.12	0.062	Sports Category	−0.03	0.31	0.916
FFM(kg)	0.66	0.07	<0.01	FFM(kg)	0.17	0.03	<0.01	FFM (kg)	0.83	0.07	<0.01
FM (kg)	−0.03	0.06	0.645	FM (kg)	0.10	0.03	<0.01	FM (kg)	0.07	0.06	0.286
Age	−0.12	0.05	0.017	Age	0.003	0.02	0.859	Age	−0.114	0.05	0.017
Men	β	SE	p	**Men**	β	SE	p	**Men**	β	SE	p
Xc(Ω)	0.08	0.03	0.010	Xc(Ω)	−0.12	0.02	<0.01	Xc(Ω)	−0.03	0.03	0.306
Height (cm)	−0.24	0.03	<0.01	Height (cm)	0.06	0.02	0.003	Height (cm)	−0.18	0.03	<0.01
Sports Category	0.20	0.34	0.562	Sports Category	0.45	0.19	0.020	Sports Category	0.65	0.30	0.031
FFM (kg)	0.71	0.05	<0.01	FFM (kg)	0.12	0.03	<0.01	FFM (kg)	0.83	0.04	<0.01
FM (kg)	0.16	0.05	0.002	FM (kg)	0.03	0.03	0.294	FM (kg)	0.19	0.04	<0.01
Age	−0.08	0.05	0.091	Age	−0.02	0.03	0.611	Age	−0.10	0.05	0.025

Model adjusted for height, sports category, fat free mass, fat mass, and age; Abbreviations: Xc, reactance; TBW, total-body water; ECW, extracellular water; ICW, intracellular water; FM, fat mass; FFM, fat-free mass; SE, standard error, β, regression coefficient.

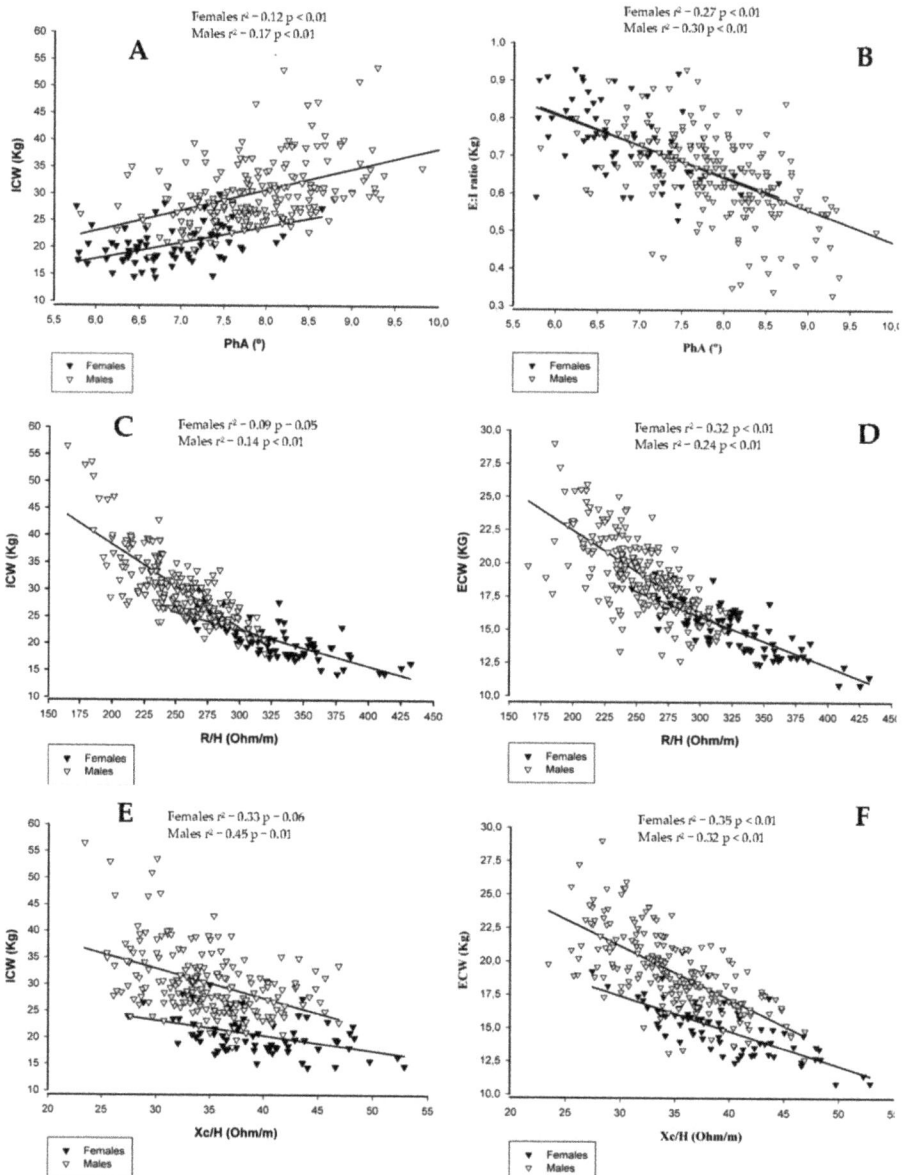

Figure 1. The independent association of BI parameters with fluid-related variables assessed through dilution techniques. Panel (**A**): PhA vs ICW; Panel (**B**): PhA vs E:I ratio; Panel (**C**): R/H vs ICW; Panel (**D**): R/H vs ECW; Panel (**E**): Xc/H vs ICW; Panel (**F**): Xc/H vs ECW. Abbreviations: PhA, phase angle; R/H, ratio between resistance and height (m); E:I ratio, ratio between extra-to-intracellular water; Xc/H, ratio between reactance and height (m); ECW, extracellular water; ICW, intracellular water.

4. Discussion

The main findings of this study conducted in athletes included: (i) athletes with higher PhA values were those presenting higher values of TBW, particularly at the ICW compartment and, consequently, lower E:I ratio (representing body fluid distribution); (ii) higher Xc values predicted lower ECW and higher ICW; and (iii) R is strongly associated with water compartments. The role of these BI parameters on fluid compartments remained significant regardless of FM, FFM, age, height and sports category. The adjustment for the covariates was performed since FM, FFM, age, height [11], and sport category [26] were shown to have an impact on the variables under study.

In a recent study, a strong association between E:I ratio and PhA in healthy people was observed [11]. Few studies [4,17] explored associations between BI measurements and reference determinations of fluid volumes in athletes using tracer dilution methods. Marini and colleagues [17] confirmed in athletes that PhA detected E:I differences in both sexes, with lower PhA values in subjects with higher E:I ratio, independently of age and sports category. However, the authors did not adjust these associations for body composition.

Regarding R, in this study, it was found that the males presented significantly lower values than the females (329.0Ω/m ± 39.6 and 251.8Ω/m ± 31.8, respectively). These values extend results observed in other studies performed in athletes [6,17]. R refers to the opposition offered by the human body to the passage of an electric current. In short, the conductivity of the tissues is proportional to the amount of body water and electrolytes [8]. Men presented significantly higher values of TBW than women, which means that the electric current flows more freely in the male body than in the female body. In addition, women presented higher FM values than men. FM has a poor conducting ability due to its low water constitution. In both sexes, as expected, the lowest R values are found in athletes who have higher TBW, ICW and ECW after adjusting for covariates.

Reactance has been associated with cellular integrity. Theoretically, in biological conductors, high reactance values are expected from a BI measurement in healthy membranes with higher integrity. The healthy cell membranes act as capacitors by storing the current and releasing it. For example, it was found a Xc decrease after muscle injury (greater decline in major lesions) attributable to the muscle cell damage [12]. As a result, PhA also decreased. Thus, Xc is proportional to cell membrane integrity with Xc and PhA decrements occurring when the cell membrane is compromised. According to Liedtke [27], Xc is a measure of the volume of cell membrane capacitance and an indirect measure of the intracellular volume. In our study, higher Xc values explained higher ICW values in both sexes, regardless of height, FFM, FM, age and sports category.

In addition, we observed that Xc was a predictor of ECW values in males and females. Marini and colleagues [17] found similar results. The negative relationship between Xc and ECW in both sexes may be a possible biological justification for the high values of Xc in this study when compared to a clinical population [28,29]

Concerning PhA, in this study males presented a mean value of 7.9° ± 0.7 and females a mean value of 6.9° ± 0.6. These values are similar to those found in other studies conducted in athletes or active young population [6,17,24,30,31]. However, the values found in present study are slightly below those proposed by Barbosa-Silva and colleagues [32] according to gender and age for healthy adult population. As shown previously, men have higher PhA values than women [11,17,24,32], despite in the present study the Xc values were higher in females than in males (39.5 Ω/m ± 5.4 and 34.8 Ω/m ± 4.9, respectively), the lower R in the male group may be part of the explanation for a larger PhA in men relative to women. Indeed, PhA is a significant predictor of ICW in females and males, regardless of the covariates. It is sufficiently clear how important ICW is in increasing performance in athletes. For example, Silva and colleagues [2] observed in elite judo athletes that there is a decrease in the upper limbs power, in athletes that decreased the ICW compartment. In addition, ICW appears to be a good predictor of the risk of lower grip strength in elite judo athletes [3], essential for attack and defense techniques. It has long been postulated that a larger intracellular volume is an anabolic signal promoter according to "The Cell Swelling Theory" and consequent increase in cell volume. In fact, cell swelling leads to anabolism, whereas cell shrinkage promotes catabolism [33,34]. Considering the above-mentioned information, it seems plausible that PhA a predictor of ICW in athletes.

PhA was also considered a significant predictor of TBW in males. There is currently robust scientific evidence regarding the importance of TBW in biological performance, and only a small reduction in the hydration state may limit some of the body's physiological processes, namely, power, muscular strength and endurance [2,35]. Although the amount of TBW is of extreme importance, focusing on this parameter alone can be limiting. Ribeiro and colleagues [30] in a study conducted in a non-athletic population, found that despite unchanged TBW, strength training contributed to a greater expansion of ICW, resulting in a reduction of the E:I ratio and an increased PhA. A better understanding of how TBW is distributed through its water compartments is required.

The E:I ratio has previously been studied in a healthy non-athletic adult population [10] by using labeled tritium dilution (^3H_2O) to determine TBW, total body potassium for ICW and ECW estimated by the difference between TBW and ICW. The authors verified that E:I was considered a predictor of PhA. Our results extend the aforementioned findings as the PhA was considered a strong predictor of the E:I ratio in athletes independently of height, FM, FFM, age and sports category.

Lower E:I values are often found in athletes. For example, Marini and colleagues [17] found E:I values of 0.6 ± 0.1 in men and 0.7 ± 0.1 in women. On the other hand, higher values were found in a study by Gonzales and colleagues [11] conducting in healthy non-athletic adults. These authors found E:I values of 1.03 in women and 0.79 in men. We can speculate that athletes have well-defined water regulation mechanisms at the level of cell membranes preserving a greater amount of ICW.

In Marini's study the raw parameters of the BIA were evaluated by means of a single BIA frequency (BIA 101 Anniversary, Akern, Florence, Italy). This method utilizes a phase-sensitive impedance that introduces a constant, low-level alternating current, enabling direct measurement of PhA and Z and then R and Xc can be calculated. In our study BIS was used to measure resistance R and reactance Xc while impedance and PhA were calculated at each measured frequency (in this case 50kHz which is reported as a standard constant current condition, commonly used by most studies). In a recent study by Silva and colleagues [25], a comparison between single and multi-frequency devices (Akern and BIS) was conducted in a highly active population. The authors found that the both devices were highly related in measuring raw BIA parameters at a frequency of 50kHz but a lack of agreement was observed at the individual level. In the aforementioned study, the BIS instrument provided significantly lower values of R and Xc but higher values of PhA at 50kHz.

Thus, we should address as a limitation of this study the fact that the use of a non-phase sensitivity BIA equipment may not be free of a latent model error prediction in the calculation of PhA, though reference techniques were used to determine water and its compartments. In addition, this study presented a cross-sectional design limiting the inference for longitudinal relationships. Thus, further studies should be carried out using a longitudinal approach to explore how raw BIA measures impact fluid-related changes, especially in light of the high physical damage resulting from a large volume of training and competitions during the sport season.

In conclusion, athletes with higher values of PhA have a lower value of E:I ratio and a higher value of ICW and TBW, regardless of height, body composition, sports category, and age. As expected, R values were predictors of TBW, ECW and ICW. Lower R values are observed in athletes who present higher TBW and its extra and intracellular water compartments. In both sexes, higher values of Xc are associated with a lower ECW expansion and with a higher ICW pool. The practical applicability of this study is clear for coaches, physicians, nutritionists, and exercise physiologists: new methods to assess hydration status that are time-efficient, simple, safe, precise, accurate and reliable are needed and the usefulness of raw BI parameters in the assessment water compartments and fluid distribution of elite athletes was highlighted in this study.

Author Contributions: Formal analysis, D.A.S.; investigation, R.F., C.N.M. and D.A.S.; methodology, D.A.S.; supervision, A.M.S.; writing—original draft, R.F., C.N.M., C.M. and A.M.S.; writing—review and editing, F.C., P.R., S.B.H., H.L., L.B.S. and A.M.S. All authors have read and agreed to the published version of the manuscript.

Funding: This research received no external funding.

Acknowledgments: We would like to express our gratitude to the athletes for their time and effort.

Conflicts of Interest: The authors declare no conflicts of interest.

References

1. Campa, F.; Gatterer, H.; Lukaski, H.; Toselli, S. Stabilizing Bioimpedance-vector-analysis measures with a 10-minute cold shower after running exercise to enable assessment of body hydration. *Int. J. Sports Physiol. Perform.* **2019**, *14*, 1–13. [CrossRef] [PubMed]
2. Silva, A.M.; Fields, D.A.; Heymsfield, S.B.; Sardinha, L.B. Body composition and power changes in elite judo athletes. *Int. J. Sports Med.* **2010**, *31*, 737–741. [CrossRef] [PubMed]
3. Silva, A.M.; Fields, D.A.; Heymsfield, S.B.; Sardinha, L.B. Relationship between changes in total-body water and fluid distribution with maximal forearm strength in elite judo athletes. *J. Strength Cond. Res.* **2011**, *25*, 2488–2495. [CrossRef] [PubMed]
4. Campa, F.; Matias, C.N.; Marini, E.; Heymsfield, S.B.; Toselli, S.; Sardinha, L.B.; Silva, A.M. Identifying athlete body-fluid changes during a competitive season with bioelectrical impedance vector analysis. *Int. J. Sports. Physiol. Perform.* **2019**, *11*, 1–21. [CrossRef]
5. Matias, C.N.; Judice, P.B.; Santos, D.A.; Magalhaes, J.P.; Minderico, C.S.; Fields, D.A.; Sardinha, L.B.; Silva, A.M. Suitability of bioelectrical based methods to assess water compartments in recreational and elite athletes. *J. Am. Coll. Nutr.* **2016**, *35*, 413–421. [CrossRef]
6. Matias, C.N.; Monteiro, C.P.; Santos, D.A.; Martins, F.; Silva, A.M.; Laires, M.J.; Sardinha, L.B. Magnesium and phase angle: a prognostic tool for monitoring cellular integrity in judo athletes. *Magnes. Res.* **2015**, *28*, 92–98. [CrossRef]
7. Campa, F.; Silva, A.M.; Toselli, S. Changes in phase angle and handgrip strength induced by suspension training in older women. *Int. J. Sports Med.* **2018**, *39*, 442–449. [CrossRef]
8. Kyle, U.G.; Bosaeus, I.; de Lorenzo, A.D.; Deurenberg, P.; Elia, M.; Gomez, J.M.; Heitmann, B.L.; Kent-Smith, L.; Melchior, J.C.; Pirlich, M.; et al. Bioelectrical impedance analysis—part I: Review of principles and methods. *Clin. Nutr.* **2004**, *23*, 1226–1243. [CrossRef]
9. Kyle, U.G.; Bosaeus, I.; de Lorenzo, A.D.; Deurenberg, P.; Elia, M.; Manuel, G.J.; Lilienthal, H.B.; Kent-Smith, L.; Melchior, J.C.; Pirlich, M.; et al. Bioelectrical impedance analysis-part II: Utilization in clinical practice. *Clin. Nutr.* **2004**, *23*, 1430–1453. [CrossRef]
10. Garlini, L.M.; Alves, F.D.; Ceretta, L.B.; Perry, I.S.; Souza, G.C.; Clausell, N.O. Phase angle and mortality: A systematic review. *Eur. J. Clin. Nutr.* **2019**, *73*, 495–508. [CrossRef]
11. Gonzalez, M.C.; Barbosa-Silva, T.G.; Bielemann, R.M.; Gallagher, D.; Heymsfield, S.B. Phase angle and its determinants in healthy subjects: influence of body composition. *Am. J. Clin. Nutr.* **2016**, *103*, 712–716. [CrossRef] [PubMed]
12. Nescolarde, L.; Yanguas, J.; Lukaski, H.; Alomar, X.; Rosell-Ferrer, J.; Rodas, G. Localized bioimpedance to assess muscle injury. *Physiol. Meas.* **2013**, *34*, 237–245. [CrossRef] [PubMed]
13. Toso, S.; Piccoli, A.; Gusella, M.; Menon, D.; Bononi, A.; Crepaldi, G.; Ferrazzi, E. Altered tissue electric properties in lung cancer patients as detected by bioelectric impedance vector analysis. *Nutrition* **2000**, *16*, 120–124. [CrossRef]
14. Miura, T.; Matsumoto, Y.; Kawaguchi, T.; Masuda, Y.; Okizaki, A.; Koga, H.; Tagami, K.; Watanabe, Y.S.; Uehara, Y.; Yamaguchi, T.; et al. Low phase angle is correlated with worse general condition in patients with advanced cancer. *Nutr. Cancer* **2019**, *71*, 83–88. [CrossRef]
15. Kang, S.H.; Choi, E.W.; Park, J.W.; Cho, K.H.; Do, J.Y. Clinical significance of the edema index in incident peritoneal dialysis patients. *PLoS ONE* **2016**, *11*. [CrossRef]
16. Yamazoe, M.; Mizuno, A.; Niwa, K.; Isobe, M. Edema index measured by bioelectrical impedance analysis as a predictor of fluid reduction needed to remove clinical congestion in acute heart failure. *Int. J. Cardiol.* **2015**, *201*, 190–192. [CrossRef]
17. Marini, E.; Campa, F.; Buffa, R.; Stagi, S.; Matias, C.N.; Toselli, S.; Sardinha, L.B.; Silva, A.M. Phase angle and bioelectrical impedance vector analysis in the evaluation of body composition in athletes. *Clin. Nutr.* **2019**. [CrossRef]
18. Tanner, J. The development of the reproductive system. *Growth at adolescence* **1962**, 28–39.
19. Lohman, T.G. Applicability of body composition techniques and constants for children and youths. *Exerc. Sport Sci. Rev.* **1986**, *14*, 325–357. [CrossRef]
20. Casa, D.J.; Clarkson, P.M.; Roberts, W.O. American college of sports medicine roundtable on hydration and physical activity: Consensus statements. *Curr. Sports Med. Rep.* **2005**, *4*, 115–127. [CrossRef]

21. Silva, A.M.; Santos, D.A.; Matias, C.N.; Minderico, C.S.; Schoeller, D.A.; Sardinha, L.B. Total energy expenditure assessment in elite junior basketball players: A validation study using doubly labeled water. *J. Strength Cond. Res.* **2013**, *27*, 1920–1927. [CrossRef] [PubMed]
22. Prosser, S.J.; Scrimgeour, C.M. High-precision determination of 2H/1H in H2 and H2O by continuous-flow isotope ratio mass spectrometry. *Anal. Chem.* **1995**, *67*, 1992–1997. [CrossRef]
23. Matias, C.N.; Silva, A.M.; Santos, D.A.; Gobbo, L.A.; Schoeller, D.A.; Sardinha, L.B. Validity of extracellular water assessment with saliva samples using plasma as the reference biological fluid. *Biomed. Chromatogr.* **2012**, *26*, 1348–1352. [CrossRef] [PubMed]
24. Campa, F.; Matias, C.; Gatterer, H.; Toselli, S.; Koury, J.C.; Andreoli, A.; Melchiorri, G.; Sardinha, L.B.; Silva, A.M. Classic bioelectrical impedance vector reference values for assessing body composition in male and female athletes. *Int. J. Environ. Res. Public Health* **2019**, *16*. [CrossRef]
25. Silva, A.M.; Matias, C.N.; Nunes, C.L.; Santos, D.A.; Marini, E.; Lukaski, H.C.; Sardinha, L.B. Lack of agreement of in vivo raw bioimpedance measurements obtained from two single and multi-frequency bioelectrical impedance devices. *Eur. J. Clin. Nutr.* **2019**, *73*, 1077–1083. [CrossRef]
26. Silva, A.M. Structural and functional body components in athletic health and performance phenotypes. *Eur. J. Clin.Nutr.* **2019**, *73*, 215–224. [CrossRef]
27. Liedtke, R.J. *Principles of Bioelectrical Impedance Analysis*; RJL Systems Inc.: Clinton, MI, USA, 1997.
28. Van Lettow, M.; Kumwenda, J.J.; Harries, A.D.; Whalen, C.C.; Taha, T.E.; Kumwenda, N.; Kang'ombe, C.; Semba, R.D. Malnutrition and the severity of lung disease in adults with pulmonary tuberculosis in Malawi. *Int. J. Tuberc. Lung. Dis.* **2004**, *8*, 211–217.
29. Maggiore, Q.; Nigrelli, S.; Ciccarelli, C.; Grimaldi, C.; Rossi, G.A.; Michelassi, C. Nutritional and prognostic correlates of bioimpedance indexes in hemodialysis patients. *Kidney Int.* **1996**, *50*, 2103–2108. [CrossRef]
30. Ribeiro, A.S.; Nascimento, M.A.; Schoenfeld, B.J.; Nunes, J.P.; Aguiar, A.F.; Cavalcante, E.F.; Silva, A.M.; Sardinha, L.B.; Fleck, S.J.; Cyrino, E.S. Effects of single set resistance training with different frequencies on a cellular health indicator in older women. *J. Aging Phys. Act.* **2018**, *26*, 537–543. [CrossRef]
31. Campa, F.; Toselli, S. Bioimpedance vector analysis of elite, subelite, and low-level male volleyball players. *Int. J. Sports Physiol. Perform.* **2018**, *13*, 1250–1253. [CrossRef]
32. Barbosa-Silva, M.C.; Barros, A.J.; Wang, J.; Heymsfield, S.B.; Pierson, R.N., Jr. Bioelectrical impedance analysis: Population reference values for phase angle by age and sex. *Am. J. Clin. Nutr.* **2005**, *82*, 49–52. [CrossRef] [PubMed]
33. Haussinger, D.; Lang, F.; Gerok, W. Regulation of cell function by the cellular hydration state. *Am. J. Physiol.* **1994**, *267*, 343–355. [CrossRef]
34. Haussinger, D.; Roth, E.; Lang, F.; Gerok, W. Cellular hydration state: an important determinant of protein catabolism in health and disease. *Lancet* **1993**, *341*, 1330–1332. [CrossRef]
35. Judelson, D.A.; Maresh, C.M.; Anderson, J.M.; Armstrong, L.E.; Casa, D.J.; Kraemer, W.J.; Volek, J.S. Hydration and muscular performance: Does fluid balance affect strength, power and high-intensity endurance? *Sports Med.* **2007**, *37*, 907–921. [CrossRef] [PubMed]

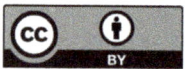

© 2020 by the authors. Licensee MDPI, Basel, Switzerland. This article is an open access article distributed under the terms and conditions of the Creative Commons Attribution (CC BY) license (http://creativecommons.org/licenses/by/4.0/).

Article

Overweight in Young Athletes: New Predictive Model of Overfat Condition

Gabriele Mascherini [1,*], **Cristian Petri** [1], **Elena Ermini** [1], **Vittorio Bini** [2], **Piergiuseppe Calà** [3], **Giorgio Galanti** [1] and **Pietro Amedeo Modesti** [1]

1. Dipartimento di Medicina Sperimentale e Clinica, Università degli Studi di Firenze, 50134 Firenze, Italy
2. Dipartimento di Medicina, Università di Perugia, 06156 Perugia, Italy
3. Sector "Health and Safety in the Workplace and Special Processes in the Field of Prevention", Directorate of Citizenship Rights and Social Cohesion, 50139 Firenze, Italy
* Correspondence: gabriele.mascherini@unifi.it; Tel.: +393396895925

Received: 18 November 2019; Accepted: 14 December 2019; Published: 16 December 2019

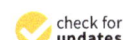

Abstract: The aim of the study is to establish a simple and low-cost method that, associated with Body Mass Index (BMI), differentiates overweight conditions due to a prevalence of lean mass compared to an excess of fat mass during the evaluation of young athletes. 1046 young athletes (620 male, 426 female) aged between eight and 18 were enrolled. Body composition assessments were performed with anthropometry, circumferences, skinfold, and bioimpedance. Overweight was established with BMI, while overfat was established with the percentage of fat mass: 3.5% were underweight, 72.8% were normal weight, 20.1% were overweight, and 3.5% were obese according to BMI; according to the fat mass, 9.5% were under fat, 63.6% were normal fat, 16.2% were overfat, and 10.8% were obese. Differences in overfat prediction were found using BMI alone or with the addition of the triceps fold (area under the receiver operating characteristics curve (AUC) for BMI = 0.867 vs. AUC for BMI + TRICEPS = 0.955, $p < 0.001$). These results allowed the creation of a model factoring in age, sex, BMI, and triceps fold that could provide the probability that a young overweight athlete is also in an overfat condition. The calculated probability could reduce the risk of error in establishing the correct weight status of young athletes.

Keywords: Triceps skinfold; overweight; youth; obese; child; adolescent

1. Introduction

The definition of overfat is necessary in order to accurately specify the problem of excess body fat that directly affects health and physical fitness [1]. Excess body fat is a public health problem and is considered an independent risk factor for several non-communicable chronic diseases [2]. Body Mass Index (BMI, expressed in kg/m^2) is the main parameter in clinical practice of classifying the subject's weight status. However, the limitation of this method is clearly established. In order to establish the overfat condition, the use of adequate tools for the evaluation of the fat mass (FM) in addition to the BMI value is recommended [3]. This aspect should be considered in particular during the evaluation of an athlete due to greater muscle mass with the same body weight [4].

In the pediatric population, the assessment of weight status is an aspect that the World Health Organization is continuously evaluating, because childhood obesity is associated with a higher chance of obesity, premature death, and disability in adulthood [5]. In addition, for pediatric ages, BMI has low sensitivity to establish excess adiposity, and 25% of children fail to identify their own correct weight status [6]. This difference is particularly evident in the evaluation of young athletes' obesity [7].

There are numerous techniques and equations in order to quantify FM [8]. The reference methods in this field have some inherent problems, such as the time needed for evaluations, the financial costs involved, or the unnecessary exposure to radiation, in particular with young people [9].

During clinical practice or in sports fields, a simple and low-cost procedure is required to discriminate overweight with low levels of FM from overweight with overfat. For this reason, Junior [10] recommended the use of waist circumferences (WC) and waist-to-height ratio (WTHR) in addition to BMI in order to body fat discriminators in children and adolescents in both sexes.

However, to date it is unknown whether these parameters can be used with the same efficacy even in young athletes. Therefore, the purpose of the present study is to establish a simple and low-cost method that, associated with BMI, provides the discriminating factor between overweight conditions due to a prevalence of lean mass compared to that due to an excess of FM during the evaluation of young athletes.

2. Materials and Methods

2.1. Subjects

A group of young athletes was enrolled before pre-participation screening for sport eligibility in the Sports Medicine Department. In Italy, the sport eligibility certification is 12 months long but may not coincide with the start of the competitive season; therefore, the athletes were evaluated during the regular season.

We have analyzed data from 1046 young athletes (620 male and 426 female) aged between 8 and 18 years (mean age 13.9 ± 2.4 years for male and 12.7 ± 2.3 years for female). Inclusion criteria for the subjects included being Caucasian, practicing sports at a competitive level, and not having any contraindications to sports eligibility. Exclusion criteria in the analyses were age outside the range of ±6 months compared to the average age of its own stratum, and abnormal values for weight and height (5 kg below the third or 30 kg above the 97th percentile; 5 cm below the third or 5 cm above the 97th percentile) [11].

Written informed consent from both parents or guardians was retrieved for children under the age of 18. After receiving consent, all subjects underwent a voluntary assessment of body composition. The study was carried out in conformity with the ethical standards laid down in the 1975 declaration of Helsinki and was approved by the local ethics committee. This study is part of a project of the Tuscany Region called "Sports Medicine to support regional surveillance systems"; it was approved by the Regional Prevention Plan 2014–2018 with the code O-Range18. Informed consent was obtained from all the participants before inclusion in the study.

2.2. Body Composition Assessment

Technical staff trained in data integration of anthropometry, circumferences, skin fold thickness, and bioelectric impedance analysis (BIA) [12] performed total body composition assessments.

Anthropometry and circumferences.

Weight was measured to the nearest 0.1 kg and height to the nearest 0.1 cm (Seca GmbH & Co.). BMI was calculated as body mass divided by height squared (kg/m^2). Circumference measures were made with a tape metric (Holtain Limited, 1.5 m Flexible Tape) at waist, hip, and biceps:

1. Waist is taken at the narrowest level, or if this is not apparent, at the midpoint between the lowest rib and the top of the hip bone (iliac crest).
2. Hip is taken over minimal clothing at the greatest protrusion of the gluteus muscles. The subject stands erect with their weight evenly distributed on both feet and legs slightly parted without tensing the muscles.
3. Bicep circumference, with the arms relaxed, is taken at the level of the midpoint between the acromion and the olecranon processes.

Skin fold thickness.

Skin fold measurements are widely utilized to assess body FM. Measurements were taken in eight different anatomical sites around the body using calipers (Holtain, Limited Tanner/Whitehouse Skinfold Caliper): triceps, biceps, sub scapula, supra ilium, mid axilla, pectoral, abdominal, and quadriceps (expressed as mm). In addition to the values of the single folds, the sum of all eight folds and the FM percentages derived from skinfold thickness were reported [12,13].

Bioelectric impedance analysis (BIA).

Body impedance is generated in lean tissues as an opposition to the flow of an injected alternate current. Bioelectrical impedance was measured with a phase-sensitive impedance plethysmograph (BIA 101 Sport Edition, Akern, Florence, Italy). The device emits an alternating sinusoidal electric current of 800 mA at an operating single frequency of 50 kHz; standard whole-body tetra polar measurements were performed according to manufacturer guidelines [14]. Resistance (Rz, Ω) is the opposition to the flow of an injected alternating current; reactance (Xc, Ω) is the dielectric or capacitive component of cell membranes and organelles; and phase angle (PA, in degrees) is defined as the ratio between Rz and Xc or between intra and extracellular volumes [15]. In addition, the percentages of FM (FM%) as suggested by McCarthy were recorded [16].

2.3. Statistical Analysis

In order to establish underweight, normal weight, overweight, or obese conditions, a subdivision according to BMI, age, and gender was adopted with the International Obesity Task Force (IOTF) guidelines for children and adolescents [17]. In order to establish under fat, normal fat, overfat, or obese conditions, a subdivision according to FM percent, age, and gender was adopted with the body fat reference curves for children developed by McCarthy [16].

The Shapiro–Wilk test was used to assess the normal distribution of variables. The Chi-square test with Yate's continuity correction was used for comparisons of categorical variables, and the Mann–Whitney's U-test was used for comparisons of non-normally distributed continuous variables. Multivariate logistic regression models were fitted for the prediction of the dichotomized FM (under fat/normal fat = 0; overfat/obese condition = 1), incorporating to the base model (age, gender, BMI) one at a time in separate models and all the anthropometric variables. To decrease the overfit bias and internally validate our results, all regressions were subjected to 200 bootstrap resamples, and the goodness-of-fit of logistic models were checked using the Hosmer and Lemeshow test. The predictive accuracy of logistic regression models was quantified as the area under the receiver operating characteristics (ROC) curve (AUC), and AUCs were compared using the DeLong method [18]. Odds ratios (ORs) with 95% confidence intervals were also calculated. Furthermore, multivariate logistic regression coefficients were used to develop an FM-based nomogram (Orange software, version 3.4.2, 2017; https://orange.biolab.si/) [19].

All statistical analyses were performed using IBM-SPSS® version 23.0 (IBM Corp., Armonk, NY, USA, 2015). In all analyses, a two-sided *p*-value < 0.05 was considered significant.

3. Results

Anthropometrics, skin fold, and bioelectric impedance parameters of the sample with a gender comparison are shown in Table 1.

The prevalence of the weight status of the 1046 subjects depends on which classification is used. Following the IOTF classification (based on BMI) 3.5% were underweight, 72.8% were normal weight, 20.1% were overweight, and 3.5% were obese, compared to 9.5% under fat, 63.6% normal fat, 16.2% overfat, and 10.8% obese, according to the FM. Figure 1 shows the prevalence of the weight status differences between sexes based on the subdivision by BMI or by FM. The division into weight classes carried out by the BMI shows no differences between genders (p = 0.375); FM stratification shows a different prevalence (p < 0.001), in particular for the overweight condition.

Table 1. Anthropometrics, skin fold and bioimpedance parameters of the whole sample of young athletes. Data for reading simplicity are expressed as mean ± SD.

Variable	Male (n = 620)	Female (n = 426)	p Value
Age (y)	13.87 ± 2.42	12.74 ± 2.33	<0.001
Height (m)	1.64 ± 0.14	1.55 ± 0.12	<0.001
Weight (kg)	55.71 ± 15.24	48.97 ± 13.19	<0.001
BMI (kg/m^2)	20.23 ± 3.33	20.04 ± 3.33	0.076
Waist circ. (cm)	68.34 ± 8.88	64.22 ± 8.67	<0.001
Hip circ. (cm)	85.18 ± 10.07	83.85 ± 13.41	0.057
Hip/waist	0.807 ± 0.14	0.809 ± 0.46	<0.001
WHR	0.52 ± 0.04	0.54 ± 0.07	<0.001
Biceps Circ. (cm)	24.40 ± 4.30	25.08 ± 29.41	0.001
Biceps fold (mm)	6.07 ± 3.50	8.54 ± 3.87	<0.001
Triceps fold (mm)	11.57 ± 5.48	16.47 ± 5.74	<0.001
Subscapular fold (mm)	9.16 ± 5.18	12.28 ± 8.11	<0.001
Supra iliac fold (mm)	11.08 ± 7.06	15.10 ± 7.37	<0.001
Axilla fold (mm)	8.06 ± 5.25	10.68 ± 6.81	<0.001
Pectoral fold (mm)	7.85 ± 4.96	11.03 ± 5.05	<0.001
Abdomen fold (mm)	12.51 ± 8.02	17.14 ± 7.98	<0.001
Quadriceps fold (mm)	15.29 ± 9.54	22.10 ± 6.51	<0.001
Sum fold (mm)	81.58 ± 42.66	91.25 ± 38.95	<0.001
Fat Mass from Skinfold (%)	16.85 ± 7.22	23.62 ± 7.56	<0.001
RZ (Ω)	566.85 ± 89.97	623.62 ± 69.18	<0.001
XC (Ω)	61.62 ± 8.07	66.22 ± 25.74	<0.001
PA (°)	6.29 ± 0.92	6.08 ± 2.17	<0.001
Fat Mass from BIA (%)	18.25 ± 7.00	25.11 ± 6.34	<0.001
Fat Mass (Kg)	10.43 ± 6.20	12.92 ± 6.35	<0.001
Free Fat Mass (Kg)	45.28 ± 11.79	36.08 ± 7.72	<0.001

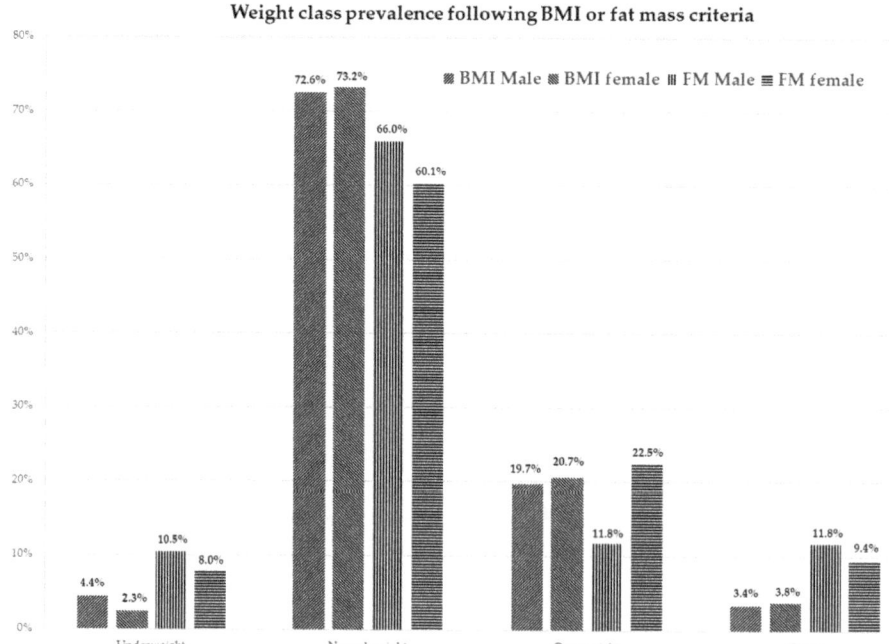

Figure 1. Differences in prevalence weight status between gender in the sample of young athletes based on the subdivision by Body Mass Index (BMI) or by fat mass (FM).

The results of the logistic regression analysis considering the parameters of age, sex, and BMI show a coverage of the AUC equal to 0.867 ± 0.013. Table 2 shows the results of the AUC in the case of the addition of a fourth anthropometric variable to the BMI, age, and gender variables. Triceps, abdominal fold, and skinfold sum have achieved the highest results.

Table 2. Area under the curve (area under the receiver operating characteristics curve (AUC) ± SE) results with the addition the fourth anthropometric variable to the BMI, age and gender in young athletes.

Anthropometric Variable	Area under the curve (%)
Waist circumference	0.877 ± 0.011
Waist/height	0.882 ± 0.013
Waist/hip	0.867 ± 0.013
Biceps circumference	0.867 ± 0.013
Triceps fold	0.955 ± 0.008
Sub scapula fold	0.920 ± 0.010
Supra ilium fold	0.938 ± 0.009
Mid axilla fold	0.944 ± 0.009
Pectoral fold	0.946 ± 0.008
Abdominal fold	0.960 ± 0.007
Quadriceps fold	0.938 ± 0.008
Skinfolds sum	0.976 ± 0.006

Differences in overfatness prediction were found using BMI alone or with the addition of the triceps fold value (AUC: 0.867 vs 0.955, $p < 0.001$, Figure 2).

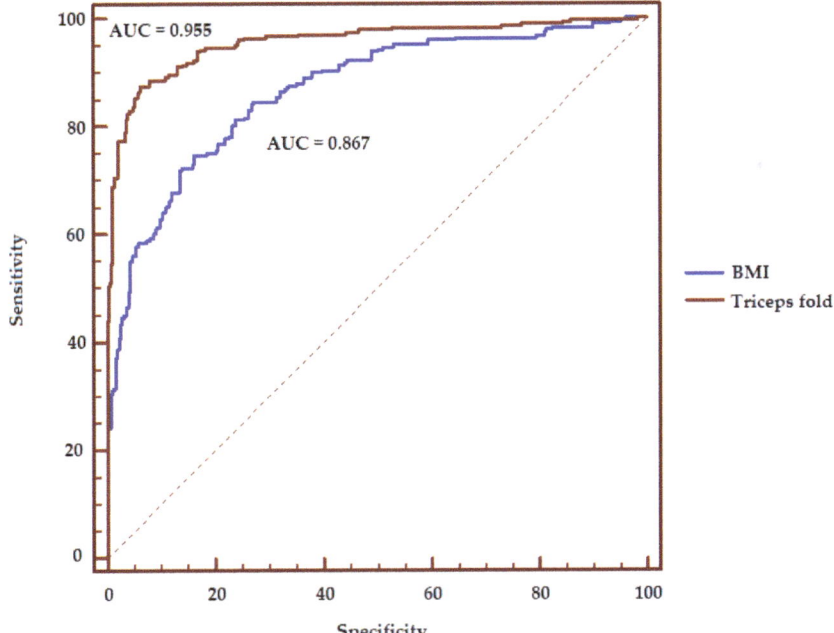

Figure 2. Receiver operating characteristics (ROC) curve, assessment of the accuracy of overfatness prediction using BMI alone (AUC = 0.867) or with the addition of the triceps fold value (AUC = 0.955) in young athletes. Statistical difference were found $p < 0.001$.

This result allowed the authors to create a model with age, sex, BMI, and triceps fold variables that could provide the probability that an overweight child is also in an overfat condition (Figure 3).

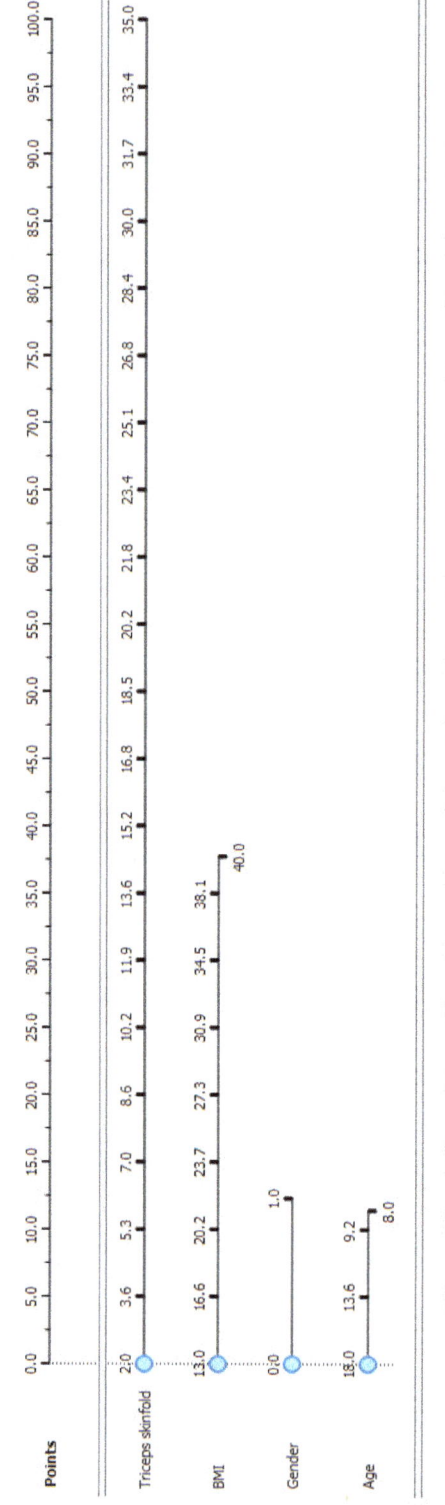

Figure 3. Probabilities that an overweight young athlete is also in overfat condition. Triceps skinfold, BMI, gender, and age are the four variables that give the probability of having an excess of fat mass in addition to the overweight condition. At the top of the figure there is a scores scale corresponding to the values of these four variables. At the bottom of the figure there is a scale that corresponds to the sum of the scores obtained from the four variables (Total) corresponds to a probability (%) that the subject is in an overfat condition. Gender: 0 = Female, 1 = Male.

4. Discussion

The objective of this study was to provide a practical and simple solution, applicable in a clinical or in a field setting, to differentiate the excess weight due to FM from that due to muscle mass in young athletes.

The review performed by Junior [10] concludes that BMI, waist circumference, and waist-to-height ratio are body fat discriminators in children and adolescents with low operational costs. Another study performed by Sardinha [20] suggests that triceps fold gives the best result in order to define the relationship between BMI and percentage of body fat in healthy boys and girls aged 10 to 15 years, whereas BMI and upper arm girth are reasonable second choices. Both studies suggest specific cutoffs by age group and sex; however, these parameters should be utilized with caution in the evaluation of young athletes [10].

Athletes are subjected to remodeling of the proportions of FM compared to the whole body; these modifications are particularly evident when young athletes are compared to untrained young people [21]. This process occurs due to the different movements and training regimens required by the sport practiced. Therefore, body shape of the athletes could be classified into three categories: muscular and well-balanced type (running, volley, soccer, cycling, and swimming); rich muscular and large-built type (canoeing and rugby); and rich muscular and long-torso type (weight lifting) [22]. Our study enrolled exclusively young athletes. The waist circumference, waist-to-height ratio, and biceps circumference results reached lower statistical power compared to skinfold parameters. Our results suggest using only the triceps fold in order to simplify the assessment: upper arm is easily accessible for detection purposes, and the difference in comparison with abdominal fold (that gave a higher AUC value) is not statistically significant. The evaluation of adiposity in young athletes, unlike non-sporting young people, should include the use of more specific tools that allow a direct assessment of the concerned body compartment.

Currently, the main clinical techniques for the measurement of adiposity in youth are BMI and circumferences, which enable the use of growth centile charts [23]. Skinfold thickness measurement and the use of standardized equations involve some limitations in the estimation of the adiposity in the pediatric population. These biases were particularly high with increasing fatness and were affected by age [24], reaching an error rate of over 5% [25]. Our study did not use any equation for FM estimation but only the triceps fold value [26], expressed in mm.

The prediction model proposed by this study does not provide an absolute certainty of the overfatness condition of a young overweight athlete. However, it provides a probability that further action to promote the health of the young athlete should be considered starting from the value of 50%. Figure 3 describes the procedures that health professionals should follow after pinching the tricep folds of young athletes. This value should be recorded in addition to the age, sex, and BMI values; each value corresponds to a score at the top of the figure. At the bottom of the figure, there is the sum of the scores that provides a probability that the subject is in an overfat condition in addition to overweight.

The skinfold technique requires measurement expertise, and in order to achieve the best results possible, health professionals should undergo training in this technique before carrying it out in order to reach a good reliability and accuracy [27].

Data concerning anthropometrics and body composition, as well as the percentage of body fat, of the present study are in agreement with well-documented sex-related differences in body composition between males and females [28].

The prevalence of overweight and obesity is in line with previous studies [29,30]. However, the weight status analyzed with FM results shows some differences in comparison with BMI results. In particular, the prevalence of the obesity rises from about 3–4% to around 10% in both sexes. In males, the status of overweight is transferred into obesity status, while in females there is a transfer from the state of normal weight in favor of obesity. This differentiation also affects an adequate assessment of cardiorespiratory fitness of young athletes, which in fact is mainly influenced by the FM rather than by the BMI [31]. This is significant because high levels of cardiorespiratory fitness may attenuate the association between excessive adiposity and risks of cardiovascular and metabolic diseases.

The present study shows some strengths. Firstly, the number of subjects that underwent the body composition assessment is in line with those present to date. Secondly, all subjects regularly perform organized sport. Finally, the same expert operator in young athlete evaluation carried out all the anthropometric and skinfold assessments.

The authors are aware that a limitation of the study is the use of BIA to evaluate the percentage of FM, but they followed the study by McCarthy et al. [16] to establish the prevalence of weight status based on FM in a sample of athletes aged eight to 18 of both sexes. This study did not distinguish children and adolescents by maturation phase; it could be inferred that the sample heterogeneity could alter the accuracy of the results. However, the objective of the study does not predict the evaluation following stages of growth, because this aspect involves a further variable that would not allow the creation of a simple tool applicable in a clinical setting or in the field.

This paper should be considered as a preliminary proposal for a new work tool that needs validation on a larger population. At the same time, a future study direction could be extending the possibility of this evaluation to other races as well.

5. Conclusions

In summary, obesity during youth is a public health problem that is constantly on the rise worldwide. Participation in organized sports during youth is a widely used activity in western countries because it brings many benefits to children. Among these advantages, there is also weight control. However, it has been shown that BMI has some inherent limitations in assessing adiposity, especially in young athletes. The authors therefore suggest a new predictive model to determine when excess weight is due to excess fat mass. This practice could be used as an additional assessment of young athletes during physical examinations conducted by the sports medicine physicians or physical fitness evaluations conducted by the athletic trainers.

Author Contributions: C.P. and E.E. carried out the evaluation; G.M. and P.A.M. drafted the manuscript; V.B. performed statistical analysis; G.M. and G.G. perform the design of the study. G.M., P.A.M. and P.C. conceived the study. All authors approved the final version of manuscript.

Funding: This research received no external funding.

Conflicts of Interest: The authors declare no conflict of interest.

References

1. Maffetone, P.B.; Rivera-Dominguez, I.; Laursen, P.B. Overfat and Underfat: New Terms and Definitions Long Overdue. *Front Public Health.* **2016**, *4*, 279. [CrossRef] [PubMed]
2. Goossens, G.H. The Metabolic Phenotype in Obesity: Fat Mass, Body Fat Distribution, and Adipose Tissue Function. *Obes. Facts.* **2017**, *10*, 207–215. [CrossRef] [PubMed]
3. De Lorenzo, A.; Gratteri, S.; Gualtieri, P.; Cammarano, A.; Bertucci, P.; Di Renzo, L. Why Primary obesity is a Disease? *J. Transl. Med.* **2019**, *17*, 169. [CrossRef] [PubMed]
4. Jonnalagadda, S.S.; Skinner, R.; Moore, L. Overweight athlete: fact or fiction? *Curr. Sports Med. Rep.* **2004**, *3*, 198–205. [CrossRef] [PubMed]
5. WHO, Obesity Fact Sheet. Available online: https://www.who.int/news-room/fact-sheets/detail/obesity-and-overweight (accessed on 18 September 2019).
6. Javed, A.; Jumean, M.; Murad, M.H.; Okorodudu, D.; Kumar, S.; Somers, V.K.; Sochor, O.; Lopez-Jimenez, F. Diagnostic Performance of Body Mass Index to Identify Obesity as Defined by Body Adiposity in Children and Adolescents: A Systematic Review and Meta-Analysis. *Pediatr. Obes.* **2015**, *10*, 234–244. [CrossRef] [PubMed]
7. Petri, C.; Mascherini, G.; Bini, V.; Anania, G.; Calà, P.; Toncelli, L.; Galanti, G. Integrated Total Body Composition Versus Body Mass Index in Young Athletes. Available online: https://europepmc.org/article/med/27057821 (accessed on 14 December 2019).

8. Borga, M.; West, J.; Bell, J.D.; Harvey, N.C.; Romu, T.; Heymsfield, S.B.; Dahlqvist, L.O. Advanced Body Composition Assessment: from Body Mass Index to Body Composition Profiling. *J. Investig. Med.* **2018**, *66*, 1–9. [CrossRef]
9. Ackland, T.R.; Lohman, T.G.; Sundgot-Borgen, J.; Maughan, R.J.; Meyer, N.L.; Stewart, A.D.; Müller, W. Current Status of Body Composition Assessment in Sport: Review and Position Statement on Behalf of the Ad Hoc Research Working Group on Body Composition Health and performance, Under the Auspices of the I.O.C. Medical Commission. *Sports Med.* **2012**, *42*, 227–249. [CrossRef]
10. Alves Junior, C.A.; Mocellin, M.C.; Gonçalves, E.C.A.; Silva, D.A.; Trindade, E.B. Anthropometric Indicators as Body Fat Discriminators in Children and Adolescents: A Systematic Review and Meta-Analysis. *Adv. Nutr.* **2017**, *8*, 718–727. [CrossRef]
11. Roberts, C.; Freeman, J.; Samdal, O.; Schnohr, C.W.; de Looze, M.E.; Nic Gabhainn, S.; Iannotti, R.; Rasmussen, M.; International HBSC Study Group. The Health Behavior in School-Aged Children (HBSC) Study: Methodological Developments and Current Tensions. *Int. J. Public Health* **2009**, *54*, 140–150. [CrossRef]
12. Mascherini, G.; Petri, C.; Galanti, G. Integrated Total Body Composition and Localized Fat-Free Mass Assessment. *Sport Sci. Health* **2015**, *11*, 217. [CrossRef]
13. Stewart, A.D.; Marfell-Jones, M.; Olds, T.J.; De Ridder, H. *Skinfolds in International Standards for Anthropometric Assessment*; International Society for the Advancement of Kinanthropometry: Glasgow, UK, 2011.
14. Kyle, U.G.; Bosaeus, I.; De Lorenzo, A.D.; Deurenberg, P.; Elia, M.; Gómez, J.M.; Heitmann, B.L.; Kent-Smith, L.; Melchior, J.C.; Pirlich, M.; et al. Bioelectrical Impedance Analysis—Part I: Review of Principles and Methods. *Clin. Nutr.* **2004**, *23*, 1226–1243. [CrossRef] [PubMed]
15. Marini, E.; Campa, F.; Buffa, R.; Stagi, S.; Matia, C.N.; Toselli, S.; Sardinha, L.S.; Silva, A.M. Phase Angle and Bioelectrical Impedance Vector Analysis in the Evaluation of Body Composition in Athletes. *Clin. Nutr.* **2019**. [CrossRef] [PubMed]
16. McCarthy, H.D.; Cole, T.J.; Fry, T.; Jebb, S.A.; Prentice, A.M. Body Fat Reference Curves for Children. *Int. J. Obes. (Lond.)* **2006**, *30*, 598–602. [CrossRef] [PubMed]
17. Cole, T.J.; Lobstein, T. Extended International (IOTF) Body Mass Index Cut-Offs for Thinness, Overweight and Obesity. *Pediatr. Obes.* **2012**, *7*, 284–294. [CrossRef] [PubMed]
18. Swets, J.A. Measuring the Accuracy of Diagnostic Systems. *Science* **1998**, *240*, 1285–1293. [CrossRef]
19. Demsar, J.; Curk, T.; Erjavec, A.; Gorup, C.; Hocevar, T.; Milutinovic, M.; Možina, M.; Polajnar, M.; Toplak, M.; Starič, A.; et al. Orange: Data Mining Toolbox in Python. *J. Mach. Learn. Res.* **2013**, *14*, 2349–2353.
20. Sardinha, L.B.; Going, S.B.; Teixeira, P.J.; Lohman, T.G. Receiver Operating Characteristic Analysis of Body Mass Index, Triceps Skinfold Thickness, and Arm Girth for Obesity Screening in Children and Adolescents. *Am. J. Clin. Nutr.* **1999**, *70*, 1090–1095. [CrossRef]
21. Hoshikawa, Y.; Muramatsu, M.; Iida, T.; Uchiyama, A.; Nakajima, Y.; Kanehisa, H. Event-Related Differences in the Cross-Sectional Areas and Torque Generation Capabilities of Quadriceps Femoris and Hamstrings in Male High School Athletes. *J. Physiol. Anthropol.* **2010**, *29*, 13–21. [CrossRef]
22. Tsunawake, N.; Tahara, Y.; Yukawa, K.; Katsuura, T.; Harada, H.; Kikuchi, Y. Classification of Body Shape of Male Athletes by Factor Analysis. *Ann. Physiol. Anthropol.* **1994**, *13*, 383–392. [CrossRef]
23. Horan, M.; Gibney, E.; Molloy, E.; McAuliffe, F. Methodologies to Assess Paediatric Adiposity. *Ir. J. Med. Sci.* **2015**, *184*, 53–68. [CrossRef]
24. Reilly, J.; Wilson, J.; Durnin, J. Determination of Body Composition From Skinfold Thickness: A Validation Study. *Arch. Dis. Child.* **1975**, *73*, 305–310. [CrossRef]
25. Sinning, W.E.; Dolny, D.G.; Little, K.D.; Cunningham, L.N.; Racaniello, A.; Siconolfi, S.F.; Sholes, J.L. Validity of "Generalised" Equations for Body Composition Analysis in Male Athletes. *Med. Sci. Sports Exerc.* **1985**, *17*, 124–130.
26. Wells, J.C. A Critique of the Expression of Paediatric Body Composition Data. *Arch. Dis. Child.* **2001**, *85*, 67–72. [CrossRef]
27. Krebs, N.F.; Himes, J.H.; Jacobson, D.; Nicklas, T.A.; Guilday, P.; Styne, D. Assessment of Child and Adolescent Overweight and Obesity. *Pediatrics* **2007**, *120*, S193–S228. [CrossRef]
28. Mascherini, G.; Castizo-Olier, J.; Irurtia, A.; Petri, C.; Galanti, G. Differences between the Sexes in Athletes' Body Composition and Lower Limb Bioimpedance Values. *Muscles Ligaments Tendons J.* **2018**, *7*, 573–581. [CrossRef]

29. Mascherini, G.; Petri, C.; Calà, P.; Bini, V.; Galanti, G. Lifestyle and Resulting Body Composition in Young Athletes. Available online: https://europepmc.org/article/med/28006893 (accessed on 18 November 2019).
30. Petri, C.; Mascherini, G.; Bini, V.; Toncelli, L.; Armentano, N.; Calà, P.; Galanti, G. Evaluation of Physical Activity and Dietary Behaviors in Young Athletes: A Pilot Study. *Minerva Pediatr.* **2017**, *69*, 463–469. [CrossRef]
31. Fairchild, T.J.; Klakk, H.; Heidemann, M.S.; Andersen, L.B.; Wedderkopp, N. Exploring the Relationship between Adiposity and Fitness in Young Children. *Med. Sci. Sports Exerc.* **2016**, *48*, 1708–1714. [CrossRef]

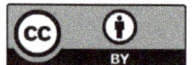

© 2019 by the authors. Licensee MDPI, Basel, Switzerland. This article is an open access article distributed under the terms and conditions of the Creative Commons Attribution (CC BY) license (http://creativecommons.org/licenses/by/4.0/).

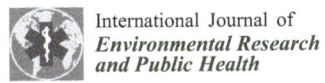

Article

Classic Bioelectrical Impedance Vector Reference Values for Assessing Body Composition in Male and Female Athletes

Francesco Campa [1], Catarina Matias [2], Hannes Gatterer [3], Stefania Toselli [1,*], Josely C. Koury [4], Angela Andreoli [5], Giovanni Melchiorri [5], Luis B. Sardinha [2] and Analiza M. Silva [2]

1. Departments of Biomedical and Neuromotor Sciences, University of Bologna, 40121 Bologna, Italy
2. Exercise and Health Laboratory, CIPER, Faculdade de Motricidade Humana, Universidade de Lisboa, 1499-002 Cruz Quebrada, Portugal
3. Institute of Mountain Emergency Medicine, Eurac Research, 40121 Bolzano, Italy
4. Department of Basic and Experimental Nutrition, Nutrition Institute, State University of Rio de Janeiro, Rio de Janeiro 20550-900, Brazil
5. Department of Systems Medicine, University of Tor Vergata, 00175 Rome, Italy
* Correspondence: stefania.toselli@unibo.it; Tel.: +390512094195

Received: 15 November 2019; Accepted: 10 December 2019; Published: 12 December 2019

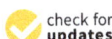

Abstract: Bioimpedance standards are well established for the normal healthy population and in clinical settings, but they are not available for many sports categories. The aim of this study was to develop reference values for male and female athletes using classic bioimpedance vector analysis (BIVA). In this study, 1556 athletes engaged in different sports were evaluated during their off-season period. A tetrapolar bioelectrical impedance analyzer was used to determine measurements of resistance (R) and reactance (Xc). The classic BIVA procedure, which corrects bioelectrical values for body height, was applied, and fat-free mass, fat mass, and total body water were estimated. In order to verify the need for specific references, classic bioelectrical values were compared to the reference values for the general male and female populations. Additionally, athletes were divided into three groups: endurance, velocity/power, and team sports. In comparison with the general healthy male and female populations, the mean vectors of the athletes showed a shift to the left on the R–Xc graph. Considering the same set of modalities, BIVA confidence graphs showed that male and female endurance athletes presented lower body fluids, fat mass, and fat-free mass than other sets of modalities. This study provides BIVA reference values for an athletic population that can be used as a standard for assessing body composition in male and female athletes.

Keywords: BIVA; confidence ellipses; phase angle; R–Xc graph; tolerance ellipses

1. Introduction

The analysis of body composition (BC) is a critical component in the sports field, given its relationship to physical performance [1]. Several techniques are used to assess BC in athletes. These include underwater weighing (densitometry), dual energy X-ray absorptiometry (DXA), bioelectrical impedance analysis (BIA), and anthropometric measurements. Although densitometry and DXA are the most accurate methods to evaluate BC, they are expensive and impractical for field use because they require large, specialized equipment. In recent years, bioimpedance vector analysis (BIVA) has received attention in the sports science field as a method to obtain a qualitative assessment of BC [2].

BIA data (i.e., resistance (R) and reactance (Xc)), through BIVA, are used to evaluate cellular function and body fluid content. This method plots the impedance parameters standardized for the subject's height as a single vector on the R–Xc graph [3,4]. Recently, different studies compared BIVA, dual X-ray absorptiometry, and body fluid measurements obtained by dilution technique. The studies demonstrated the ability of BIVA to evaluate BC changes in athletes by studying the vector displacements and BC variables (i.e., total body water (TBW), percentage of fat mass (%FM), and the intracellular/extracellular water (ICW/ECW) ratio) [5,6]. The ICW/ECW ratio is identified by the bioelectrical phase angle (PA), which is calculated as the arctangent of Xc/R × 180°/π [5–7]. An increase in ICW/ECW can be a consequence of gain in muscle mass due to physical activity [8–11]. However, the analysis of only the PA leads to interpretation errors. In fact, groups of athletes characterized by a similar PA may show different TBW or %FM. BIVA goes beyond this limitation because it takes into consideration the relationship between ICW and ECW (determined by the vector slope in the R–Xc graph) in addition to the TBW amount (which is represented by the vector length) [5].

Recent studies conducted on athletes have highlighted the need for sport-specific BIVA references by establishing data from sets of sports such as soccer, volleyball, or cycling [12–14]. In the absence of appropriate references for each sport category, researchers continue to use reference values from the general healthy population [15–18]. A characteristic and innovative aspect of BIVA is that it provides soft tissue classification (under, normal, and over) and ranking (more or less than before intervention), comparing the position of an individual vector to a reference population. For this reason, the application of BIVA can be compromised if inappropriate reference R–Xc graphs are used, leading to evaluations that are difficult to interpret. Furthermore, to the best of our knowledge, no reference values are available for female athletes.

The use of appropriate R–Xc graphs allows for the correct interpretation of BIVA patterns in the assessment of BC, adding useful information regarding the influence of BC on somatic maturation in young athletes [19]. While specific references do not exist for every single sport, establishing BIVA references for the general male and female athlete populations may be useful even if values may differ slightly between individual sports. Considering the importance of the use of BIVA for the athletic population, the present study aimed to generate bioimpedance reference values for male and female athletes.

2. Materials and Methods

2.1. Subjects

This was a cross-sectional observational study on 1556 athletes (men: n = 1116, age 23.1 ± 6.8 y; women: n = 440, age 26.9 ± 6.6 y). The athletes participated in 23 sport modalities: athletics (men = 78 and women = 19), badminton (men = 5 and women = 4), basketball (men = 117 and women = 53), boxing (women = 9), cross-country skiing (men = 4), CrossFit (men = 26 and women = 33), cycling (men = 15), field hockey (men = 12), handball (men = 43 and women = 4), judo (men = 78 and women = 28), karate (men = 29 and women = 5), kick boxing (men = 48 and women = 20), marathon (men = 49 and women = 24), pentathlon (men = 33 and women = 21), rowing (women = 13), rugby (men = 102), rhythmic gymnastics (women = 28), soccer (men = 67), short-distance swimming (men = 85 and women = 49), tennis (men = 26 and women = 15), triathlon (men = 64 and women = 18), volleyball (men = 176 and women = 79), and water polo (men = 59 and women = 17).

The control groups were represented by the healthy male and female general populations [20]. The athletes were sorted into three groups: endurance (cycling, marathon, pentathlon, cross-country skiing, rowing, and triathlon), velocity/power (athletics including jumping, throwing, short-distance running; badminton; boxing; CrossFit; judo; karate; kickboxing; rhythmic gymnastics; swimming including short-distance swimming; and tennis), and team sports (basketball, field hockey, handball, rugby, soccer, volleyball, and water polo).

Medical screening indicated that all subjects were in good health. The following inclusion criteria were used: (1) a minimum of 10 to a maximum of 13 h of training per week; (2) tested negative for performance-enhancing drugs; and (3) not taking any medications. All subjects were informed of the study procedures before they gave written consent to participate. All procedures were approved by the Bioethics Committee of the University of Bologna and were conducted in accordance with the Declaration of Helsinki for human studies (Ethical Approval Code: 25027; dated 13.03.2017).

2.2. Procedures

All measurements were performed in resting conditions during the off-season period (9:00 a.m.) at the athletes' training centers. The impedance measurements were performed with BIA (BIA 101 Anniversary, Akern, Florence, Italy), which applies an alternating current of 800 µA at a single frequency of 50 kHz. Measurements were made using four electrical conductors. The subjects were in the supine position with a leg opening of 45° compared to the median line of the body and the upper limbs positioned 30° away from the trunk. After cleansing the skin with alcohol, two Ag/AgCl low-impedance electrodes (Biatrodes, Akern Srl, Florence, Italy) were placed on the back of the right hand and two electrodes on the corresponding foot, with a distance of 5 cm between each other [4,21] (Figure 1). To avoid disturbances in fluid distribution, athletes were instructed to abstain from food and drink for ≥4 hours before the test.

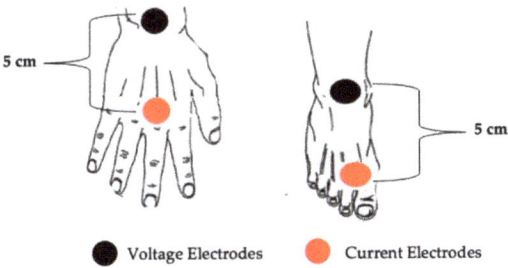

Figure 1. Hand and foot electrode positioning.

The bioelectrical PA was calculated as the arctangent of $Xc/R \times 180°/\pi$. Total body water (TBW), fat-free mass (FFM) and fat mass (FM) were determined according to Kotler et al. [22]. The vector length (Z/H) was calculated as the hypotenuses of individual impedance normalized values. Height was measured to the nearest 0.1 cm using a stadiometer. Body weight was determined to the nearest 0.1 kg using a mechanical scale. Body mass index (BMI) was calculated as total body mass (kilograms) divided by height (meters) squared.

2.3. Statistical Analysis

Results are presented as mean ± SD. Normal distribution of data was evaluated using the Shapiro–Wilk test. A univariate analysis of variance (ANOVA) with Bonferroni post-hoc tests for multiple comparisons was performed. The two-sample Hotelling T^2 test was used to compare the differences in the mean impedance vectors between groups. The 50%, 75%, and 95% tolerance ellipses were generated using the BIVA software [23]. Statistical significance was predetermined as $p < 0.05$. IBM SPSS 23.0 (SPSS, Chicago, IL, USA) was used for all statistical calculations.

3. Results

Characteristics of the athletes, sorted into three groups by sex and ANOVA results, are reported in Table 1. Male team-sports athletes showed higher values of height, weight, BMI, FM, FFM, and TBW than those for male endurance and male velocity/power athletes ($p < 0.01$). Female team-sports athletes showed higher values of weight, FFM, and TBW than female endurance and female velocity/power athletes ($p < 0.01$). FM was higher in female team-sports athletes than in female velocity/power athletes. For both sexes, bioelectrical variables were lower in team-sports athletes, except for PA, which was similar for all groups.

Table 1. Descriptive and comparative statistics for anthropometric, bioelectrical, and body composition variables for the athletes according to sex and sports categories.

Variable	Male					Female				
	Endurance n = 165	Velocity/Power n = 375	Team Sports n = 576	ANOVA p	All n = 1116	Endurance n = 76	Velocity/Power n = 177	Team Sports n = 187	ANOVA p	All n = 440
Age (years)	23.5 ± 6.2	23.6 ± 7.4	22.7 ± 6.5	0.098	23.1 ± 6.8	27.4 ± 7.0	26.2 ± 5.5	27.5 ± 7.4	0.116	26.9 ± 6.6
Weight (kg)	69.8 ± 8.1 #§	74.7 ± 9.8 *§	84.7 ± 13.8 *#	<0.001	79.5 ± 13.5	61.2 ± 8.4 §	62.5 ± 7.9 §	68.5 ± 9.1 *#	<0.001	65.4 ± 9.2
Height (cm)	175.9 ± 6.2 #§	178.3 ± 7.5 *§	185.9 ± 11.2 *#	<0.001	181.9 ± 10.4	169.2 ± 7.7 §	167.2 ± 7.9 §	176.1 ± 9.9 *#	<0.001	171.4 ± 9.8
BMI (kg/m²)	21.9 ± 4.1 #§	23.5 ± 2.5 *	24.4 ± 4.4 *	<0.001	23.7 ± 4.0	21.4 ± 2.3	22.1 ± 1.8	22.1 ± 2.3	0.087	21.9 ± 2.1
R/H (ohm/m)	267.2 ± 28.0 #§	253.3 ± 32.4 *§	246.2 ± 32.3 *#	<0.001	251.6 ± 32.5	337.5 ± 42.9 §	321.0 ± 46.9 §	305.6 ± 37.6 *#	<0.001	318.1 ± 42.8
Xc/H (ohm/m)	35.5 ± 4.7 §	34.2 ± 5.5 *§	32.9 ± 4.8 *#	<0.001	33.9 ± 4.8	40.1 ± 5.5 §	38.0 ± 7.4 §	36.3 ± 5.3 *#	<0.001	38.3 ± 6.4
Z/H (ohm/m)	269.6 ± 28.1 #§	255.6 ± 32.3 *§	248.4 ± 32.4 *#	<0.001	253.8 ± 32.7	338.5 ± 42.9 §	326.1 ± 44.8 §	307.8 ± 37.7 *#	<0.001	320.4 ± 43.1
PA (degree)	7.6 ± 0.8	7.7 ± 0.8	7.6 ± 0.8	0.446	7.7 ± 0.8	6.8 ± 0.8	7.0 ± 0.8	6.8 ± 0.8	0.060	6.9 ± 0.8
FM (kg)	10.4 ± 3.6 §	11.6 ± 4.2 §	15.7 ± 5.8 *#	<0.001	13.7 ± 5.6	12.8 ± 6.3	12.6 ± 4.5 §	14.3 ± 5.6 #	0.015	13.6 ± 5.5
FM (%)	14.6 ± 3.5 §	15.2 ± 3.5 §	18.1 ± 3.8 *#	<0.001	16.7 ± 4.1	20.2 ± 8.8	19.8 ± 5.6	20.5 ± 6.2	0.719	20.2 ± 6.7
FFM (kg)	59.4 ± 5.3 #§	63.2 ± 6.2 *§	68.9 ± 8.8 *#	<0.001	65.7 ± 8.5	48.4 ± 5.5 §	49.9 ± 5.5 §	54.6 ± 6.2 *#	<0.001	51.9 ± 6.4
TBW (L)	43.9 ± 4.5 #§	47.3 ± 5.3 *§	51.8 ± 7.5 *#	<0.001	49.3 ± 7.3	35.2 ± 4.2 §	36.6 ± 4.4 §	39.8 ± 4.8 *#	<0.001	38.0 ± 4.9

ANOVA: analysis of variance; BMI: body mass index; FM: fat mass; FFM: fat-free mass; TBW: total body water; R/H: resistance standardized for height; Xc/H: reactance standardized for height; Z/H: vector length standardized for height; PA: phase angle. * Differences ($p < 0.017$) compared with the endurance group. # Differences compared with the velocity/power group. § Differences compared with the team-sports group. All post hoc Bonferroni test, 1-way ANOVA.

Figure 2 shows the mean impedance vectors with the 95% confidence ellipses for all athletes compared to the 95% ellipses for the general healthy reference populations [20]. Compared to the general populations, the vectors of both male and female athletes shifted to the left.

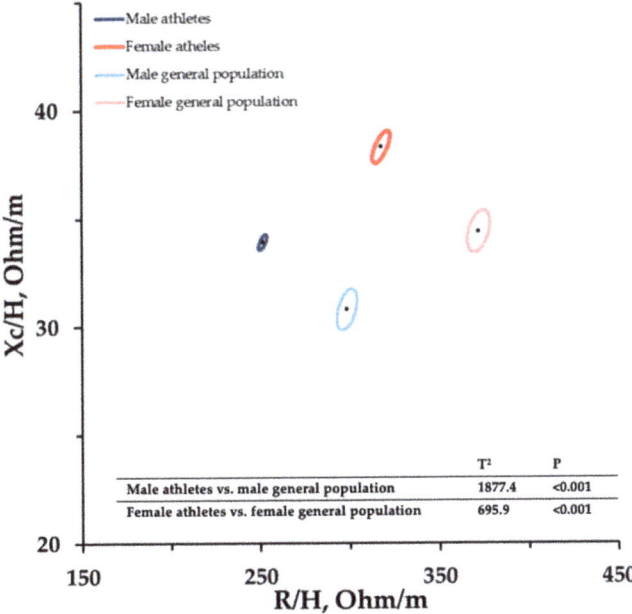

Figure 2. Mean impedance vectors with the 95% confidence ellipses for athletes and the general healthy populations. The Hotelling T^2 test results are included.

The mean impedance vectors of the three categories of athletes showed significant differences between each other ($p < 0.01$). Similarly, male and female endurance athletes showed longer impedance vectors than the athletes included in the velocity/power and team-sports groups, which were respectively lower in the R–Xc graph (Figure 3B,D).

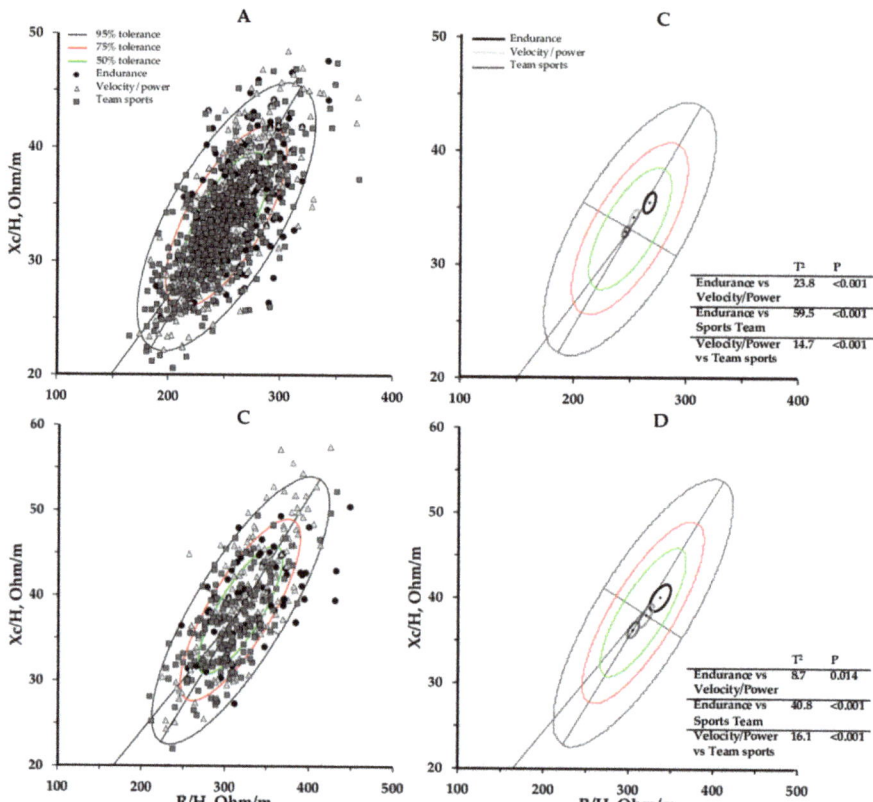

Figure 3. Scattergrams of the individual (**A,C**) and mean (**B,D**) impedance vectors, divided by sports categories and plotted on the new tolerance ellipses, for male (**A,B**) and female (**C,D**) athletes. The Hotelling T² test results are included.

The new 50%, 75%, and 95% tolerance ellipses calculated for all athletes and for the three groups are shown in Figure 4 for males and in Figure 5 for females.

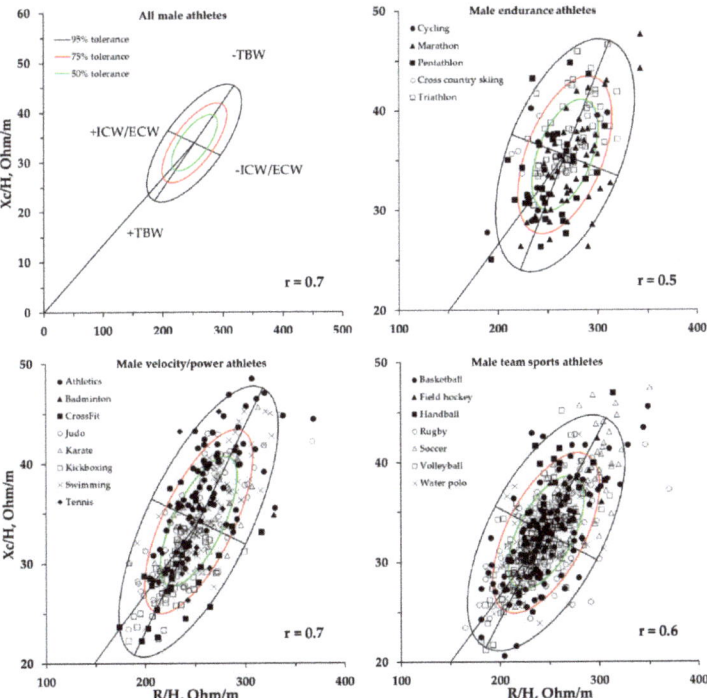

Figure 4. New 50%, 75%, and 95% tolerance ellipses of the entire male athlete population and for the endurance, velocity/power, and team-sports categories with the single athletes' vectors. r = correlation coefficient between R/H and Xc/H. ICW/ECW: intracellular/extracellular water ratio.

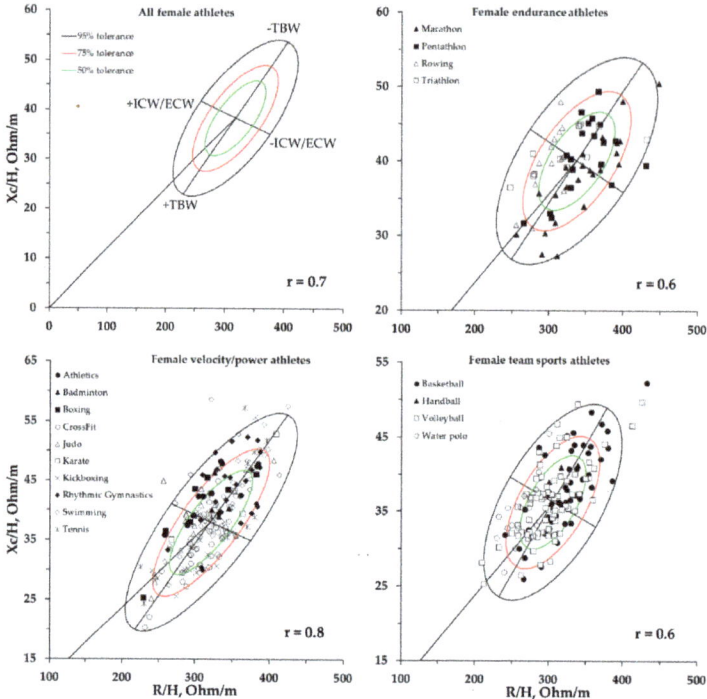

Figure 5. New 50%, 75%, and 95% tolerance ellipses of the entire female athlete population and for the endurance, velocity/power, and team-sports categories with the single athletes' vectors. r = correlation coefficient between R/H and Xc/H.

The 95% confidence ellipses for the mean impedance vectors of elite male soccer players [12] (n = 219, R/H = 252.1, SD = 23.1, Xc/H = 33.9, SD = 4.1, r R/H; Xc/H = 0.69), volleyball players [14] (n = 75, R/H = 232.1, SD = 24.1, Xc/H = 31.5, SD = 4.3, r R/H; Xc/H = 0.81), and cyclists [13] (n = 79, R/H = 284.5, SD = 31.4, Xc/H = 34.9, SD = 4.1, r R/H; Xc/H = 0.56) plotted on the new reference tolerance ellipses are shown in Figure 6. Separate 95% confidence ellipses indicate a significant vector difference ($p < 0.05$).

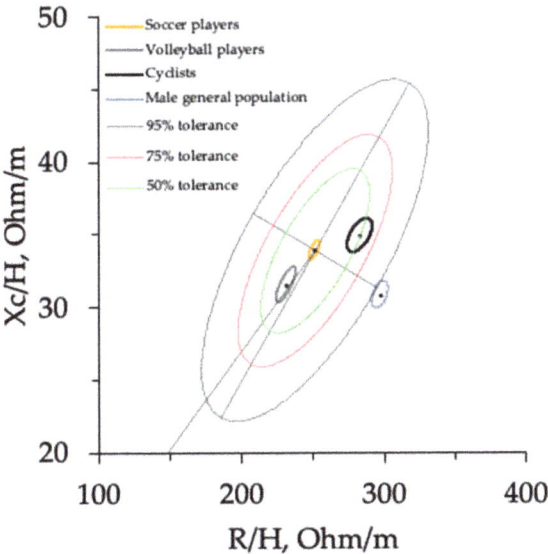

Figure 6. The 95% confidence ellipses for the mean impedance vectors of elite male soccer players [12], volleyball players [14], cyclists [15], and for the general population [19] plotted on the new reference tolerance ellipses.

4. Discussion

The present study, for the first time, generates BIVA reference data for the male and female athlete populations and for endurance, velocity/power, and team-sports athletes. The different distributions of the athletes' bioelectrical values compared to the general population is indicative of the athletes' BC peculiarities and shows the need for athlete-specific reference values. The differences in the BIVA distributions between athlete groups and the general healthy population might reflect the sport- and training-specific adaptation of body masses and composition. In fact, the athletes' lower R/H and higher Xc/H values compared to the general population indicate a higher ICW/ECW ratio and FFM, which is typical for athletes [24,25].

Additionally, the comparison of the 95% confidence ellipses of the mean impedance vectors of the three groups (endurance, velocity/power, and team sports) shows that each athlete group had a slightly different vector distribution on the R–Xc graph. As previously noted, in addition to having morphological and BC differences compared to the general population [24,25], athletes also differ according to the sport that they practice [26–28]. In particular, compared to the velocity/power and team-sports athletes, endurance athletes showed a longer mean impedance vector on the R–Xc graph, indicating less body fluids, which is most likely due to lower body weight. On the contrary, athletes practicing in team sports are positioned at the lowest points on the R–Xc graph compared to the other two group categories.

Our results show that there were no existing PA differences among the three groups of athletes. Recently, a literature review conducted by Di Vincenzo et al. [29] suggested that the PA is a reliable indicator of the ICW/ECW ratio, and that it decreases with age and varies by sex [30]. However, the authors highlighted that it is still uncertain to what extent the PA varies between different sports. Our results show significant differences among the three groups of athletes assessed by BIVA, in both sexes. The BIVA vector position, whose slope is determined by the PA and whose length is determined by the TWB amount, improves the categorization of athletes practicing different sports by overcoming the limitation of evaluating only the PA. In fact, the reference data of the elite categories of soccer [12], volleyball [14], and cycling showed different vector displacements on the R–Xc graph when assessed by BIVAR–. In particular, if we consider the reference values of the PA in soccer players and volleyball players, they were closely similar (7.7 ± 0.6 and 7.7 ± 0.7, respectively). However, as shown in the R–Xc graph (Figure 6), the vector length was lower in volleyball players than in soccer players. This indicates an increased quantity of fluids due to a heavier body mass with similar ICW/ECW ratio. In this regard, as shown in a cross-sectional study by Campa et al. [31], high-level volleyball and soccer players present similar calf and thigh muscle areas, but upper muscle area and body mass are greater in athletes who play volleyball. As studied previously, BIVA has already shown effectiveness in discriminating between division levels within the same sport [12–14]. This is due to the fact that athletes competing at elite levels, in addition to better technical abilities, have a different BC with higher muscle masses and a lower %FM [12,31,32].

A strength of this study is the large sample size of 1116 males and 440 female athletes (in comparison to the 354 male and 372 female subjects proposed as reference for the general population by Piccoli et al. [20]). Additionally, subjects considered in this study were measured in the same conditions and during the same off-season period. This is noteworthy when comparing BIVA measurements because vector changes occur during the competitive season [6,15,33]. Future research should provide sport-specific BIVA references, including samples of different division categories, with a focus on the vector changes throughout the competitive period.

Some limitations of this study should also be acknowledged. Our results are only applicable when using bioimpedance devices operating at a single frequency of 50 kHz. Additionally, the proposed references are specific to the population that was tested in this study. Even though using these BIVA references might constitute an advantage to the use of the general population data, it still might not be the optimal solution for each individual sport.

5. Conclusions

This study proposes new BIVA references that will be useful in assessing BC in male and female athletes. The research shows that vector distributions of endurance, velocity/power, and team-sport athletes differ from the general healthy population and among themselves, due to their different BCs. The BIVA vector, whose position is due to the PA and vector length values, provides additional information with respect to the interpretation of the PA alone. This allows for the assessment of soft tissues (e.g., ICW/ECW) in relation to TBW.

Author Contributions: Conceptualization, F.C.; Formal analysis, F.C.; Investigation, F.C., S.T., A.A., and G.M.; Methodology, F.C., S.T., and A.M.S.; Project administration, A.M.S.; Supervision, H.G. and A.M.S.; Writing—original draft, C.M., H.G., S.T., and A.A.; Writing—review and editing, J.C.K., L.B.S., and A.M.S.

Funding: This research received no external funding.

Acknowledgments: The authors thank the subjects whose participation made this study possible.

Conflicts of Interest: The authors declare no conflict of interest.

References

1. Silva, A.M. Structural and functional body components in athletic health and performance phenotypes. *Eur. J. Clin. Nutr.* **2019**, *73*, 215–224. [CrossRef] [PubMed]
2. Castizo-Olier, J.; Irurtia, A.; Jemni, M.; Carrasco-Marginet, M.; Fernández-García, R.; Rodríguez, F.A. Bioelectrical impedance vector analysis (BIVA) in sport and exercise: Systematic review and future perspectives. *PLoS ONE* **2018**, *13*, e0197957. [CrossRef] [PubMed]
3. Piccoli, A.; Rossi, B.; Pillon, L.; Bucciante, G. A new method for monitoring body fluid variation by bioimpedance analysis: The RXc graph. *Kidney Int.* **1994**, *46*, 534–539. [CrossRef] [PubMed]
4. Lukaski, H.C.; Piccoli, A. Bioelectrical impedance vector analysis for assessment of hydration in physiological states and clinical conditions. In *Handbook of Anthropometry*; Preedy, V., Ed.; Springer: Berlin, Germany, 2012; pp. 287–305.

5. Marini, E.; Campa, F.; Buffa, R.; Stagi, S.; Matias, C.N.; Toselli, S.; Sardinha, L.B.; Silva, A.M. Phase angle and bioelectrical impedance vector analysis in the evaluation of body composition in athletes. *Clin. Nutr.* **2019**. [CrossRef]
6. Campa, F.; Matias, C.N.; Marini, E.; Heymsfield, S.B.; Toselli, S.; Sardinha, L.B.; Silva, A.M. Identifying athlete body-fluid changes during a competitive season with bioelectrical impedance vector analysis. *Int. J. Sports Physiol. Perform.* **2019**. [CrossRef]
7. Gonzalez, M.C.; Barbosa-Silva, T.G.; Bielemann, R.M.; Gallagher, D.; Heymsfield, S.B. Phase angle and its determinants in healthy subjects: Influence of body composition. *Am. J. Clin. Nutr.* **2016**, *103*, 712–716. [CrossRef]
8. Campa, F.; Silva, A.M.; Toselli, S. Changes in phase angle and handgrip strength induced by suspension training in older women. *Int. J. Sports Med.* **2018**, *39*, 442–449. [CrossRef]
9. Ribeiro, A.S.; Avelar, A.; Dos Santos, L.; Silva, A.M.; Gobbo, L.A.; Schoenfeld, B.J.; Sardinha, L.B.; Cyrino, E.S. Hypertrophy-type resistance training improves phase angle in young adult men and women. *Int. J. Sports Med.* **2017**, *38*, 35–40. [CrossRef]
10. Souza, M.F.; Tomeleri, C.M.; Ribeiro, A.S.; Schoenfeld, B.J.; Silva, A.M.; Sardinha, L.B.; Cyrino, E.S. Effect of resistance training on phase angle in older women: A randomized controlled trial. *Scand. J. Med. Sci. Sports* **2017**, *27*, 1308–1316. [CrossRef]
11. Mundstock, E.; Amaral, M.A.; Baptista, R.R.; Sarria, E.E.; Dos Santos, R.R.G.; Filho, A.D.; Rodrigues, C.A.S.; Forte, G.C.; Castro, L.; Padoin, A.V.; et al. Association between phase angle from bioelectrical impedance analysis and level of physical activity: Systematic review and meta-analysis. *Clin. Nutr.* **2019**, *38*, 1504–1510. [CrossRef]
12. Micheli, M.L.; Pagani, L.; Marella, M.; Gulisano, M.; Piccoli, A.; Angelini, F.; Burtscher, M.; Gatterer, H. Bioimpedance and impedance vector patterns as predictors of league level in male soccer players. *Int. J. Sports Physiol. Perform.* **2014**, *9*, 532–539. [CrossRef] [PubMed]
13. Giorgi, A.; Vicini, M.; Pollastri, L.; Lombardi, E.; Magni, E.; Andreazzoli, A.; Orsini, M.; Bonifazi, M.; Lukaski, H.; Gatterer, H. Bioimpedance patterns and bioelectrical impedance vector analysis (BIVA) of road cyclists. *J. Sports Sci.* **2018**, *36*, 2608–2613. [CrossRef] [PubMed]
14. Campa, F.; Toselli, S. Bioimpedance vector analysis of elite, subelite, and low-level male volleyball players. *Int. J. Sports Physiol. Perform.* **2018**, *13*, 1250–1253. [CrossRef] [PubMed]
15. Pollastri, L.; Lanfranconi, F.; Tredici, G.; Schenk, K.; Burtscher, M.; Gatterer, H. Body fluid status and physical demand during the Giro d'Italia. *Res. Sports Med.* **2016**, *24*, 30–38. [CrossRef]
16. Carrasco-Marginet, M.; Castizo-Olier, J.; Rodríguez-Zamora, L.; Iglesias, X.; Rodríguez, F.A.; Chaverri, D.; Brotons, D.; Irurtia, A. Bioelectrical impedance vector analysis (BIVA) for measuring the hydration status in young elite synchronized swimmers. *PLoS ONE* **2017**, *12*, e0178819. [CrossRef]
17. Piras, A.; Campa, F.; Toselli, S.; Di Michele, R.; Raffi, M. Physiological responses to partial-body cryotherapy performed during a concurrent strength and endurance session. *Appl. Physiol. Nutr. Metab.* **2019**, *44*, 59–65. [CrossRef]
18. Campa, F.; Gatterer, H.; Lukaski, H.; Toselli, S. Stabilizing bioimpedance-vector-analysis measures with a 10-minute cold shower after running exercise to enable assessment of body hydration. *Int. J. Sports Physiol. Perform.* **2019**, *14*, 1006–1009. [CrossRef]
19. Campa, F.; Silva, A.M.; Iannuzzi, V.; Mascherini, G.; Benedetti, L.; Toselli, S. The role of somatic maturation on bioimpedance patterns and body composition in male elite youth soccer players. *Int. J. Environ. Res. Public Health* **2019**, *16*, 4711. [CrossRef]
20. Piccoli, A.; Nigrelli, S.; Caberlotto, A.; Bottazzo, S.; Rossi, B.; Pillon, L.; Maggiore, Q. Bivariate normal values of the bioelectrical impedance vector in adult and elderly populations. *Am. J. Clin. Nutr.* **1995**, *61*, 269–270. [CrossRef]
21. Khalil, S.F.; Mohktar, M.S.; Ibrahim, F. The theory and fundamentals of bioimpedance analysis in clinical status monitoring and diagnosis of diseases. *Sensors* **2014**, *14*, 10895–10928. [CrossRef]
22. Kotler, D.P.; Burastero, S.; Wang, J.; Pierson, R.N. Prediction of body cell mass, fat-free mass, and total body water with bioelectrical impedance analysis: Effects of race, sex, and disease. *Am. J. Clin. Nutr.* **1996**, *64*, 489S–497S. [CrossRef] [PubMed]
23. Picocli, A.; Pastori, G. *BIVA Software*; University of Padova: Padua, Italy, 2002.

24. Koury, J.C.; Trugo, N.M.F.; Torres, A.G. Phase angle and bioelectrical impedance vectors in adolescent and adult male athletes. *Int. J. Sports Physiol. Perform.* **2014**, *9*, 798–804. [CrossRef] [PubMed]
25. Meleleo, D.; Bartolomeo, N.; Cassano, L.; Nitti, A.; Susca, G.; Mastrototaro, G.; Armenise, U.; Zito, A.; Devito, F.; Scicchitano, P. Evaluation of body composition with bioimpedance. A comparison between athletic and non-athletic children. *Eur. J. Sport Sci.* **2017**, *17*, 710–719. [CrossRef] [PubMed]
26. Campa, F.; Piras, A.; Raffi, M.; Toselli, S. functional movement patterns and body composition of high-level volleyball, soccer, and rugby players. *J. Sport Rehabil.* **2019**, *28*, 740–745. [CrossRef]
27. Nakagawa, Y.; Hattori, M. Intramyocellular lipids of muscle type in athletes of different sport disciplines. *Open Access J. Sports Med.* **2017**, *8*, 161–166. [CrossRef]
28. Mala, L.; Maly, T.; Zahalka, F.; Bunc, V.; Kaplan, A.; Jebavy, R.; Tuma, M. Body composition of elite female players in five different sports games. *J. Hum. Kinet.* **2015**, *45*, 207–215. [CrossRef]
29. Di Vincenzo, O.; Marra, M.; Scalfi, L. Bioelectrical impedance phase angle in sport: A systematic review. *J. Int. Soc. Sports Nutr.* **2019**, *16*, 49. [CrossRef]
30. Mattiello, R.; Amaral, M.A.; Mundstock, E.; Ziegelmann, P.K. Reference values for the phase angle of the electrical bioimpedance: Systematic review and meta-analysis involving more than 250,000 subjects. *Clin. Nutr.* **2019**, *19*, 30286–30289. [CrossRef]
31. Campa, F.; Semprini, G.; Judice, P.B.; Messina, G.; Toselli, S. Anthropometry, physical and movement features, and repeated-sprint ability in soccer players. *Int. J. Sports Med.* **2019**, *40*, 100–109. [CrossRef]
32. Toselli, S.; Campa, F. Anthropometry and functional movement patterns in elite male volleyball players of different competitive levels. *J. Strength Cond. Res.* **2018**, *32*, 2601–2611. [CrossRef]
33. Mascherini, G.; Gatterer, H.; Lukaski, H.; Burtscher, M.; Galanti, G. Changes in hydration, body-cell mass and endurance performance of professional soccer players through a competitive season. *J. Sports Med. Phys. Fit.* **2015**, *55*, 749–755.

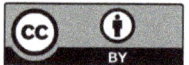

© 2019 by the authors. Licensee MDPI, Basel, Switzerland. This article is an open access article distributed under the terms and conditions of the Creative Commons Attribution (CC BY) license (http://creativecommons.org/licenses/by/4.0/).

MDPI
St. Alban-Anlage 66
4052 Basel
Switzerland
Tel. +41 61 683 77 34
Fax +41 61 302 89 18
www.mdpi.com

International Journal of Environmental Research and Public Health Editorial Office
E-mail: ijerph@mdpi.com
www.mdpi.com/journal/ijerph

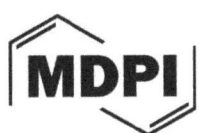